SECOND

BREASTFEEDING ANSWERS
Pocket Guide

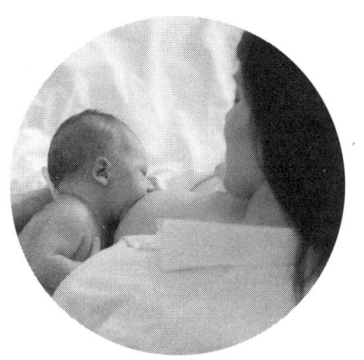

Nancy Mohrbacher, IBCLC, FILCA

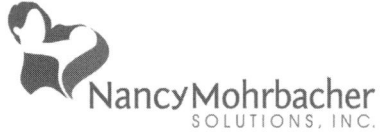

Arlington Heights, Illinois

Breastfeeding Answers Pocket Guide, Second Edition
Nancy Mohrbacher, IBCLC, FILCA

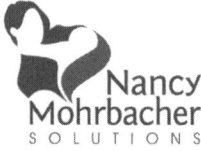

Nancy Mohrbacher Solutions, Inc.
Arlington Heights, IL
630-336-9525
info@nancymohrbacher.com
www.NancyMohrbacher.com

Copyright ©2021 by Nancy Mohrbacher Solutions, Inc.

All rights reserved. No part of this publication may be reproduced or transmitted in any form by any means, electronic or mechanical, including photocopy, recording, or any information storage and retrieval system, without written permission from the publisher.

Executive Editor: Nancy Mohrbacher
Proofreading: Heather Behles
Indexer: Gina Guilinger, Weight of the Word LLC
Cover and Text Design: Nelly Murariu

BREASTFEEDING ANSWERS POCKET GUIDE, Second Edition

ISBN: 978-1-7345239-4-2
Library of Congress Control Number: 2021906830
Printed in the United States of America

CONTENTS

Introduction	*vii*
Chapter 1 Basic Nursing Dynamics	**1**
Baby's Inborn Feeding Behaviors	1
What Supports and Undermines Baby	2
Helping Nursing Couples Get in Sync	3
Positioning Basics	5
How Feeds End	15
Digital Resources	16
Chapter 2 Birth, Early Nursing, and Nursing Norms	**17**
Birth Practices and Early Nursing	17
Establishing Nursing	17
The Older Baby	21
Pacifiers/Dummies	23
Sleep and Night Feeds	24
Digital Resources	26
Chapter 3 Breast or Chest Issues	**27**
Engorgement	27
Mastitis	29
Deep Breast Pain	35
Breast Lumps	37
Blood in the Milk or Nipple Discharge	39
Unusual Breast Development	40
Breast or Chest Surgery or Injury	43
Digital Resources	51
Chapter 4 Challenges with Latching and Nursing	**53**
Safeguarding Nursing	53
Struggles During the Early Weeks	54
Struggles After the Early Weeks	63
Not Latching to One or Both Sides	68
Chapter 5 Contraception	**75**
Lactation, Sexuality, and Fertility	75
Nursing and Contraception	76
Chapter 6 Emergencies and Infant Feeding	**83**
Risks of Non-Human Milks	83
Support Optimal Nursing Practices	83
Give Formula Only to Those Not Fully Nursing	85
Follow International Formula Guidelines	86
Digital Resources	87
Chapter 7 Employment	**89**
Length of Parental Leave and Nursing	89
Priorities During Parental Leave	89
Returning to Work	96

Chapter 8 Health and Anatomy Issues: Baby   101
Oral Anatomy of the Nursing Baby   101
Illness in the Nursing Baby   112
Chronic Conditions in the Nursing Baby   117
Hospitalization of the Nursing Baby   130
Digital Resources   133

Chapter 9 Health Issues: Nursing Parent   135
Nursing with Health Issues   135
Bacterial Illnesses   135
Viral Infections   137
Cancer   145
Cardiac Issues/Hypertension   147
Depression, Anxiety, and Mental Health   147
Endocrine, Metabolic, and Autoimmune Disorders   151
Headaches and Lactation   160
Hospitalization and Surgery   160
Physical Impairment or Challenge   162
Digital Resources   165

Chapter 10 Hypoglycemia and Jaundice   167
Newborn Hypoglycemia   167
Newborn Jaundice   170
Digital Resources   178

Chapter 11 Making Milk   179
Anatomy of the Mammary Gland   179
Milk Ejection   180
Milk Production   181
Digital Resources   206

Chapter 12 Milk Expression and Storage   207
Milk Expression Basics   207
Milk Expression Methods   210
Milk Expression Strategies   210
Milk Storage and Handling   216
Digital Resources   220

Chapter 13 Nipple Issues   221
Nipple Pain   221
Bacterial, Fungal and Viral Nipple Infections   226
Other Skin Problems   229
Nipple Blisters and Blebs   231
Nipple Types and Procedures   232
Digital Resources   236

Chapter 14 Nutrition, Exercise, and Lifestyle Issues   237
Nutrition for Nursing Parents   237
Exercise   242
Grooming: Hair Care, Tanning, and Piercings   242
Substance Use During Lactation   243
Digital Resources   249

Chapter 15 Pregnancy and Tandem Nursing — 251
Nursing During Pregnancy — 251
Tandem Nursing — 252

Chapter 16 Preterm Baby — 255
Parents' Role in the Preemie's Care — 255
Nursing the Preterm Baby — 256
The Late-Preterm and Early-Term Baby — 268
Preterm Twins, Triplets, and More — 269
Digital Resources — 270

Chapter 17 Relactation and Induced Lactation — 271
Definitions and Goals — 271
Strategies to Increase Milk Production — 272
Transitioning Baby to Nursing — 276
Co-Nursing with Partners — 280
Digital Resources — 282

Chapter 18 Vaccines, Vitamins, and Other Supplements — 283
Vaccines — 283
Vitamins and Other Supplements — 284

Chapter 19 Weaning from Nursing — 289
Recommendations — 289
The Decision to Wean — 289
Weaning Dynamics — 290

Chapter 20 Weight Gain and Growth — 297
Normal Growth — 297
Slow Weight Gain — 298
Rapid Weight Gain — 306
Digital Resources — 308

Appendices — 309
Appendix A: Breast Compression — 309
Appendix B: Feeding Methods — 311
Appendix C: Latching Techniques — 319
Appendix D: Milk-Expression Techniques — 323
Appendix E: Nipple Shields — 329
Appendix F: Reverse Pressure Softening (RPS) — 333

Index — 335

INTRODUCTION

How does *Breastfeeding Answers Pocket Guide, Second Edition* differ from its gigantic cousin, *Breastfeeding Answers, Second Edition*? Of course, the size difference is enormous. The original is a dictionary-sized tome that weighs in at more than six pounds, while this slim volume is small and lightweight enough to carry in a tote, purse, or, yes, even a pocket. Obviously, there must be other differences, too.

What's missing in this *Pocket Guide*? Gone from its pages are the citations of thousands of articles and books and the summaries of their contents. Also gone are the sometimes lengthy explanations for its suggested strategies. What remains are the strategies themselves and the basic background information needed when helping nursing families in a vast range of common and unusual circumstances.

Unlike its huge predecessor, this companion volume is intended to be used as an easy reference while you assist nursing parents. Its purpose is to provide quick and portable answers to the questions: "What do I need to remember in this situation?" and "What should I try next?"

A note about some language changes in this edition: Because the families who come to us for lactation help—and indeed also some of our colleagues—include those who are not heterosexual and cisgender, it's important to widen our worldview and for the language in this book to be appropriately inclusive. I don't think the words "mother" or "mother's milk" will ever go out of style, so you'll continue to find them in these pages. (After all, many transgender women happily embrace these words, along with many cisgender women.) But I also use other, more inclusive terms throughout, such as "birthing parent" and "nursing parent." My hope is that by using these broader terms, it will help us all remember that our work has expanded to include a wider range of loving and nurturing families, which—for me at least—is a cause for celebration.

Regarding the use of pronouns, in the first edition, the nursing parent was always presumed to be "she" and baby was referred to as "he." In this edition, you'll see the word "parents" used more often with the pronoun "they" and baby's gender will alternate by chapter, with odd chapters using "he" and even chapters using "she."

I hope this book is a useful tool as you join families on their lactation journey. Please accept my thanks for the lives you touch and for the invaluable help you give.

Nancy Mohrbacher, IBCLC, FILCA
Chicago suburbs
April 2021

CHAPTER 1   BASIC NURSING DYNAMICS

Think of nursing not as a skill to be taught, but rather as part of the intimate relationship between parent and child. With each new baby, families learn what works with that baby and then tailor their responses accordingly. A good first step is a basic understanding of what nature builds into babies and how to use this to make early nursing easier.

BABY'S INBORN FEEDING BEHAVIORS

Under the right conditions, like all mammal newborns, healthy term humans emerge from the womb with the innate behaviors needed to get to their food source and feed, known as the breast crawl.

THE BREAST CRAWL   After birth, the breast crawl is how newborns make their way to the nipple, latch, and feed. Comprised of nine "instinctive stages" (p. 18), on average the time from birth to nursing is 60 minutes. These newborn movements increase the parents' blood levels of oxytocin, which strengthens the parent-child bond and triggers milk ejection. After birth, when compared with babies who do not do the breast crawl, babies who do the breast crawl at their first feed have fewer nursing struggles and much less weight loss. Their nursing parents have earlier milk increase and less nipple pain.

Once thought to be fragile and short-lived, these inborn feeding behaviors can be triggered for months and even years. Supporting baby's feeding behaviors during nursing attempts can prevent and overcome common problems. When both parents and babies take an active role, this simplifies the latching process and enhances their relationship. Positive experiences reinforce effective feeding.

PRIMITIVE NEONATAL REFLEXES   Researchers identified 20 primitive neonatal reflexes (PNRs), like hand-to-mouth, arm and leg cycling, and head lifting, which are components of the breast crawl and are seen in preemies as young as 29 weeks. Their main functions are to help baby find the nipple and latch and once latched to transfer milk. The specific PNRs used vary from feed to feed and position to position, with semi-reclined positions (p. 6) triggering more PNRs than others. The reflexes identified in human newborns indicate our babies are hardwired to feed most easily resting on their abdomens rather than with pressure applied to their back.

NORMAL ROOTING, SUCKING, AND SWALLOWING   Latching and sucking occur in a predictable sequence of actions: baby finds the nipple (usually by rooting), the touch of the baby's chin on the gland stimulates a wide-open mouth (gape), and finally, baby drops his tongue, extending its tip over his lower lip as he attaches and sucks.

Swallowing is easier if the baby's head is tilted back slightly, known as the ***instinctive feeding position***. While nursing, the baby draws milk through a combination of tongue and jaw movements. While milk is flowing, the front of baby's tongue moves as a rigid body with the cycling movement of baby's lower jaw, and the back of baby's tongue moves in the wavelike motion needed for swallowing. The vacuum generated by the back of the tongue dropping plays a major role in milk transfer.

Depth of latch often affects comfort, active feeding, and milk transfer. A shallow latch (with the nipple pressed against baby's hard palate) contributes to nipple pain and slow milk flow. If flow is slow enough, the baby may gain weight poorly, suck less actively, or fall asleep quickly. With a deep latch, which usually leads to comfortable and effective nursing, the nipple extends on average to within about 4 to 5 mm of the junction of the baby's hard and soft palates.

WHAT SUPPORTS AND UNDERMINES BABY

TRIGGERS OF INBORN FEEDING BEHAVIORS Touch is the primary trigger and maintainer of a newborn's innate feeding behaviors, specifically the full-frontal contact of the baby against the adult's body. It also helps orient baby so he can focus on feeding. Foot contact with the parent or something else helps baby orient, so he can move to the nipple more easily.

Hearing, smell, and sight also play a role in orienting the baby to the nipple. Hunger and thirst can trigger feeding behaviors, too. The rooting reflex (when a baby's cheek is touched, he turns his head in that direction) can help or hinder nursing. Baby may turn away if his cheek is touched by accident.

THE IMPORTANCE OF POSITIONAL STABILITY Babies need to feel physically stable before they can focus on feeding. For better head-and-neck coordination during nursing, young babies need a stable midsection (core) and equal use of both sides of their body. Resting tummy down on the parent's body provides a stable place for feeding.

FACTORS THAT UNDERMINE BABY Several physical dynamics can lead to feeding struggles: gaps forming between a hungry newborn and the parent, causing the loss of full-frontal contact, pushing on the back of baby's head can cause baby to push back, baby latching chin-to-chest rather than head tilted back makes swallowing more difficult, and pushing baby's nose into the mammary tissue, obstructing baby's breathing.

HELPING NURSING COUPLES GET IN SYNC

Getting in sync with a newborn is a part of responsive parenting, which produces the best physical and emotional outcomes for both children and parents. Nursing makes this process easier. Getting in sync involves keeping baby's stress levels low by nursing on cue rather than on a schedule and responding consistently to baby's needs for milk and comfort. Parents need to experiment with different calming strategies to find what works best for that baby.

BABY'S STATE, READINESS, AND ENGAGEMENT A baby's state of alertness affects his feeding behaviors and his ability to nurse. The Neonatal Behavior Assessment Scale describes six infant states: deep sleep, light sleep, drowsy, quiet alert, fussy, and crying. Innate feeding behaviors can be triggered and babies can nurse when they are in quiet alert, drowsy, and light sleep states. When possible, suggest nursing before baby starts crying. If the baby is crying, begin by calming him. Eye contact, touch, and talking to baby calms him and improves coordination during feeding attempts.

Signs baby is ready to feed include increased alertness, activity, mouthing (including hand to mouth), and rooting. Especially during the early weeks, suggest nursing whenever the baby will suck. The more time spent nursing, the more quickly it becomes automatic and the more milk is made.

THE NURSING PARENT: INSTINCTS AND LEARNING For parents, nursing may be partly learned and partly innate. Like newborns, birthing parents have biological triggers and innate responses. During skin-to-skin contact, a parent's body helps regulate a baby's body temperature. Oxytocin release during skin-to-skin contact and nursing increases parents' desire to touch and stroke their baby.

While newborns' feeding behaviors are entirely reflex-driven, adults can overthink nursing. Unlike other mammals, in human parents, intellect can overrule innate behaviors. Engaging nursing parents' intellect unnecessarily can alter their hormonal state, disconnecting them from their body's response.

THE ROLE OF THE HELPER Effective lactation help can boost families' "breastfeeding self-efficacy" (BSE), their level of confidence in their ability to meet their nursing goals, a key influencer of nursing initiation, exclusivity, and duration.

APPROACHES TO LACTATION HELP Effective lactation help involves more than knowledge and clinical skills. Attitude and approach also matter in how families feel about our help. Lactation supporters usually use one of two basic approaches. With the first approach, which many parents consider undermining, milk transfer is the top priority and the nursing parent is seen as a novice who needs training in a mechanical skill. With the second approach, which parents find supportive, the parent-child relationship is the top priority and the nursing parent is considered the expert on their baby and their own needs.

Parents consider lactation helpers most supportive when they project trust and connectedness and are empathetic. These helper-parent discussions include realistic expectations and are sufficiently detailed and specific to be helpful. Conversations are two-way, not one-way "information dumps."

Helpers perceived as undermining are viewed as dogmatic, giving standard information not appropriate to the situation. Parents consider them rushed and may feel criticized. Their conversations are one-way, with little listening, and families describe feeling pressured to do things the helper's way rather than feeling empowered to find their own best way. When hands-on help is provided, parents report it often feels intrusive and rough.

KEEP EARLY LACTATION HELP SIMPLE Brain changes during pregnancy and after delivery make following instructions and remembering facts difficult for birthing parents. They also, however, increase brain plasticity, which makes adjusting to parenthood easier.

Simplified lactation help is more than just a better fit for birthing parents' physiology. It makes it easier for families to respond to their baby and focus on their relationship. Learning to nurse by feel allows parents to be guided by the physical responses that draw parent and baby to one another. These body responses are why they love to look at each other, touch, and interact. These parent-baby behaviors spring naturally from the emotions triggered by the hormones of birth and nursing.

Parents need to know that there is no one right way to nurse. Display confidence that nursing will work. Encourage parents to talk to their baby and maintain eye contact. Reassure them that their baby's actions are normal. The main message is that parents' job is not to learn to nurse or to make their baby nurse. Their job is to get comfortable themselves, make sure the baby is well supported, and help the baby stay calm, relaxed, and comfortable.

Teaching specific feeding positions can make nursing seem unnecessarily complicated and put the focus in the wrong place: on "doing it right" rather than being guided by their own and their baby's responses. Nursing parents and babies come in different shapes and sizes and are not limited to just a few positions. It boosts new parents' confidence to find comfortable positions on their own.

Keep the focus on creating a conducive environment rather than giving instructions. Early nursing ideally occurs in a place that enhances parents' hormonal response to their baby, a place that includes privacy, warmth, and comfort, respect for parents' choices and acknowledgement of what they do right, and enhances parents' feelings of competence by minimizing information/teaching.

POSITIONING BASICS

Encourage families to keep an open mind about feeding positions, using comfort as the guide. A basic understanding of what nature builds into babies and parents is also helpful. When considering feeding positions, the baby's age also matters. During the first 4 to 6 weeks, newborns have little head-and-neck control. That's why some approaches to positioning may be easier than others.

There is no reason to vary positions at every feed, unless there is a special need. In the past, based on the faulty premise that normal nursing causes nipple pain, it was thought that varying positions would make nursing more comfortable. But now this is recommended only when even with a deep latch nursing is painful, such as untreated symptomatic tongue-tie or an unusually shaped palate.

Approaches to positioning fall into two main categories: those in which baby primarily drives the latching process and those in which the parent is primarily in charge of latching. The baby-driven approach is especially well-suited to newborns.

Primarily baby-driven approach to positioning. The inborn feeding behaviors described previously are more likely to lead to successful nursing when the parent leans back into a semi-reclined position and baby rests tummy down on top. These *starter positions* (next section) include many variations that allow families to tailor them to their unique anatomies and preferences.

Primarily parent-driven approach to positioning. This second approach includes the upright feeding positions that lactation supporters once taught: the cradle hold, the cross-cradle hold, and the football/rugby or clutch hold, as well as side-lying. While these positions may work well for older babies and some newborns, during the early weeks Table 1.1 describes their drawbacks.

Table 1.1 How Parent-Driven and Baby-Driven Positioning Affect Early Feeding Dynamics

	Parent-Driven Upright Holds	**Baby-Driven Starter Positions**
Full frontal contact	Requires effort	Automatic
Positional stability	Requires effort	Automatic
Effect of gravity on baby's reflexes	May act as barriers to latching	Leads to more successful latching
Managing milk flow	More challenging	Easier
Who controls latching?	Parent	Baby
Instructions needed	Detailed	Simple
Pressure on perineum	Yes	No
Physical effort needed	Possible muscle strain	Can relax, rest
Effect of gravity on depth of latch	May make it shallower	Deepens latch

Adapted from **NaturalBreastfeeding.com**

STARTER POSITIONS: THE EARLY WEEKS During the first 4 to 6 weeks, starter positions—which use a primarily baby-driven approach to early positioning—are easier for many new families than upright holds. These semi-reclined positions offer many variations, and because most newborns can latch and feed more easily, their use prevents nipple pain and other early feeding problems. Starter positions are compared with upright holds in Table 1.1.

In starter positions (Figure 1.1), nursing parents relax into a well-supported, semi-reclined position with a body slope between about 15 and 65 degrees (Figure 1.2). With good head, arm, and body support, parents can relax all their muscles and rest and recover while baby feeds. Baby lies tummy down, hands free on the parent's body with easy access to the nipple. Nursing parents' arms act as guardrails to keep baby safely in place and, as needed, to provide baby with head support.

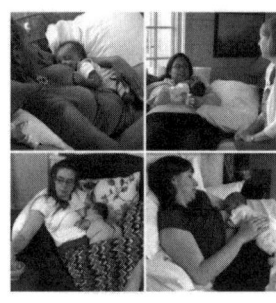

Figure 1.1
Starter positions

These positions are especially well-suited to young babies with nursing challenges such as tongue-tie or a small or receding lower jaw, because gravity pulls their tongue and chin forward.

For lactation helpers, starter positions save time and reduce job-related back pain. But helpers more familiar with upright nursing holds may need to acquire new skills and use a different vocabulary to help families customize starter positions to their anatomy and preferences. The following simplified vocabulary is not copyrighted or trademarked, so these terms can be used freely. The three basic adjustments are: ***adjust your body, adjust your baby,*** and ***adjust your breast***. See the Table 1.2 checklist, and see them in action in the free video at **NaturalBreastfeeding.com**.

ADJUST YOUR BODY refers to the adjustments used by parents to get comfortable and support the baby and includes the following.

- **Parent's body slope** The body slope most effective at triggering feeding reflexes is between 15 and 65 degrees (Figure 1.2). Nursing parents need to be reclined enough so the baby's weight is fully supported by their body, not their arms or hands. If parents raise their hands, the baby stays in place. Parents' torso needs to be elevated enough so baby's face is easily visible without neck strain. Avoid lying fully supine (flat on their back) to prevent baby's breathing from becoming obstructed.

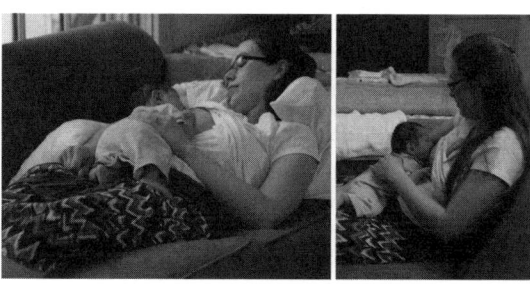

Figure 1.2 Starter positions involve a body slope between 15° and 65°.

- **Parent's body support**. To get enough support so parents can relax all their muscles, try putting pillows behind their back, under their arms, and/or behind their head. To gauge if more support is needed, stand back and look for a raised shoulder or tense muscles.

- **Parents' arms and hands** are used differently than in upright holds. Baby's weight rests fully on the parent's body, not in arms. Baby self-attaches, so parents don't pull baby on deeply during latch. Instead, their hands are often free and their arms are used as guardrails to help keep baby safely on their body and as head support during feeds. Depending on their arm length and mammary size, baby may rest his head on their upper or lower arm for support.

- **Arm adjustments to safeguard baby's breathing.** If baby does a face plant into the mammary tissue and breathing is obstructed, suggest slightly lowering the arm supporting baby's head (Figure 1.3), or adjust baby's body position (see next section). A small adjustment may be all that's needed for more breathing space.

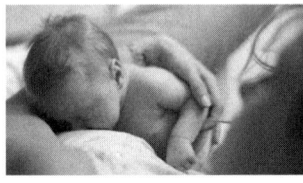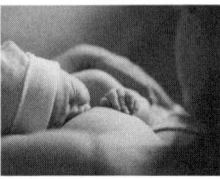

Figure 1.3 Left: Face plant. Right: Mother's left arm lowered slightly to create breathing space

- **Support the mammary gland.** Nursing is usually easier when the mammary gland lays at its natural level. But in some cases, support may help (see later section, "Adjust Your Breast").

ADJUST YOUR BABY refers to several adjustments of baby's body position, including:

- **Baby's body direction.** Baby can approach the nipple from many directions. If you think of the gland as a clock face and baby's body like the hands on a clock, in most cases, babies approach the nipple between 3 and 9 o'clock, vertically, horizontally, or diagonally (Figure 1.4). After a cesarean birth, avoid a vertical lie to prevent pressure on the incision. Also, baby may be supported at the parent's side or over the shoulder.

- **Baby's hands are free and uncovered.** Babies use their hands to calm, stabilize, and orient themselves, find the nipple, and stimulate oxytocin release.

- **Frog legs.** To help baby orient and find the nipple, he needs to be fully tummy down on the parent's body. To make sure his hips are not twisted, lift slightly with a hand under baby's groin area. If baby's legs are splayed apart (like frog legs), this ensures full frontal contact.

- **Baby's head higher than bottom.** Most babies feel unstable when held in a head-down position, and rather than focusing on feeding, try to get stable. If baby's head is lower than his bottom, suggest parents readjust their body until baby's head is higher than his bottom.

- **Foot contact.** Baby orients more easily if the tops or soles of his feet touch the nursing parent or something else. If baby's feet are out in thin air, try rolling a small cloth and wedge it under his feet or shift baby's body until his feet touch the parent.

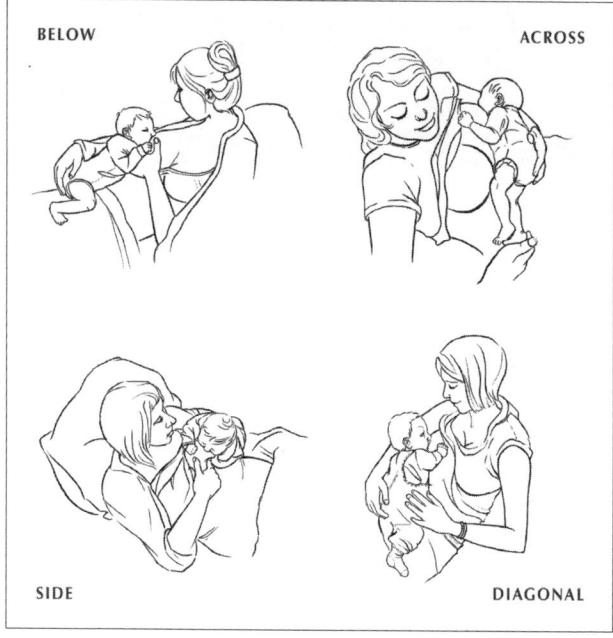

Figure 1.4 Some of baby's many lie options
©2021 Nancy Mohrbacher Solutions, Inc.

ADJUST YOUR BREAST is not always needed, but if baby still struggles to latch after the other adjustments are made, some gentle shaping may help baby get his mouth around the gland for a deeper latch, especially with engorged or naturally taut mammary tissue.

To shape the mammary tissue, place the fingers far enough back from the areola so they aren't in baby's way (Figure 1.5). Then squeeze gently. Make sure the oval runs in the same direction as baby's lips. If the oval is opposite to baby's lips, it makes latching harder, like trying to take a bite out of a sandwich held vertically rather than horizontally in front of your mouth. One way to describe this is to suggest shaping it "like a hamburger, not a taco," illustrating with hand motions.

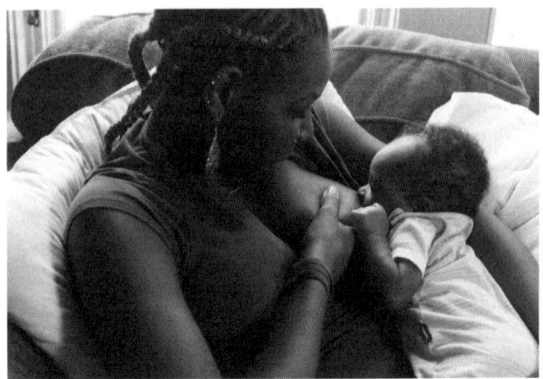

Figure 1.5 If baby struggles to latch, gentle shaping of the mammary tissue can sometimes help.

Table 1.2 Starter Positions Checklist

ADJUSTMENTS TO TRY	YES	NO
Is the baby upset and needs to be calmed first?		
Is the nursing parent semi-reclined (body slope between 15° and 65°) and fully supported and relaxed?		
When the nursing parent's hands are raised, does baby stay in place?		
Is baby fully tummy down in a frog-legs position?		
Is baby's head higher than his bottom?		
Have they tried varying the direction of baby's lie?		
Are baby's feet in contact with the parent or something else?		
Have they tried shaping the mammary tissue (hamburger not taco)?		
If baby's breathing is blocked, have they tried slightly lowering the arm that supports baby's head or varying the direction of baby's lie?		

Adapted from **NaturalBreastfeeding.com**

Some strategies commonly used with upright holds are best avoided with starter positions.

- **Nursing pillows** support baby's weight in upright holds, but in starter positions, unless used to support the parent, they get in the way.

- **Pressure on baby's back or shoulders during latch** is needed in upright holds to latch deeply, but is not needed in starter positions. Some babies react badly to being pushed on.

- **Asymmetrical latch** (p. 319) makes a deep latch easier in upright positions. In starter positions, baby can adjust the latch as needed.

- **After latch, checking baby's lips** often makes a deep latch shallower. Instead, gauge a deep latch by its comfort and baby's active jaw movements. When both are present, ignore baby's lips.

- **Covering or restraining baby's hands.** Swaddling baby or pinning his arms is often recommended in upright positions. But when gravity works in harmony with baby's reflexes in starter positions, this is unnecessary and can cause feeding struggles.

- **Touching or pushing on the back of baby's head.** Baby may push back and struggle.

BASIC BODY DYNAMICS IN ANY POSITION No one positioning strategy works with all families all the time, so be ready with alternatives when:

- **The parent does not want to use starter positions.** Some prefer upright or side-lying. Affirming what feels right to parents is a vital aspect of supportive lactation help.

- **After trying all the adjustments, the baby still struggles to nurse.** After previous negative attempts, some babies become upset when near the nipple. Some struggle due to an undiagnosed health problem or other factors.

As babies grow, most parents want to try other holds. Knowing something about inborn infant feeding behaviors can make nursing easier in any position. The same dynamics that make starter positions work can be used in other positions, for example:

- **Positional stability** with baby's head higher than bottom helps him focus on feeding.

- **Full frontal contact** with no gaps helps baby orient more easily.

- **Foot and eye contact.** Foot contact (tops or soles of feet) helps baby orient. If needed, tuck a small, rolled cloth against his feet. Eye contact improves baby's coordination.
- **Nose to nipple with baby's head slightly tilted back** for easier swallowing.
- **Chin touching the mammary tissue to trigger a wide gape.**
- **Asymmetrical latch** (p. 319). During latch, position baby's lower jaw far from the nipple so the nipple can extend deeper into baby's mouth. (Not needed in starter positions.)
- **Gentle pressure behind baby's shoulders during latch, avoiding the back of baby's head.** If head support is needed, position a palm on baby's back with thumb and index finger behind baby's ears (p. 319).
- **Continued gentle pressure on baby's shoulders** to prevent gaps from forming while nursing for greater core stability and coordination. (Not needed in starter positions.)

SIDE-LYING is often used for night nursing, so parents can rest while baby feeds, and is a good second choice for newborns, because the surface provides positional stability.

In side-lying positions, parent and baby lie on their sides facing one another. When used with a newborn, the parent needs to help baby latch with a palm on baby's upper back. Babies older than 6 weeks or so may have enough head-and-neck control to latch by themselves. Try these variations until parent and baby find their own best fit:

- Baby's head lies flat on the surface with parent's lower arm out of the way or cradling baby.
- Baby's head is supported by the parent's lower arm.
- To keep a newborn on his side and in close, either place the hand of the upper arm on baby's back or wedge a rolled cloth behind baby's back, leaving his head free to tilt back (Figure 1.6).
- When switching sides, either hold baby to chest while rolling over or lean over so baby can latch to the upper side in the same position
- Try adding pillows for support under parents' head and upper knee. Depending on the size of the mammary tissue and the nipple location, try leaning back slightly into a pillow.

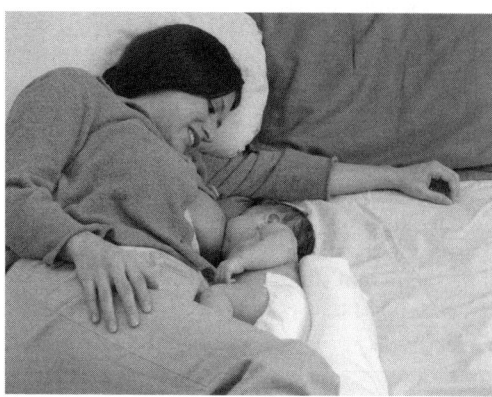

Figure 1.6 Pillows provide this mother with head and knee support. A rolled cloth wedged behind baby's back keeps him in place while allowing his head to tilt back.

UPRIGHT HOLDS The most commonly taught upright holds are the cradle, cross-cradle, and football/rugby or clutch holds. The football/rugby hold is often recommended after a cesarean birth to keep baby away from the incision. The best way to achieve positional stability in these holds is for nursing parents to keep baby's entire front gently pressed against their body.

In upright positions, keeping baby at nipple height and his body touching can feel awkward, tiring, and lead to muscle strain. Try pillows to support the baby at a level that is not too high, which makes getting a deep latch challenging, and not too low, which may lead to back or neck pain from bending over. Without body support, a deep latch may become shallower as the feed progresses and baby drops lower. If the cross-cradle hold is helpful during latch, to increase comfort, latch baby in the cross-cradle hold and then relax back into a semi-reclined position, with baby's full weight resting on the parent's body.

As with other positions, tailor upright holds to the nursing parents' anatomy and baby's response.

SUPPORTING OR SHAPING MAMMARY TISSUE Some nursing parents use their hand to support their mammary tissue during feeds; others do not; and some vary this from feed to feed. Depending on body shape, feeding position, and nipple location, a nursing parent may or may not support their gland. Leave this to the parent. When supporting mammary tissue in upright positions, suggest keeping it at or near its natural level, which involves less work. If nursing is easier with support, focus on supporting just the section near the areola.

POSITIONING FOR SPECIAL SITUATIONS can sometimes be helpful in unusual circumstances. Here are some examples.

THE STRADDLE HOLD may work well for babies with a cleft palate or those who feed better with more body flexion (hip dysplasia or low muscle tone) or head extension (an airway abnormality). In a straddle hold—either upright or semi-reclined (Figure 1.7)—parent and baby face each other with baby supported on the parent's lap and baby's legs straddling the parent's leg. Its upright version can be tiring, as it requires parents use their hands and arm muscles to keep baby close.

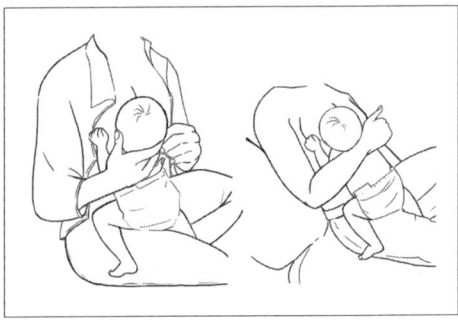

Figure 1.7 Left: A more upright straddle hold.
Right: A semi-reclined straddle hold

OVER-THE-SHOULDER HOLD (Figure 1.8) is not used often, because it is awkward, makes eye contact impossible, and reduces body contact. But it may work after a cesarean birth, help relieve a plugged duct, or when unresolved nipple pain creates a need to vary positions regularly.

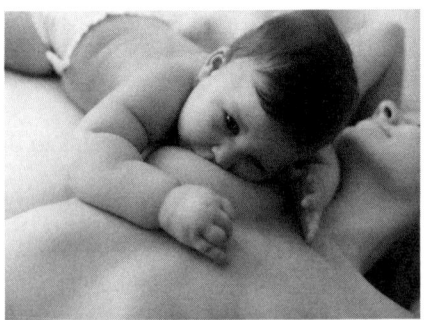

Figure 1.8 The over-the-shoulder hold

ALL-FOURS DANGLE (HANDS-AND-KNEES) POSITIONS
These positions may resolve a plugged duct faster than other holds. They involve getting up on hands and knees and

dangling the gland into baby's mouth, with baby's chin or nose pointing toward the plug (Figure 1.9).

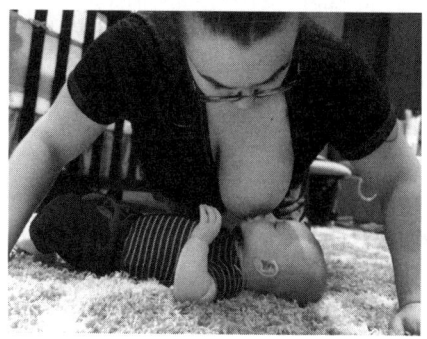

Figure 1.9 The all-fours-dangle position

NURSING TWO BABIES AT THE SAME TIME Parents of multiples often prefer to nurse two babies together at some feeds and separately at others. Nursing two babies together can save time and may be better at increasing milk production in the early weeks. It can also be helpful when one baby nurses more effectively than the other baby. Figure 1.10 illustrates some options.

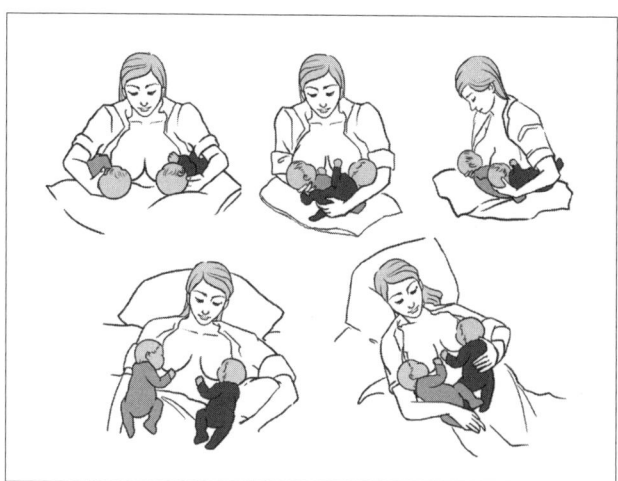

Figure 1.10 Some ways to position two babies at once.

HOW FEEDS END

When nursing is going well, suggest nursing on one side until the baby comes off on his own and then offer the other side. Not all babies drop off when finished, but they will usually eventually release the nipple. If unsure if baby is done, suggest wriggling or gently moving the mammary tissue. If baby had enough milk, he will come off. If baby is thriving, there is no advantage to timing feeds or switching sides after a specific number of minutes. If the baby falls asleep while nursing on the first side and comes off, offer the other side when he awakens. When taking baby off before he's finished, to avoid nipple pain, suggest first breaking the suction.

DIGITAL RESOURCES

GlobalHealthMedia.org/videos—A large selection of free, downloadable videos. **bit.ly/BA2-Attaching** is excellent.

NaturalBreastfeeding.com—A free video demo of the starter positions and their adjustments. The "Professionals" tab offers licensing rights for educational use of videos, images, and a digital lactation course for families.

YouTube.com/NancyMohrbacher—Free short videos of diverse women with different body types using starter positions with their newborns.

CHAPTER 2 BIRTH, EARLY NURSING, AND NURSING NORMS

Nursing norms are affected by both biology and culture. They include how often and how long baby nurses at a session, whether baby takes one side or more, the day and night changes in feeding frequency, and how these variables change over time as baby matures.

BIRTH PRACTICES AND EARLY NURSING

Practices that prolong labor or make birth more stressful or traumatic can undermine early nursing and delay milk increase. These practices include keeping laboring parents immobile and lying on their backs, leaving them alone to labor, withholding food and drink, induction of labor by drugs, using forceps and/or vacuum extractors, and performing cesarean deliveries.

When parents perceive a birth as traumatic, some develop posttraumatic stress disorder (PTSD), which may affect their intention to nurse. After a traumatic birth, some parents are less likely to nurse while others find nursing gives them a welcome respite from their trauma.

Extra lactation support is needed when labor medications are used (even synthetic oxytocin during the third stage of labor), because they may affect baby's alertness, inborn feeding behaviors, and feeding effectiveness. Emotional support received during labor is associated with earlier nursing, which is associated with better long-term nursing outcomes.

A cesarean birth puts exclusive nursing at risk. For earlier milk increase and more comfortable feeds after a surgical delivery, families need support and help in finding a comfortable feeding position. Other interventions that support nursing after a cesarean include immediate skin-to-skin contact, hand expressing after nursing and feeding baby this "dessert" by spoon (see **firstdroplets.com**), help with night nursing, knowledge about normal nursing patterns, and accurate information on the compatibility of medications with nursing. It is unclear from the research whether the surgery itself affects the timing of milk increase after birth or whether other factors (IV fluids during the surgery, differences in hormonal responses, longer time to first feed, and/or fewer feeds per day) lead to greater newborn weight loss and delayed milk increase after a surgical delivery.

ESTABLISHING NURSING

The early weeks after birth are a vulnerable time for nursing and for the family's relationship with their new baby. Post-delivery practices should be tailored to support—rather than undermine—the natural forces at work.

THE FIRST 2 HOURS AFTER BIRTH is a sensitive period. Nursing goes more smoothly and infant stability is greater when the birthing parent and baby stay together in skin-to-skin contact in a relaxed, warm, private place. Suctioning and even a short separation can interfere with the first feed.

When newborns experience the nine instinctive stages of the breast crawl (Table 2.1) at the first feed, research found fewer feeding problems (latching struggles, excess weight loss, nipple pain, delayed milk increase) during the hospital stay. When the first nursing occurs within the first hour or two after birth, there is greater infant survival, earlier increase in milk production, and fewer feeding problems. See the breast crawl in action at: **bit.ly/BA2-BF1stHours**.

Table 2.1 Nine Instinctive Stages after Birth

Stages of the Breast Crawl		Description
Stage 1	Birth cry	The intense crying after birth
Stage 2	Relaxation phase	A period of recovery where there is no movement of baby's mouth, head, arms, legs, or body
Stage 3	Awakening phase	Signs of activity, such as head movements, small movements of limbs and shoulders
Stage 4	Active phase	More determined movements of head and limbs, pushing and rooting with no shifting of body
Stage 5	Crawling phase	Pushing, which shifts body position
Stage 6	Resting phase	More resting, this time with some movements of mouth or sucking on hand
Stage 7 phase	Familiarization	After reaching areola/nipple, brushing and licking activities
Stage 8	Sucking phase	Taking nipple in mouth and sucking
Stage 9	Sleeping phase	Closed eyes

THE FIRST FEW DAYS AFTER BIRTH is a critical period for infant stability, as well as for establishing both nursing and strong relationships. During their first 24 hours, newborns consume on average about 7 mL of colostrum per nursing session, with an average daily intake of 37 mL. By the second day, the average milk intake per feed is 14 mL. When nursing is going normally, each day during the first week of life, the baby takes more milk as the milk production increases.

For the newborn, small feeds have advantages over larger feeds. Newborns have small stomachs, which at birth hold on average about 20 mL of milk. During the first 24 hours, newborn stomachs don't stretch. Supplementing with large volumes of milk can contribute to nursing problems because they raise baby's expectations, leaving her dissatisfied with average nursing volumes. Also, consistent overfeeding during the first week increases weight gain to a level during this critical period that is associated with increased risk of obesity later in life.

During the following days, a greater number of effective nursing sessions in the first 24 hours is associated with more milk intake and a lower risk of excess weight loss. More feeds during the first 4 days are associated with a lower risk of exaggerated newborn jaundice.

One early practice associated with better nursing outcomes is 24-hour rooming-in, which keeps parent and baby together around the clock. Another is more time spent in parent-baby full-frontal contact, which stimulates inborn feeding behaviors and more nursing sessions. Among sleepy babies and those who seem disinterested in feeding, this physical contact—either in skin-to-skin contact or lightly dressed—is especially important in triggering baby's feeding behaviors. Newborns can nurse effectively even in light sleep.

Sleeping arrangements in the birthing facility and the attitude conveyed by the staff about night rooming-in affect nursing outcomes, too. Sleeping arrangements that give the parent easy access to the baby—such as side-cars—result in more nursing and reduce safety risks. Rooming in during the first 48 hours is associated with significantly more total sleep in new parents. If hospital staff conveys a negative attitude about parent and baby staying together at night, parents are less likely to keep their babies with them.

Unnecessary newborn supplementation is common worldwide and can interfere with frequent nursing. The most common reason parents supplement unnecessarily is unfamiliarity with newborn behavior and nursing norms. If supplements are given, make their volumes per feed based on baby's age and consistent with the average volumes consumed during nursing. For example, on the first day, no more than 7 to 10 mL, on the second day, no more than 15 to 20 mL, and on the third day, no more than 30 mL (1 oz.). When supplements are given, the first choice is expressed mother's own milk. The second choice is donor human milk. And the third choice is non-human milks, such as infant formula.

Early exposure to non-human milks puts newborns at greater risk of allergy sensitization, unhealthy changes in the infant gut microbiome, and a longer period of intestinal permeability, which increases their vulnerability to illness.

With significant increases in milk production around the third or fourth day, nursing patterns often change, with feeds becoming shorter and babies being satisfied for some longer stretches. Stool color should change from black meconium to green transitional stools by around Day 3 and to yellow by Day 4 or 5. An earlier-than-usual transition to yellow stools is a reliable sign that nursing is going especially well, which usually means less weight loss and earlier weight gain. See p. 297 for the normal range of weight loss after birth.

SLEEP PATTERNS DURING THE EARLY WEEKS Most babies are born with their days and nights mixed up and feed more often at night than during the day. If new parents are unaware that frequent night feeds are common during this time, they may mistakenly assume it's a sign of inadequate milk or another nursing problem, which can lead to unnecessary supplementation.

THE FIRST 40 DAYS During the first weeks after birth, newborns usually nurse intensively as they establish full milk production. Hormones play a role in initiating milk production, but when hormones are at normal levels, the main driver of milk production is the rhythm and effectiveness of milk removal from the mammary glands, either by nursing or expressing milk. This dynamic is known as *autocrine control* (or local control) of milk production. When a baby nurses effectively, her feeding rhythm is the most influential factor in terms of rate of milk production. With normal nursing dynamics, by the end of the first 40 days, the nursing parent produces nearly as much milk as the baby will ever need. During this time, expect the baby to nurse at irregular intervals, "clustering" or bunching her feeds close together during some parts of the day.

The first week. With frequent nursing, by the end of the first week, milk production increases more than 10-fold—from an average of a little more than 1 ounce (37 mL) per day total on the first day to about 10 to 19 ounces (280 to 576 mL) per day by Day 7. During this same time, the baby's stomach expands and can comfortably hold about 1 to 2 ounces (30 to 59 mL) of milk at a feed. Baby's stomach grows along with milk production.

The second and third weeks. With frequent feeds, milk production continues to build. Now baby consumes about

2 to 3 ounces (59 to 89 mL) per feed and takes about 20 to 25 ounces (591 to 750 mL) of milk per day. At this stage, babies often increase the number and length of feeds to boost milk production to meet her growing needs. Periods of longer, more frequent feeds are sometimes called **growth spurts** or **frequency days**.

The fourth and fifth weeks. Babies now take an average of about 3 to 4 ounces (89 to 118 mL) per feed, and daily milk intake increases to an average of about 25 to 30 ounces (750 to 900 mL) per day. At 1 month, most nursing parents produce nearly as much milk per day as their nursing baby will ever need. Because babies' growth and metabolic rate slow as they age, they continue to need about the same daily volume of milk from 1 month to 6 months of age. But not every baby is average. Some need more and some need less to gain the expected weight.

When parents expect intensive nursing during the first 40 days, they can plan ahead to get help with meals, household chores, and any older children. With a good understanding of normal nursing patterns, they will be less likely to assume something is wrong because the baby wants to nurse so often.

THE OLDER BABY

BIOLOGY AND CULTURE Some expect the nursing baby to feed significantly less often as she grows, but that is not consistent with human biology. Compared with other mammals, human babies are born very immature, and human milk is among the lowest in fat and protein content of all mammalian milks. This puts humans in the category of "carry" or "continuous contact" mammals, which are meant to be carried constantly and fed often around the clock.

Many nursing babies do not conform to feeding and sleeping expectations of Western cultures, which were based on research on formula-fed babies. In Western societies, babies are often expected to stay full for hours after feeds and to sleep alone for long stretches at night. While some nursing babies follow these patterns, many do not. When the natural feeding patterns of a nursing baby are in conflict with cultural beliefs, this creates anxiety among many new parents.

Feeding schedules are more compatible with bottle-feeding norms and are part of an approach to child-rearing sometimes referred to as "scientific mothering." This approach became popular in the early 20th century and was based on the beliefs of early behaviorist psychologists. Despite being disproved by science, some of its basic tenets are a part of Western cultural beliefs and undermine nursing.

DAILY FEEDING PATTERNS As newborns become more in tune with the rest of the family, they may nurse less at night so milk accumulates in the mammary gland. After the first few weeks, many nursing babies feed more often in the evening and less often in the morning.

FOREMILK AND HINDMILK No matter what the time intervals between feeds, babies consume about the same amount of fat over the course of a day. This is because the baby who nurses more often gets foremilk higher in fat and hindmilk lower in fat than the baby who nurses less often. Whatever the feeding rhythm, total daily milk intake is what's most important to a baby's growth. On average, babies between 1 and 6 months of age consume about 25 to 30 ounces (750 to 900 mL) per day. As far as growth is concerned, it doesn't matter if a baby takes 1 ounce (30 mL) every hour or 3 ounces (89 mL) every 3 hours, as long as she receives enough milk overall. Whether babies practice the very frequent feeds of the hunter-gatherers (several feeds per hour) or the longer intervals between feeds of Western societies, nursing babies take about the same amount of milk each day.

Variables that affect feeding patterns over time include baby's stomach size and the nursing parent's storage capacity, or how much milk baby's stomach can hold and how much milk is available at each feed from the mammary gland. Baby's stomach size is determined in part by age and weight.

The term ***storage capacity*** refers to the maximum volume of milk available to the baby when the mammary gland is at its fullest time of the day. Because this volume of milk varies—sometimes greatly—among nursing parents, this concept helps explain why feeding rhythms can vary so much from one nursing couple to another. Storage capacity can range from 74 to 606 mL (2.6 to 20.5 oz.) per side. It is not related to the size of the mammary gland, which is usually determined mainly by the amount of fatty tissue present. Parents with smaller mammary glands may have a large storage capacity and parents with large mammary glands may have a small storage capacity.

With a large storage capacity, babies may thrive on one side per feed and fewer feeds per day. With a small storage capacity, to gain weight as expected, baby may need to take both sides per feed and feed more times each day. That's why it's best to feed nursing babies on cue rather than imposing a feeding schedule. On average, babies take one side at some feeds and both sides at some feeds.

MILK INTAKE AS BABY GROWS At around 5 weeks, a nursing baby reaches her peak daily milk intake of about 25 to 30 ounces (750 to 900 mL) of milk per day, and this stays roughly the same until she begins solid foods at 6 months and her need for milk begins to decrease. Because babies' growth and metabolic rate slow as they age, even as they get bigger and heavier, they continue to need about the same volume of milk from 1 month to 6 months of age. For more details, see p. 188.

On average, formula-fed babies consume much more milk per feed and per day compared with nursing babies: 15% more milk at 3 months, 23% more at 6 months, 20% more at 9 months, and 18% more at 12 months.

After 1 year, feeding rhythm varies from child to child and from place to place. Where nursing older babies is the norm, parents average more feeds per day and greater milk production than in places where nursing older babies is not the norm.

PACIFIERS/DUMMIES

Pacifiers/dummies are not recommended for healthy term infants during the first month of nursing. They are used to help settle fussy babies and prolong the intervals between feeds. But during the intense first 40 days of nursing, fussy newborns should ideally be settled by nursing, which also helps establish healthy milk production. Regular, frequent use of a pacifier during this critical time can decrease the number of feeds per day, potentially undermining milk production. Research on the effects of pacifier use on nursing outcomes is mixed and may be affected by the parent's motivation to nurse.

Pacifiers can be an appropriate tool in some situations, such as to soothe babies when the nursing parent is not present or nursing is not possible, to speed the transition of preterm babies from tube feeding to oral feeds, to help some low-tone babies overcome feeding problems, and during painful procedures when nursing is not an option.

Based on few studies, one U.S. health organization recommends all nursing babies older than 1 month be given a pacifier while going to sleep to prevent Sudden Infant Death Syndrome (SIDS). This organization recommends nursing families wait to start the pacifier until after milk production is firmly established, usually after the first 3 to 4 weeks. In the Netherlands, however, pacifiers are only recommended for bottle-fed babies while going to sleep.

Using pacifiers to keep baby calm instead of nursing lowers progesterone levels, contributing to an earlier return to fertility. Higher postnatal progesterone levels are associated with delayed menstruation, while the use of pacifiers and infant formula are associated with earlier return to menstruation.

SLEEP AND NIGHT FEEDS

SLEEP PATTERNS Most babies are born with their days and nights mixed up. This means many newborns wake to feed more often at night and sleep for longer stretches during the day. One long 4- to 5-hour sleep stretch is not unusual and is not a problem, as long as baby fits in at least 8 or more nursing sessions each 24-hour period. This longer sleep stretch may be more likely during daylight hours. Parents don't need to wake the baby during this long daytime sleep stretch unless they want to encourage the baby to sleep more at night. The exception is the baby who feeds fewer than 8 times in 24 hours, who needs to be stimulated to feed more.

To gently shift a baby's longest sleep period from day to night, suggest parents start by reducing all sensory stimulation at night. This involves keeping lights low and sound and movements to a minimum. Change diapers only when baby is soaked or passed a stool.

To get more rest, encourage nursing parents to sleep when their baby sleeps and find a feeding position, that allows them to safely doze during feeds.

Exclusively nursing parents sleep more deeply and get either the same amount or more sleep per night than parents who mixed-feed or formula feed. Feeding newborns formula at night resulted in parents and partners getting less sleep because preparing and feeding bottles disrupted the sleep of the nursing parents, as well as those doing the night feeds. Giving nursing babies formula so they sleep longer may undermine milk production and increase risk of SIDS. Research is mixed on whether feeding solids before 6 months helps babies sleep longer at night.

The nursing parent's storage capacity may affect the baby's need to nurse at night. Storage capacity affects the number of night feeds needed for a baby to grow and gain weight as expected, as well as the length of the longest interval between feeds. A large storage capacity may make it possible for baby to sleep longer at night at a younger age without compromising weight gain and growth. A small storage capacity may require continued night feeds for a longer period.

Average sleep patterns vary among nursing and formula-fed babies, but their total time spent asleep over 24 hours is the same. Nursing babies wake more often at night but fall back asleep faster. Formula-fed babies sleep deeper and longer, but this puts them at increased risk for SIDS. Nursing families who know about normal sleep patterns in nursing babies and receive support for meeting their baby's needs at night report feeling less stressed than those with unrealistic expectations.

Reliable information about normal sleep patterns in nursing babies is available in the free Infant Sleep Info app available from the App Store and Google Play.

Sleep-training disrupts parent-baby synchrony, has the potential to undermine nursing outcomes, and may encourage a more unresponsive parenting style. To learn more, see the website created by the sleep researchers at the University of Durham at **bit.ly/BA2-SleepTrain**

WHERE SHOULD BABIES SLEEP? To prevent SIDS, a U.S. health organization recommended that for the first 6 to 12 months, baby should sleep in the parents' room. This is an advantage in terms of total sleep because parents will hear the baby stir before she is fully awake and starts to cry. Most parents and babies fall back to sleep faster if they have not been fully awakened. Some sleep arrangements make night feeds easier.

- A bassinet or cradle next to the parents' bed
- Baby's crib attached to the parents' bed as a "side-car"
- A co-sleeper bed that attaches to the parents' bed
- Baby nurses to sleep on a pallet or mattress on the floor away from the walls and furniture in the parents' room, so nursing parents can lie down and sleep while feeding the baby and return to their bed if desired after the baby goes back to sleep.
- Baby sleeps in the parents' bed, either for all or part of the night

The free Infant Sleep Info app created by the U.K. sleep researchers at the University of Durham describes safe sleeping options. Encourage families to do what works best for them while following safe sleeping practices.

Bed-sharing among nursing families is common worldwide and is associated with more sleep and longer and more exclusive nursing. Bed-sharing is common even in cultures that caution against it. Unlike recommendations about sleep position, bed-sharing is part of some ethnic and cultural norms, so it is not an infant-care behavior that is easily changed by simple recommendations.

Attempts to avoid bed-sharing can inadvertently lead to dangerous sleeping practices, such as falling asleep on a sofa, a recliner, or an adult bed not made safe for infants. An alternative to issuing a blanket recommendation against bed-sharing is to recommend parents adopt safer bed-sharing practices. In its 2020 Clinical Protocol #6 (**bfmed.org/protocols**), the Academy of Breastfeeding Medicine makes the scientific case that the best way to decrease infant deaths during sleep is to openly discuss the specific ways parents who bed-share (intentionally or unintentionally) can reduce risk.

DIGITAL RESOURCES

basisonline.org.uk—Website of Baby Sleep Info Source from the University of Durham in the U.K., which features information and free downloadable handouts for parents on normal infant sleep and research on sleep strategies, as well as resources for professionals.

bit.ly/BA2-BF1stHours—Free 10-minute video on **GlobalHealthMedia.org** showing the 9 instinctive stages of the breast crawl in action.

firstdroplets.com—Free videos for parents by U.S. pediatrician Jane Morton show how to avoid excess newborn weight loss, maximize milk production, and increase self-confidence by learning hand expression before birth and using it in the first days after birth to provide newborns with "dessert" by spoon after nursing.

Infant Sleep Info app available free from the App Store and Google Play. Created for parents by the U.K. sleep researchers at the University of Durham. Includes a sleep log that tracks and displays baby's sleep patterns on a chart depicting the range of normal sleep at different ages, a bed-sharing decision guide, and a guide to safe sleep.

CHAPTER 3 BREAST OR CHEST ISSUES

ENGORGEMENT

Between the 2nd and 6th day after birth, the mammary glands usually start to feel tender, larger, and heavier. These normal sensations are caused by increasing milk production and increased flow of blood and lymph to the glands, which play a role in milk production. The difference between normal feelings of fullness and engorgement is a matter of degree, and there is no standard measure to differentiate them.

CAUSES OF ENGORGEMENT   If milk is removed early, often, and effectively by the baby or by milk expression, normal mammary fullness is less likely to become painful engorgement. But if nursing is delayed or the baby nurses infrequently or ineffectively and the glands stay full of milk for too long, blood circulation to the glands slows. As pressure builds from milk accumulation (***milk stasis***), the spaces between the milk-producing cells open and proteins from the blood and milk seep into the mammary tissues, causing swelling. Those giving birth for the first time are less likely to become severely engorged than others. Within 48 hours of birth, if swelling (***edema***) occurs in the mammary tissue, excess IV fluids given during labor may be the cause. Swelling from excess IV fluids—which may also cause swollen ankles—is sometimes confused with engorgement. If a parent with this type of tissue swelling also becomes engorged, this can delay the resolution of engorgement for up to 10 to 14 days.

ENGORGEMENT SYMPTOMS AND DURATION   The mammary swelling of engorgement can cause discomfort, warmth, and throbbing that may extend into the armpit area, where some milk-producing glands (the ***tail of Spence***) are located. The skin on the glands may appear taut and shiny. When pressure builds inside the gland, this causes milk production to slow. If pressure keeps building, eventually continued pressure will cause the milk-making cells known as mammary epithelial cells, or lactocytes, to shut down operations entirely and over time self-destruct. Engorgement may also cause a fever of up to 101°F/38.3°C which is sometimes confused with a post-delivery infection, resulting in unnecessary separation of the nursing couple. On average, engorgement peaks at around 5 days and with effective treatment lasts an average of 4 days.

ENGORGEMENT TYPES AND COMPLICATIONS   Engorgement may occur only in the areola (***areolar engorgement***), only in other areas (***peripheral engorgement***), or in both. It may also occur in one or both sides. Possible complications of engorgement include a shallow latch from taut mammary tissue, which may lead to latching struggles and excess weight loss in babies and nipple damage and mastitis in nursing parents. In extreme cases, unrelieved pressure can damage the milk-making tissue, which may compromise long-term milk production.

STRATEGIES TO PREVENT OR MINIMIZE ENGORGEMENT Keep the nursing couple together after birth and encourage them to nurse early, often, and effectively. If the baby sleeps for long stretches, suggest parents keep the baby on their body as much as they are comfortable. When this stimulation triggers inborn feeding behaviors, parents can help guide baby to latch, even while baby is in light sleep. When the milk is well drained from the gland, this allows blood and lymph to drain more easily, reducing tissue congestion. During nursing sessions, let baby "finish the first side first." This means waiting until baby comes off the first side on his own before offering the second side. Nursing from each side more than once drains the gland even more. After nursing, express colostrum into a spoon, and feed baby this "dessert" (see **firstdroplets.com**). As weeks pass and milk production is established, the hormones of childbirth decrease to lower levels and the glands feel softer, even with abundant milk production.

ENGORGEMENT TREATMENTS should begin as soon as fullness become uncomfortable to reduce discomfort and prevent complications. With early and effective treatments, extreme symptoms can usually be prevented or resolved within 12 to 48 hours. If not treated promptly, it may take up to 7 to 14 days or longer for symptoms to resolve completely. Basic treatment strategies involve draining the milk more often and/or more fully and reducing painful swelling. These include nursing often and long with a deep latch, using techniques that are soothing and stimulate more milk flow during nursing (brief application of heat before feeds, gentle massage), expressing milk by hand or with a pump after nursing, applying cold compresses between feeds to reduce swelling, and taking anti-inflammatory medication).

If taut, engorged glands make the nipple so flat and the areola so taut that it is difficult for baby to latch or to get a deep latch, suggest softening the areola first. Ways to do this include ***reverse pressure softening*** (p. 333), massaging and expressing a little milk, or wearing breast shells for about 30 minutes before a nursing attempt. If these don't work, the short-term use of a nipple shield (p. 329) may help. If baby still cannot latch, suggest expressing milk and feeding it to the baby. If milk expression must temporarily substitute for nursing, see p. 211-214 for effective milk-expression strategies.

Promising treatments for engorgement with low-quality evidence include acupuncture, cabbage leaves, Chinese Gua-Sha scraping therapy, and herbal compresses (using hollyhock or a mix of herbs).

Engorgement treatments found ineffective include kinesio-elastic therapeutic taping, progesterone gel, and ultrasound.

If one-sided engorgement persists despite consistent treatment, suggest seeing a healthcare provider to rule out other causes. Rarely, continued engorgement may be a warning sign of another type of health problem, such as mastitis, a cyst, or even breast cancer.

MASTITIS

The word "mastitis" means inflammation of the mammary gland. It may be mild or severe. Some define mastitis as only those cases that involve fever, body aches and lethargy. Others suggest using the term **acute mastitis** when fever and body aches are present and **subacute mastitis** for the milder, localized version sometimes called **plugged, clogged**, or **blocked ducts.** It may help to think of cases of mastitis as falling somewhere on a spectrum.

At the least severe end of this spectrum is **subclinical mastitis**, a type with no obvious symptoms that can only be detected by analyzing human milk components. In the absence of weaning, one sign of subclinical mastitis is an altered sodium/potassium ratio (abnormally high sodium and low potassium). In HIV-positive parents, subclinical mastitis increases the risk of HIV transmission to the nursing baby.

Next along the mastitis spectrum is subacute mastitis, or a plugged duct. Further along this spectrum is acute mastitis, also called a **breast infection**, which includes flu-like symptoms such as fever and may or may not involve a bacterial infection. At the most severe end of the continuum is an abscess, a pus-filled cyst that requires drainage.

Mastitis occurs in as many as 1 in 5 nursing parents and happens most often during the early weeks. Where nursing is the cultural norm, rates of mastitis are much lower than in many Western countries.

CAUSES OF MASTITIS Factors that increase the risk of mastitis include periods of overfullness (from oversupply or ineffective or irregular milk removal), nipple trauma (which provides an entry point for organisms), consistent pressure on the gland (a too-tight bra or carrier strap, sleeping on the stomach), stress, and fatigue.

Nipple trauma, stress, fatigue, and antibiotic use can alter the balance of organisms, or **microbiome**, of the mammary gland. When unhealthy organisms increase at the expense of healthy organisms, **mammary dysbiosis** may occur, a disruption of the gland's microbiome that increases risk of inflammation, pain, and mastitis.

MASTITIS SYMPTOMS include tenderness, sore areas, and lumps in the gland. In more severe cases, flu-like symptoms of fever, body aches, and fatigue may occur. Milk expressed right before or during mastitis may look thick or stringy or appear to contain a crystal or grain of sand. None of these are harmful to a term, healthy baby. Symptoms specific to a bacterial infection during mastitis include visible pus in a nipple crack or fissure, pus or blood in the milk, red streaks on the mammary gland, and any other sudden symptoms with no obvious cause, such as nausea and vomiting. When symptoms of a bacterial infection are present, suggest parents contact their healthcare provider. Severe mastitis in both sides that occurs during the first 2 weeks after birth may be a hospital-acquired infection. When mastitis develops that's caused by methicillin-resistant Staphylococcus aureus (MRSA), the baby has already been exposed to it before the parent's symptoms became obvious, so there is no reason to stop nursing unless the baby is ill or preterm.

Milk production may be slowed in the affected side for about a week, but it can be brought back to its previous level quickly with frequent milk removal.

MASTITIS TREATMENTS If symptoms during the first 24 hours are not severe, suggest starting with basic home treatments, including:

- Frequent and effective milk removal by nursing and or expressing at least every 2 hours during the day and 3 hours at night. Start with the affected side. Vary feeding positions to better drain different areas (p. 14-15).

- Before nursing or expressing milk, apply heat for a few minutes at least 3 times per day and remove any dried milk from the nipple with water. While the gland is warm, massage gently with fingertips or palm, moving from the armpit toward the nipple. (See video at **bit.ly/BA2-BolmanMassage.**)

- Loosen any tight clothing.

- Take analgesia recommended by the parent's healthcare provider.

- Apply cold between milk removals to reduce swelling.

- Rest as much as possible to boost the immune system.

If the baby balks at nursing from the affected side, express milk from that side and keep nursing on the other side.

The use of antibiotics to treat mastitis varies widely by country, and research on their effectiveness is mixed. If symptoms don't improve within 12 to 24 hours of home treatment, there is visible pus, or the parent is acutely ill or suddenly spikes a high fever, suggest parents contact their provider and consider treatment with antibiotics. A penicillinase-resistant penicillin antibiotic compatible with nursing (such as flucloxacillin, dicloxacillin) is usually given for a 10- to 14-day course. Parents taking a shorter course of antibiotics may be at greater risk of recurrence.

New treatments that require more research but may complement antibiotics include:

- **Specific probiotics.** Taking orally the specific probiotics (live beneficial organisms) found in healthy mammary glands (such as *L. fermentum*) may prevent and treat mastitis. The specific strains of probiotics studied are sold by companies in Spain (Angelini), Australia (Puremedica), and in the US (Klaire Labs).

- **Nisin solution swab after nursing.** Nisin is a food-grade antimicrobial commonly found in the milk of healthy lactating parents. A small study found after 2 weeks symptoms completely resolved in the group that swabbed a nisin solution on their nipples and areolae after feeds and continued in the control group, who swabbed a placebo solution.

- **Topical curcumin.** Curcumin is the active ingredient in turmeric, which has anti-inflammatory properties. Applying (200 mg) curcumin cream to the glands every 8 hours reduced mastitis symptoms compared with those who applied a placebo cream.

If parents do not respond to antibiotics or the other treatments within 2 days, culturing the milk may help determine if another drug would be a more appropriate treatment. Also rule out causes other than mastitis, such as cellulitis, idiopathic granulomatous mastitis, or even inflammatory breast cancer. If a breast or chest lump doesn't shrink within a week of treatment, suggest contacting a healthcare provider to rule out other causes.

WEANING SAFELY DURING MASTITIS If parents with mastitis decide to wean, help them do it gradually and safely. Weaning too quickly may worsen their mastitis or cause an abscess to develop. To avoid a more serious health problem, suggest parents wait to wean until mastitis clears, and then wean very slowly to avoid a recurrence. A slow and gradual weaning plan may involve nursing and/or milk expression.

For example, parents could drop a daily nursing session and allow several days before dropping another. If exclusively expressing milk, another option is to gradually decrease the length of each pumping by a couple of minutes and continue for several days at this level before decreasing the length again.

With any gradual weaning, whenever parents feel any fullness, they can express just enough milk to soften the glands. This makes it possible to stop milk production without pain or risk of more health problems.

RECURRING MASTITIS can be demoralizing, even to a motivated parent. To determine the cause, first ask about previous treatments, as failure to fully recover from a previous bout of mastitis is a common cause. This is especially likely if the last episode of mastitis was within the previous few weeks. If mastitis recurs after treatment with antibiotics, it is possible that the same risk factors are still present. Other possibilities include:

- A course of antibiotics shorter than 10 to 14 days
- Use of an inappropriate antibiotic
- Reinfection after finishing the medication by an organism carried in the baby's throat or nose.

A milk culture can determine if another antibiotic might be more effective. For recommendations of specific drugs and doses that parents can share with healthcare providers, see the Clinical Protocol #4 from the Academy of Breastfeeding Medicine (ABM) at **bfmed.org/protocols**.

Another possibility is that the common causes of mastitis may be contributing to its recurrences. These include periods of mammary fullness, nipple trauma, which allows entry of bacteria in the gland via nipple trauma, and sustained pressure on the gland.

Fatigue, stress, and more unusual risk factors may contribute to recurring mastitis. Examples include:

- Nipple bleb, or milk blister, blocking milk flow from one or more nipple pores (p. 231)
- Exclusive pumping, which often leads to longer periods of mammary fullness than direct nursing
- Health issues that increase parents' susceptibility to infection, such as diabetes or IgA deficiency
- Nipple shield use. Was it used because the baby nursed ineffectively, or could poor hygiene be a factor?
- Breast or chest injury from intense exercise or trauma, causing mammary swelling and blocking milk flow

- Nipple piercing, which allows bacteria to enter the gland
- Internal breast or chest abnormalities, such as scar tissue from previous surgery, abscess, cyst, or cancer that causes internal pressure on ducts and blocks milk flow

If mastitis always recurs in the same area, there may be an internal cause. Previous surgery on the breast or chest increases the risk of mastitis due to internal scarring, which can put pressure on the milk ducts. Unusual anatomy in a duct or a lump is another possible cause. Since these causes cannot be easily corrected, a parent may decide to nurse only on the unaffected side, gradually allowing milk production to stop on the affected side. Recurring mastitis in the same location is also a warning sign of possible breast cancer. If this happens, suggest seeing a healthcare provider for diagnostic imaging to rule out a serious cause.

Three possible treatments for chronic recurring plugged ducts or more severe forms of mastitis are:

- **Lecithin** supplements have long been recommended although the mechanism is unclear. Recommended dose: 3,600 to 4,800 mg per day, or one 1,200 mg capsule three to four times daily. After 1 to 2 weeks at this dose with no plugged ducts, reduce it by one capsule per day. If the plugged ducts do not return during the next 2 weeks, reduce it again by one capsule per day. If the plugged ducts return, continue taking one to two capsules per day indefinitely.
- **Ultrasound therapy** involves sending noninvasive vibrating particles into the body to treat tissues damaged by disease or injury. The dosages used varies greatly among providers.
- **Long-term, low-dose antibiotics**. If a chronic bacterial infection is a possible underlying cause of recurring mastitis, it may be possible to break the cycle with a preventive, low-dose, long-term antibiotic treatment. Begin with a 10- to 14-day course of antibiotics to treat the current bout of mastitis, which is followed by low doses of antibiotics (i.e., 500 mg. erythromycin) taken daily for 2 to 3 months to prevent recurrence.

ABSCESS Mammary abscesses are uncommon and usually occur when mastitis is not treated promptly and appropriately or doesn't respond to treatment. An abscess is a walled-off area of pus in the body with no opening for drainage. To resolve an abscess, it must be either aspirated or drained. It is a serious and often painful condition that needs immediate medical attention.

ABSCESS TYPES AND PREVALENCE Abscesses are categorized by location. ***Subareolar abscesses*** are just under the areola. ***Intrammamary unilocular abscesses*** are deeper within the mammary tissue and contain just one pocket of pus. Those that contain multiple pockets are called **multiocular abscesses**. Mammary abscesses occur in about 3% of nursing parents with a history of mastitis. In some areas, most abscesses culture positive for MRSA, an organism resistant to common antibiotics.

TO CONFIRM AN ABSCESS Often, abscesses cannot be confirmed by examination alone, especially when there's no fever or other generalized symptoms. Ultrasound is preferred over a mammogram to identify an abscess and may be used during treatment to locate it for aspiration or drainage. A mammogram cannot distinguish an abscess from other masses, such as a tumor, and the tissue squeezing involved during this procedure can be very painful. Ultrasound is more comfortable and can also distinguish an abscess from solid masses. Confirming the existence, size, and location of the abscess allows the healthcare provider to determine whether or not surgical drainage is necessary or whether a less-invasive treatment is an option.

ABSCESS TREATMENTS Most abscesses can be treated with methods that are less invasive than surgical incision and drainage and make continued nursing more likely. A combination of ultrasonic imaging to locate the abscess and aspiration and flushing with a needle, catheter, or suction device can eliminate the need for surgery. These procedures can typically be done as an outpatient, which minimizes separation of nursing couples. Culturing the aspirated fluid for organisms and treating the nursing parent with appropriate antibiotics for at least 10 days is also a vital part of this treatment.

NURSING DURING ABSCESS TREATMENT Aspiration of the contents of the abscess should not affect nursing. If a catheter or surgical incision and drainage is used near the areola, the parent can continue nursing on the unaffected side. If the catheter or surgical incision is far enough from the areola so the baby's mouth does not touch it when he nurses, nursing may continue on the affected side. An abscess that is surgically drained is not usually closed. It remains open so it can drain and heal from the inside out. Rest is a vital part of the treatment.

If nursing on the affected side is interrupted, express milk from that side often enough to stay comfortable while the incision is healing to prevent engorgement. Nursing can continue on the affected side after surgical drainage and will not prevent healing, even though milk may seep from the incision. The incision may heal more slowly, but continuing to nurse prevents the affected gland from becoming painfully full of milk, which prevents the mastitis from recurring and decreases the odds that the baby will prefer the unaffected side after healing.

DEEP BREAST PAIN

The nursing parent may feel deep breast pain at any stage of lactation, and it may occur in one or both sides during or between nursing sessions. It may be localized in one area or radiate.

CAUSES OF DEEP BREAST PAIN   Try to determine the cause before suggesting strategies. Ask the age of the baby and where and when the pain is felt, if it is localized or radiating, and whether or not there is a history of nipple trauma or mastitis, which may provide clues to its cause.

Nipple trauma allows organisms to enter the mammary gland, a risk factor for mastitis and superficial bacterial and fungal nipple infections. Nipple damage may negatively alter the microbiome of the gland. When unhealthy organisms in the mammary microbiome take the place of healthy organisms, this can cause mammary dysbiosis, which can lead to a *lactiferous duct infection*, persistent sore, tender, throbbing breasts and nipples.

MOST COMMON CAUSES OF DEEP BREAST PAIN   If the pain is in one side during or between feeds, consider these common causes:

- **Nipple trauma**—The damage may be limited to the nipples, or the pain may radiate into the gland. In this case, the pain resolves when the nipples heal.

- **Mastitis**—The pain is usually localized but may radiate. It occurs most often in the early weeks of nursing but can happen later. If the pain continues after treatment, suggest seeing a healthcare provider to rule out abscess and other issues.

- **Superficial nipple infection**—The pain may be localized or radiating. Bacterial or fungal infection may develop after nipple damage and may include visible pus or yellow scabbing or crusting. With an infection, healing is often slowed or stopped and pain may be severe.

If the pain is in both sides during feeds, consider:

- **Engorgement**—The pain is usually radiating and will resolve with the engorgement. The tissue feels taut and it usually occurs during the first 2 weeks, but it can occur later from missed feeds.

- **Strong milk ejection**—The pain is usually radiating and begins at milk ejection. It may be due to milk duct dilation. This pain usually decreases over time, disappearing within a month or so after birth.

- **Pain disorder**—Those with the condition *allodynia* feel pain even with light touch that does not usually cause pain. This unusual response may occur in parents with other pain disorders, such as irritable bowel syndrome, fibromyalgia, migraines, temporomandibular joint (TMJ) disorder, and painful intercourse.

If the pain is in both sides between feeds, consider:

- **Vasospasm or Raynaud's phenomenon**—The pain is usually radiating. The nipple may turn white (blanch) after the baby releases it. As many as 1 in 4 experience vasospasm during the early weeks. If Raynaud's phenomenon is involved, the nipple may also turn red and/or blue, and there may be a history of pain and blanching when fingers are exposed to cold. Symptoms usually begin in the early weeks of nursing.

- **Oversupply**—Sharp pain or dull, aching pain may occur as the glands become full of milk.

- **Referred pain from nipple trauma**—The pain may be localized or radiating and will resolve when nipple pain resolves. It usually occurs during the early weeks of nursing or during teething.

LESS COMMON CAUSES OF DEEP BREAST PAIN If the pain is in one side during or between feedings, consider:

- **Bacterial dysbiosis or lactiferous duct infection**. A history of nipple trauma may lead to sore, tender glands and/or nipples on both sides. Caused by a change in the mammary microbiome, it can be challenging to resolve. See the ABM Clinical Protocol #26 at **bfmed.org/protocols**. The recommended treatment is to take the appropriate oral antibiotic for 2 to 6 weeks. Share this protocol with healthcare providers.

- **Internal scarring** from previous breast or chest surgery or injury—The pain is usually localized.

- **Ruptured breast implant**—The pain is usually localized. Breast shape may change or there may be skin changes. If this is the problem, removal surgery may be needed.

- **Galactocele**—The pain is usually localized. An obvious lump within the gland can be easily moved (p. 38)

- **Duct ectasia**—The pain is usually localized and may include burning, itching, and nipple swelling (p. 40)

- **Referred pain from muscle strain or injury**—The pain may be localized or radiating and resolves when the injury heals. An injury elsewhere may be felt as breast pain if it occurs along the same nerve pathways. Early on, it may be from a birth injury. Later, it may be from any injury, joint pain, or muscle strain.

- **Breast cancer**—The pain may be localized or radiating and may be in one or both sides. If the pain does not resolve within weeks, suggest seeing a healthcare provider to rule this out. This in an early symptom in 8% to 15% of those later diagnosed with breast cancer.

If the pain is in both sides during feeds, consider:

- **Premenstrual pain**—The pain is usually radiating and peaks before a menstrual period when mammary glands swell with extra blood and lymph. It can be felt during or between feeds and includes feelings of heaviness, fullness, and tenderness. Symptoms usually resolve soon after menstruation starts. If fibrocystic breast changes are a contributing factor, eliminating caffeine may help.

If the pain is in both sides between feeds, consider:

- **Very large mammary glands** are heavy and can pull on the connective tissues above the glands, causing tenderness where the glands join the chest wall near the third rib. Try a different style or better fitting bra. Using pectoral muscle massage and stretching techniques before feeds may improve comfort.

Shooting, burning pain between feeds is unlikely to be from a ductal yeast infection and more likely to have other causes. Once it was thought that the most likely cause of shooting or burning breast pain between feeds was a secondary yeast infection in or around the milk ducts (referred to as ***mammary or ductal candidiasis***), but research was unable to confirm its existence. When parents experience burning or shooting mammary pain between feeds, before considering yeast as the likely cause, first rule out other causes, such as those listed above. If there is a history of nipple trauma, consider mammary or bacterial dysbiosis (previous page).

BREAST LUMPS

During lactation, as the milk ducts fill and empty, the mammary glands typically feel lumpier than at other times. By becoming familiar with their feel, parents can learn to distinguish normal lumpiness from a lump that might need medical attention. If a lump's size stays constant or increases after nursing, suggest it be checked.

If a lump does not decrease in size after careful home treatment for mastitis, suggest seeing a healthcare provider.

If a parent has a breast exam, suggest nursing right before to reduce the volume of milk in the glands.

DIAGNOSTIC TESTS are usually compatible with nursing. Some that may be used to diagnose a lump include:

- **X-rays.** Human milk is not affected, and it's fine to nurse right after an x-ray.
- **Imaging scans (PET, MIBI, and EIT scans, and ultrasound)** do not interfere with nursing or affect the milk. Unlike mammograms, ultrasound can distinguish solid lumps from fluid-filled cysts, galactoceles, and abscesses. The ABM Clinical Protocol #30 on breast masses and imaging (at **bfmed.org/protocols**) recommends ultrasound as the first diagnostic tool with any breast lump or mass.
- **CAT scans and MRIs** do not interfere with nursing or affect the milk. The radiopaque or radiocontrast agents sometimes injected prior to these scans are considered compatible with continued nursing, despite some package inserts, which recommended interrupting nursing.
- **Mammograms** use low-level x-rays and can be done on a lactating mammary gland. Like other x-rays, mammograms do not affect the milk, so nursing can resume immediately afterward. But mammograms are usually more difficult to read in younger patients and during lactation. If an ultrasound shows a suspicious mass, the ABM recommends a 3D mammogram known as DBT be done.
- **Fine-needle aspiration cytologic study**, a quick, nearly painless procedure can determine the nature of a fluid-filled lump (galactocele, abscess) and may be done with local anesthesia without interrupting nursing.
- **Core needle biopsy** is recommended by the ABM for a solid mass.

A breast biopsy can usually be done without interrupting nursing. The ABM recommends against weaning before a biopsy to minimize risk of a milk fistula.

FIBROCYSTIC CHANGES in the mammary gland are common; pregnancy and nursing may reduce the severity of their symptoms.

GALACTOCELES are milk-filled cysts that are uncommon and harmless. If it is painful, this round lump can be surgically removed under local anesthesia without interrupting nursing. Or fine-needle aspiration with local anesthetic can be done in an office or clinic. If it is not painful or infected, no treatment is needed.

CALCIFICATIONS, tiny deposits of calcium in the mammary gland, occur more often with aging. When they are evenly distributed in both sides, this is usually not a cause for concern. When they appear in clusters, this is a risk factor for cancer, so another mammogram is recommended within a few months.

BLOOD IN THE MILK OR NIPPLE DISCHARGE

BLOOD IN THE MILK during the early weeks after birth is common and usually disappears quickly and will not harm the baby. Its most likely causes are:

- **Rusty-pipe syndrome (*vascular engorgement*)** is common during pregnancy and early nursing. It is caused by slight internal bleeding from a combination of increased blood flow to the gland and rapid growth of milk-making tissue. It usually occurs in both sides but may occur in one side at first. Usually there is little or no discomfort and it resolves on its own within the first few weeks.

- **Intraductal papilloma**, also common, is a benign wart-like growth in a milk duct that causes bleeding as it erodes. It usually occurs in only one side, cannot be felt as a lump, and may involve discomfort. The bleeding often stops without treatment within weeks of birth. Because these benign growths can become cancerous, the ABM recommends diagnostic imaging when intraductal papilloma is suspected.

- **Fibrocystic changes** within the gland, common with aging, may cause a bloody nipple discharge.

- **Breast or nipple trauma** can cause blood in the milk when broken capillaries occur from rough handling or too-high breast pump suction levels. If a nursing parent has nipple damage, it may be difficult to determine whether the blood originates from the nipple or inside the gland.

Milk color is not always what it seems. For example, milk may appear pink when nursing parents are colonized with bacteria, such as *Serratia marcescens*. Expressed milk comes in a variety of colors—blue, green, brownish, yellow, gold, and clear—which are considered normal for both colostrum and mature milk. For more details, see p. 218.

If the blood in the milk doesn't clear within a few weeks of birth, suggest nursing parents see their healthcare provider to rule out more serious causes, such as Paget's disease and other types of breast cancer. Non-invasive tests, such as ultrasound, are recommended to help determine the cause of the bloody milk.

NIPPLE DISCHARGE that is not bloody may have a variety of causes. A yellow or green nipple discharge that seems to come from multiple ducts on both sides is considered within the normal range.

Stringy-looking milk or granules can sometimes be expressed during or just prior to a bout of mastitis. For more details, see p. 30.

A multi-colored, sticky discharge may be due to **duct ectasia**, which is caused by inflammation in a milk duct. Nursing parents with this condition may have no discomfort or they may have burning pain, itching, and nipple swelling. Over time, the affected duct may feel like a hardened tube or a mass under the nipple. Treat with warm compresses and antibiotics. If duct ectasia is painful or the discharge appears bloody, surgical removal of the duct is an option.

UNUSUAL BREAST DEVELOPMENT

EXTRA NIPPLES AND BREAST TISSUE sometimes develop, usually along the milk line, which runs from the armpits to the groin. Some parents have extra **accessory** or **supernumerary nipples** that form along the milk line as remnants from embryonic development of the mammary ridge. Extra glands and nipples may also develop elsewhere.

Up to 6% of all people have extra mammary tissue and/or nipples, but these are more common in women than men. Most commonly, this involves milk-making tissue and no nipples, but there may be extra nipples with no milk-making tissue. Some have ducts that leak milk through the skin without a nipple. Some develop multiple mammary glands. Often, extra nipples look like moles. If extra glandular tissue is present, after delivery, feelings of fullness and engorgement may occur.

NURSING WITH EXTRA GLANDS AND NIPPLES usually proceeds normally. But after birth, engorgement or even mastitis may develop. Milk-making tissue normally extends into the armpit (tail of Spence). But milk may not drain into the main ductal system from extra glands and/or nipples.

STAYING COMFORTABLE AFTER BIRTH If no glandular tissue is attached to extra nipples, no comfort measures are needed. If no nipples are attached to the extra glandular tissue, use the same comfort strategies recommended for newly delivered parents who do not plan to nurse:

- Avoid wearing clothing that constricts that area.
- Keep stimulation to a minimum.
- Apply cool or cold compresses to reduce swelling.
- Discuss anti-inflammatory medication with the healthcare provider.

When milk is not removed, the tissue will stop making milk and will quickly involute, or return to its prepregnancy state.

If extra glands have a nipple attached, milk may leak from the nipple, and it may be possible to express a little milk to relieve feelings of fullness. If they leak during nursing, suggest using pads or cloths to absorb the leaked milk. If mastitis develops in extra milk-making tissue, it may need to be treated.

UNDERDEVELOPED MAMMARY GLANDS may make it impossible to produce enough milk to exclusively nurse. The normal development of milk-making tissue happens during puberty and pregnancy, as well as after birth. But ***insufficient glandular tissue*** (IGT) or mammary hypoplasia is determined by what existed before pregnancy. There is usually an obvious lack of fullness in all or part of the gland.

If they are small, IGT breasts often look as if they never finished puberty and may be less than an A cup, with little obvious milk-making tissue. If they are larger, IGT breasts may lack the tissue that provides support, causing them to look long or tubular, or appear deflated. They may look bowed, with the nipples pointing down or away from the body. There may be obvious patches of milk-making tissue in a mostly soft gland.

Why does this condition occur? It depends on whether the hypoplasia is present at birth (congenital) or acquired later. Examples of congenital hypoplasia include Jeune and Poland syndromes and conditions occurring during fetal development that affect the torso, such as mitral-valve prolapse and scoliosis. Acquired hypoplasia may affect mammary development before or after puberty. Some that occur before puberty include chest trauma or surgery that cuts through mammary buds. In a baby or child, radiation treatments of the chest may affect mammary development later. During puberty, conditions that may affect mammary development include hypothyroidism and ovarian cysts. In some areas, a greater incidence of altered breast development was found in girls exposed in utero to agricultural chemicals in their environment.

Although supplements of donor milk and/or formula may be necessary, the baby can nurse with or without a nursing supplementer. For many of these parents, the biggest challenge is keeping the baby interested in nursing long enough to provide the necessary stimulation to grow more milk-making tissue. A nursing supplementer provides continuous flow to keep baby nursing longer. For details, see p. 315.

Depending on how much milk-making tissue is present and the nursing dynamics, parents may be able to continue to increase milk production over time and eventually exclusively nurse later babies.

To read more about how long-term mammary stimulation can grow milk-making tissue, see this author's story of her own experience of nursing with one breast that didn't develop during puberty at **bit.ly/BA2-Magical**.

The appearance and spacing of the mammary glands and lack of tissue changes during pregnancy are red flags but not completely reliable indicators of future low milk production. Among individuals, there is great variability in mammary size and shape, as well as how much of the tissue is glandular versus fatty. Some possible visual indicators among those unable to produce enough milk to fully nourish their babies include:

- Widely spaced glands (more than 1.5 inches or about 4 cm apart)
- Large differences in gland size (asymmetry)
- Tubular or cone-shaped (hypoplastic) rather than rounded glands
- Bulbous-looking areolae

Never assume from the shape of the mammary glands or lack of tissue changes during pregnancy that parents will not produce enough milk for their baby. Whenever possible, parents with these anatomical red flags should be monitored closely, without planting the seeds of doubt. Even closer follow-up is crucial if both the nursing parent and the baby have risk factors for inadequate milk intake.

RAPID MAMMARY OVERDEVELOPMENT Some mammary growth is normal, but one type of rapid growth, called *gestational gigantomastia*, is an unusual condition that falls far outside the norm. During pregnancy, this condition is triggered when the parent's mammary tissue becomes hypersensitive to pregnancy hormones and grows to double or triple their previous size (8 to 20 bra cup sizes or more), which is often completely incapacitating. Although it can occur during a first pregnancy, it usually happens first during a second or third pregnancy and occurs equally in those with small and large mammary glands. Although this condition is unusual, it is not as rare as it was in the past.

The three types of gestational gigantomastia, which have different hormonal triggers, can be distinguished by the timing of the excessive mammary growth. In the first type, which is most common and responds well to antiprolactin hormone therapy, mammary growth occurs in the beginning of pregnancy and continues through all three trimesters. In the second type, the next most common, rapid growth begins in the second trimester, lasts for 3 to 6 weeks, then slows. This second type is usually accompanied by high insulin blood levels. In the third type, the rarest, rapid growth occurs right before or right after birth and, at this writing, a hormone sensitivity has not yet been identified.

Medical therapies other than surgery are available to treat gestational gigantomastia, which typically recurs with each pregnancy. In more than 80% of cases, the mammary glands return to normal size after the baby is born, but gigantomastia recurs with each subsequent pregnancy, even if breast reduction surgery is performed. In cases of extreme incapacitation, mastectomies or breast reduction surgeries are done during pregnancy or afterward. There are some case reports of parents with this condition nursing their babies.

BREAST OR CHEST SURGERY OR INJURY

When there is a history of breast or chest surgery or injury, discuss feeding goals and options. Some types of breast surgery or injury (such as breast lifts and liposuction) are unlikely to have much effect on milk production and nursing. But others, such as breast reduction and top surgery may significantly reduce milk production. In these cases, emphasize that nursing does not have to be "all or nothing." Some nursing is almost always better than none.

FACTORS THAT AFFECT NURSING If the surgery or injury involved damage to nerves or milk ducts, it may affect the volume of milk produced. Ask about the following factors.

- **Nipple sensitivity to touch and temperature.** Intact nerve pathways allow nerve impulses to travel from the mammary gland to the brain and trigger milk ejection. If the nipple or gland has reduced sensitivity to touch or temperature, this indicates possible nerve damage, which may make normal milk flow more challenging. Another possible effect of nerve damage is altered or heightened sensation.

- **Damage to milk ducts.** Whether damaged milk ducts affect milk production depends in part on how many milk ducts with openings on the nipple existed before the surgery or injury, which is impossible to determine. With enough ducts, milk production may not be noticeably affected.

- **Complications from surgery or injury.** Changes in nipple sensation over time and scarring, infection, or any subsequent surgeries may be signs of complications, which may negatively affect milk production.

- **Time elapsed since the surgery or injury.** Milk ducts and nerves can grow back over time, so the more time elapsed since the surgery or injury, the greater the chances this may have occurred. Nerves grow back very slowly compared with milk ducts.

- **Why the surgery was performed.** If the surgery was intended to improve the appearance of glands that did not develop normally, lack of glandular tissue (rather than the surgery itself) may be the root cause of milk production problems.
- **Other health issues.** In parents with a history of breast reduction surgery, consider other health conditions that may affect milk production, such as obesity, diabetes, hypothyroidism, or polycystic ovary syndrome.

If only one side was affected by surgery or injury, full milk production is likely. The exception is the parent who had surgery on one side due to asymmetry, one sign of possible insufficient glandular tissue.

When parents are considering scheduling any type of breast or chest surgery, whatever surgery they are contemplating—tumor or cyst removal, breast lift, reduction, top surgery, augmentation—encourage them to talk to their surgeon about their desire to nurse and ask the surgeon to do everything possible to avoid damaging milk ducts and nerves. Later sections describe specific concerns with specific procedures.

PREPARING DURING PREGNANCY Discuss ways these parents can prepare for nursing.

- Learn about typical nursing patterns. It is tempting to focus only on their special situation, but without realistic expectations, they may misinterpret even normal feeding patterns as signs of low milk production.
- Locate knowledgeable and supportive healthcare providers and breastfeeding-friendly birthing facilities.
- Learn strategies for minimizing interventions during labor and birth.
- Find skilled lactation help, meet these support people during pregnancy, and save their contact information.
- Learn and practice hand expression daily during the last month of a low-risk pregnancy (**firstdroplets.com**).
- Plan for weekly weight checks of the baby during the first month.
- Learn how to know when supplements are needed and feeding options.

INITIATING NURSING Plan to nurse early, often, and effectively. After nursing sessions, hand-express colostrum and feed it to their baby by spoon. This stimulates more milk production and may help prevent excess weight loss.

Engorgement may develop in any areas of active mammary tissue where milk is unable to drain due to severed ducts.

Fortunately, milk ducts that do not connect to the nipple have a lower risk for infection. Those areas will quickly stop producing milk and revert to their prepregnancy state. Consider any tissue swelling as positive signs that the glands are making milk and use the comfort measures described on p. 28.

If nerve damage inhibits milk ejection, discuss alternative strategies to trigger milk ejection, such as the use of mental imagery, synthetic oxytocin nasal spray, and/or applying pressure to the gland during nursing.

Nipple pain, blanching, and/or feeding problems may be related to nerve damage or scarring. Sharp nipple pain may occur when scar tissue is pulled during nursing, especially with the first child nursed after surgery. But other, more common causes are more likely. First rule out shallow latch, bacterial nipple infection, vasospasm, and others. Disruption of nerves and/or blood supply may also cause nipple blanching (turning white after nursing). Whatever the cause, try the treatments recommended for vasospasm (p. 274). Difficulty latching may occur because the nipple and areola feel less "full." Try improving nursing dynamics to overcome this challenge.

If low milk production is likely, suggest strategies that maximize milk-making after birth, such as using compression or massage before and during nursing to increase milk removal, frequent nursing, taking herbal or prescribed galactogogues, and expressing milk after and/or between nursing sessions.

THE NEED FOR SUPPLEMENTATION Monitor baby's weight and diaper output to gauge whether supplements are needed. The most accurate way to determine whether supplements are needed is by regular weight checks. The normal range includes a loss of up to 10% of birth weight during the first 3 to 4 days. After that, when nursing is going well, most babies gain on average about 1 ounce (28 g) per day or about 7 ounces (198 g) per week. If the baby loses more than 10% of birth weight, supplements are needed right away. But if the baby's weight gain is slightly below average, there is time to first try milk-enhancing strategies. Stool color changes (to yellow by Day 4 or 5) and output (at least 3 to 4 per day), while not as reliable, can also be used as a rough gauge between weight checks.

Possible nursing outcomes include:

- Full milk production with no need for supplements.
- Milk production sufficient for the first few days or weeks after birth, but as hormonal levels diminish as time passes and milk production becomes more dependent on the stimulation of milk removal, supplements become necessary.

- Little to no milk production, with supplements needed soon after birth.

Even parents producing little milk may be able to exclusively nurse during the first few days. Some parents with nerve damage may find that even with frequent nursing, reduced nerve stimulation results in decreased milk production over time.

If a baby does not receive adequate milk from nursing alone, first rule out other causes, such as shallow latch, tongue-tie, and others before assuming the cause is surgery or injury. It's possible something else is the root cause.

If a baby doesn't need supplements within the first 5 or 6 weeks, chances are good supplements won't be needed. Babies' milk intake typically increases during the first 5 weeks or so, then plateaus until solid foods are started around 6 months. So unless other changes that affect milk production occur, such as decreasing feeding frequency, if a baby is still growing and thriving without supplements by 5 to 6 weeks of age, the baby probably won't need them.

When supplements are needed, if the goal is to maintain milk production at the highest possible level, this balancing act involves giving just enough milk for a healthy weight gain but not too much. One aspect of striking this delicate balance is frequent nursing and the choice of feeding method.

One feeding method that may increase nursing time, and therefore grow more milk-making tissue, is the nursing supplementer. Also known as a feeding-tube device, it can keep the baby actively nursing longer, thereby stimulating more milk production. It provides extra milk during nursing, so parents don't have to devote extra time to feeding the baby again afterward. Not all parents are comfortable using a nursing supplementer, so discuss the pros and cons of other feeding options and support them in their choice. Their decision may depend in part on whether they are close to full milk production, making some milk, or making little to no milk.

BREAST LIFT does not usually affect nursing or milk production. Also known as ***mastopexy***, a breast lift is used to reshape and reposition sagging mammary glands so they appear higher and more rounded. This procedure involves removing excess skin, but the nerves and milk-making glands are not usually affected and no mammary tissue is removed. If a breast lift is done along with a breast augmentation, the risks would be the same as the two procedures combined.

BREAST AUGMENTATION SURGERY is one of the most common types of plastic surgery performed.

Also known as **augmentation mammaplasty**, in most cases, silicone- or saline-filled sacs are inserted into a pocket that is formed either between the chest muscles and the glandular tissue or under the muscle. The incision may be in the fold under the breast, near the armpit, around the edge of the areola, or rarely, through the navel. Another technique called **biocompartmental breast lipostructuring** involves injecting the person's own fat from other parts of the body into the breasts for an increase of up to two cup sizes. Another injectable option is the injectable PAAG (polyacrylamide hydrogel), which will likely have less impact on lactation than techniques involving incisions.

Those with a history of breast augmentation surgery are less likely to exclusively nurse their babies than those without this history.

INCISION LOCATION Early studies found a link between incision location around the edge of the areola and lower milk production, but larger, more recent studies did not. If the surgical incision is made around the edge of the areola, its specific location matters. Nipple sensitivity (and therefore milk ejection) depends on an intact fourth intercostal nerve, which usually enters the areola on its outer, lower edge. But many modern surgeons consider maintaining nipple sensitivity an indicator of successful surgery and are aware of the importance of avoiding that specific area to preserve sensitivity.

IMPLANT SIZE Some research found an association between larger implants in previously small-breasted women and reduced nipple sensitivity.

IMPLANT PLACEMENT above or below the chest muscles may also affect lactation. Implants placed above the chest muscle and directly below the milk-making tissue (**subglandular**) may increase pressure on this tissue and reduce milk production or block milk flow. The alternative is to place the implant either partially covered by the chest muscle (**subpectoral**) or almost completely covered by the chest muscle (**transrectus**).

COMPLICATIONS OF SURGERY may reduce milk production. Severe scarring, known as capsular contracture, can cause discomfort during nursing or put enough pressure on the milk-producing glands, reducing milk production. When scarring is severe, it may require more surgery to remove it, which can cause damage to nerves and milk ducts.

SILICONE IN THE MILK is a common but unfounded concern. Silicone is found in foods, liquids, over-the-counter colic remedies given directly to babies, and cosmetics like lipstick. Absorption of silicone by the babies' digestive tract is considered unlikely. Formula and cow's milk contain levels of silicon (elemental silicone bonded to oxygen) more than 10 times higher than the milk of mothers with silicone implants.

BREAST REDUCTION SURGERY involves different surgical techniques, some of which affect lactation outcomes more than others. Breast reduction surgery, also known as **reduction mammaplasty**, is done to decrease breast size by removing either the fat within the mammary gland via liposuction or by surgically removing mammary tissue. Unlike top surgery (see the next section), its goal is to create a smaller, female-shaped breast.

LIPOSUCTION is the breast reduction procedure least likely to affect milk production, because only fatty tissue is removed and there is minimal scarring and nerve damage. But liposuction usually reduces breast size by no more than two cup sizes, and it is not considered the best option for younger women, because their breasts tend to contain less fatty tissue than older women.

FREE NIPPLE GRAFTS put milk production at greatest risk, because this procedure involves completely detaching the nipple and areola from the mammary gland and reattaching it elsewhere for a more symmetrical appearance. Free nipple grafts, which are less common than other procedures, sever all milk ducts, nerves, and blood vessels. But because nerves and milk ducts can regrow after this procedure, some parents produce milk and a few produce ample milk. Too little blood flow to the nipple, which can happen when blood vessels are cut, can cause tissue death, a very serious complication that can greatly reduce lactation potential.

PEDICLE TECHNIQUES protect vital arteries to the nipple and areola while mammary tissue is being removed. During surgery, a section of the gland that includes arteries, milk ducts, and nerves is kept attached down to the chest wall or is partially severed. These partially or fully intact sections are called **pedicles**, and the names of these surgical techniques (**inferior, superior, central, lateral,** and **medial** pedicle techniques) refer to the specific section of the gland used to create the pedicle. Different techniques can be used with different types and shapes of incisions, which makes it impossible to tell from the shape of a scar what type of surgery was performed.

Evaluating lactation outcomes after pedicle surgery is challenging, because researchers' definitions of lactation success are vague. Reviews of the research reported:

- Time elapsed between the surgery and nursing was less important to milk production than the surgical technique used.

- Fewer cases of nursing "success" occurred after free nipple grafts as compared with any other techniques.
- When pedicle techniques were used, the best nursing outcomes were among those who had the inferior or central pedicle surgeries, as compared with the superior, medial, and lateral pedicles.
- Full preservation of the attachment of the pedicle column to the chest wall resulted in better nursing outcomes as compared with surgeries in which the column was only partially preserved.

After breast reduction surgery, most parents produce some milk. The most significant issue is how much milk.

The number of milk ducts that existed before the surgery and the number that were cut will determine in part the effect of breast reduction surgery on milk production.

CHEST MASCULINIZATION OR TOP SURGERY is performed on those assigned as female at birth but identify on the male end of the gender spectrum. When their physical anatomy does not match their internal sense of gender identity, they may experience a type of distress or anxiety known as ***gender dysphoria***. These negative feelings motivate some to go through the process of transitioning their outer appearance to make it closer to their inner gender identity. Transitioning may involve wearing different clothes, taking testosterone, or undergoing surgeries of the chest and/or reproductive organs. Chest masculinization surgery, often referred to as ***top surgery*** or ***male chest contouring***, involves removing much of the mammary tissue to create a masculine-looking chest. This makes top surgery different from breast reduction surgery, which is intended to produce a smaller but definitely female-shaped breast. Unlike a mastectomy, not all of the mammary tissue is removed during top surgery, because doing so would leave a sunken-looking chest.

Top surgery procedures vary but may involve:

- Broad incisions under the mammary tissue, with the nipples completely removed and repositioned (much like the free nipple grafts mentioned in the previous section)
- Removal of the mammary tissue while preserving the nipple pedicle

Read about the experiences of 22 transgender men who experienced pregnancy and/or lactation, in the open-access article at **bit.ly/BA2-Transmasculine**. Top surgery is commonly performed with no guidance provided by surgeons about its effects on lactation. In those who become pregnant after top surgery, chest changes may occur. In some cases, milk-making tissue may grow back to pre-surgical size. After birth, engorgement is possible in areas of the chest that do not drain due to severed milk ducts. Some may produce ample milk. Some may need to supplement. The best approach to providing lactation care and support to these families is a nuanced one. This requires becoming knowledgeable about the type of chest care needed after top surgery.

BREAST OR CHEST INJURY In parents with a history of breast or chest injury, ask how long ago it occurred. The same basic considerations mentioned for breast or chest surgery apply here. Milk production should not be affected if the milk ducts and nerves were not damaged. Injuries that may affect lactation include:

- Breast or other cancer treatments. If the mammary gland (or in a baby or child, the chest) is exposed to radiation therapy, this damages milk-making cells, which reduces milk production significantly in the exposed gland
- Spinal cord injuries of the T3, T4, T5, and T6 vertebrae or above could affect sensitivity to temperature and touch in the nipple and gland.
- Blunt force trauma to the mammary gland or the chest, especially during infancy or childhood, when the gland has not yet developed.
- Severe chest burns

A loss of sensation on one or both glands is a sign of nerve damage. If so, milk ejection may be affected on that side. However, if only one side is affected, in most cases, it will be possible to establish full milk production on the unaffected side. If both mammary glands are affected, see the previous section "Initiating Nursing."

If one or both nipples were burned, scarring may affect milk flow and reduce skin elasticity and may cause pain during nursing and latching difficulties. Even second- and third-degree burns do not usually extend deeply enough into the mammary tissue to affect the milk-making glands. If parents' nipples were scarred by burns, their ability to nurse would depend on how many nipple pores are blocked by scar tissue. The overall effect on nursing will depend on how many milk ducts and corresponding nipple pores that parent had before the injury. Scar tissue may also make the mammary tissue less pliable, which may make latching more challenging. The ability to express colostrum during pregnancy indicates that at least some of the nipple pores are not blocked.

DIGITAL RESOURCES

BFAR.org—An informational website for parents nursing after breast reduction surgery.

bfmed.org/protocols—Free, downloadable, fully referenced clinical protocols in multiple languages are ideal for sharing with healthcare providers from the Academy of Breastfeeding Medicine:

- #4   Mastitis
- #20 Engorgement
- #26 Persistent pain with breastfeeding
- #30 Breast masses, breast complaints, and diagnostic breast imaging in the lactating woman

bit.ly/BA2-FDAImplants—A U.S. Food and Drug Administration (FDA) informational website on breast implants.

bit.ly/BA2-Transmasculine—A survey of the experiences of 22 transmasculine individuals who became pregnant, 16 of whom nursed their babies.

CHAPTER 4   CHALLENGES WITH LATCHING AND NURSING

This chapter covers ineffective nursing, difficulty latching and/or not latching at all to one or both sides. These nursing struggles can usually be overcome, but to safeguard nursing, the first priority is to feed the baby, second to protect milk production, and third to suggest strategies that are more likely to result in settled nursing.

SAFEGUARDING NURSING

Nursing struggles are stressful and demoralizing and often lead to premature weaning. Parents need an outlet to express their worries, fears, and doubts. This makes it possible for them to consider their situation more objectively. They need to know that their baby needs them now more than ever and their difficulties can be overcome.

FEED THE BABY   To determine if the baby needs supplements, ask the baby's age, weight, diaper output, and how many times each day nursing goes well and at which feeds. One of the first concerns is how to make sure the baby gets the milk she needs. This and the nursing parent's comfort are the top priorities. Being underfed can compromise a baby's nursing effectiveness. In some situations, part of getting nursing going smoothly may involve feeding the baby expressed milk, donor milk, or a substitute. Withholding milk until the baby "gets hungry enough" is in most cases an ineffective strategy and will put some young babies at risk for dehydration.

BABY'S WEIGHT GAIN   There are several ways to gauge whether the baby needs a supplement. The most reliable is the baby's weight gain. For healthy weight gain by age, see WHO's Child Growth Standards at **who.int/childgrowth/standards/en**.

STOOL COLOR AND OUTPUT DURING THE EARLY WEEKS is a less reliable gauge of milk intake but can be helpful in the newborn when combined with weight checks. During the first week, a transition to yellow stools by Day 6 or earlier is linked to acceptable levels of weight loss and weight gain. Also, after Day 4, inadequate milk intake was linked to less than three stools per day along with the birthing parent's perception that the milk had not yet increased within 72 hours post-delivery. Although stool color and output are not as accurate as weight loss and gain in determining whether a baby is getting enough milk, they can be used during the early weeks as a rough gauge between weight checks. During the first 4 to 6 weeks or so, daily stool output is even less reliable than it was during the first week, but between weight checks it can be another rough indicator of whether milk intake is adequate. An average is at least four stools the diameter of a U.S. quarter (2.5 cm) or larger. If the baby has fewer stools but is gaining weight well, this is a normal variation and not a problem. After 4 to 6 weeks of age, stool count is no longer a helpful sign because many nursing babies have fewer stools, even when getting plenty of milk.

If the baby needs to be supplemented, discuss possible supplements and feeding methods. For young babies, consider feeding with spoon, cup, bowl, eyedropper, nursing supplementer, or feeding bottle. If the baby is older than 6 to 8 months, baby can drink from a cup. The best supplement is nearly always mother's milk. If that is not available and donor milk is a local option, that is the second choice. Otherwise, suggest consulting baby's healthcare provider for a recommended supplement. On the first day of life, 7-10 mL/feed is recommended. On the second day, the typical feed is 10-15 mL. Beginning on the third day, about 30 mL (or 1 oz.) is an average feed. See Table 4.1 for volumes needed by age after Day 3.

Table 4.1. Milk Intake by Age

Baby's Age	Average Milk Per Feeding	Average Milk Per Day
First week (after Day 3)	1-2 oz. (30-60 mL)	10-20 oz. (300-600 mL)
Weeks 2 and 3	2-3 oz. (60-90 mL)	15-25 oz. (450-750 mL)
Months 1-6	3-4 oz. (90-120 mL)	25-30 oz. (750-900 mL)

PROTECT MILK PRODUCTION If a newborn is not nursing or is nursing ineffectively, suggest expressing milk at least 8 times per day. This can help keep the nursing parent comfortable and establish milk production during the newborn period. How often to express and what expression method to use depends on the situation. If the baby is older, suggest expressing milk at least as often as the baby was nursing. If the baby is nursing well at some feeds, tailor the expression plan to the need.

STRUGGLES DURING THE EARLY WEEKS

GATHERING BASIC INFORMATION Before suggesting strategies to address nursing struggles, first try to determine the cause(s). Babies with a medical problem—such as an ear infection or thrush—may need diagnosis and treatment. Sometimes more than one factor is at work. When a strategy is tried and improvement is seen, be sure the problem is completely resolved. More detective work may be needed.

Ask questions in a calm, relaxed manner, and affirm nursing families for what they are doing right. Emphasize that individual differences in parents and babies create a wide range of reactions to the same factor.

Ask the baby's age now, her age when the nursing struggles started, and at what point during the feed the problem starts. Knowing this provides clues to its cause(s). See Box 4.1 for an overview of causes of nursing struggles starting at birth and Box 4.2 for an overview of causes of feeding problems that start Day 2 to 5. Knowing when during the feed the problem starts may also help in determining the cause.

Box 4.1 Factors Contributing to Nursing Struggles That Start at Birth

Interactive Factors
- Post-delivery practices that interfere with inborn feeding behaviors, such as labor medications, suctioning, unnecessary formula supplements, and separation
- Positioning issues and/or shallow latch
- Poor fit (large nipple/small mouth)

Baby Factors
- Pain from birth injury
- Feeding aversion from rough suctioning or rough handling during latch
  - Oral anatomy variations (tongue-tie, unusually shaped palate, etc.)
  - Health problems (i.e., cardiac defect, prematurity, illness, etc.)
  - Neurological impairment (Down syndrome, etc.)

Parent Factors
- Birth-related pain or trauma
- Naturally taut mammary tissue
- Anatomical variations of nipple or mammary anatomy

If the problem starts before milk ejection, consider:

- Positioning issues causing discomfort or shallow latch
- Shallow latch caused by positioning issues or taut mammary tissue
- Pain from a birth injury, medical procedure, or other causes
- Oral anatomical variations in the baby
- Health problems, such as prematurity, airway abnormality, or neurological impairment

Coughing or gasping at milk ejection may mean baby has a problem coping with milk flow. If so, try a semi-reclined starter position (see p. 6, which gives baby more control over milk flow. Other contributing factors could be abundant milk production, variations in baby's oral anatomy, airway abnormality, or neurological impairment.

If the problem starts later in the feed, baby may simply need to burp or pass a stool. Or low milk production may be the cause.

INTERACTIVE FACTORS are those to which both parent and baby contribute.

POSITIONING   Ask what nursing positions they tried and the results. Nursing in upright positions is often more challenging in the early weeks due to the lack of newborn head-and-neck control. This is not an issue for the baby older than about 6 weeks. In upright feeding positions, a newborn needs much more help. Nursing parents must support baby's weight, keep baby's body pressed against theirs, and keep baby well-aligned to the nipple. A first-time nursing parent may be unaware of how much support their newborn needs in upright positions, which can lead to a shallow latch, latching struggles, and other challenges. The starter positions described in Chapter 1 make early nursing easier for most families because the baby can use their inborn feeding behaviors to self-attach. Suggest trying these starter positions and experiment by using the three basic adjustments described in Chapter 1 (adjust your body, adjust your baby, adjust your breast) until they find their own best fit. (See the free video featuring these adjustments at **NaturalBreastfeeding.com**.) In any position, the nursing parent needs enough body support to nurse with relaxed neck and shoulder muscles and maintain the position comfortably for at least 30 to 60 minutes.

NIPPLE PAIN may indicate a shallow latch or abnormal tongue movements due to oral variations or early use of artificial nipples/teats.

BIRTH AND POST-DELIVERY PRACTICES, such as a medicated birth, suctioning after birth, delaying the first feed, the use of bottles and pacifiers, and separation can contribute to nursing struggles in some babies.

POOR FIT is the combination of a nursing parent with very wide or long nipples and a baby with a very small mouth. The baby may be able to fit only the nipple, rather than the nipple and some of the areola, in her mouth, which can lead to nipple pain and/or slow milk flow.

Box 4.2 Factors Contributing to Nursing Struggles Starting on Days 2-5

Baby Factors
- Inability to cope with greater milk flow due to anatomical variations, such as tongue tie, airway abnormality, or other health issues
- Pain from circumcision or other painful medical procedure

Parent Factors
- Newly taut mammary tissue from swelling (due to excess IV fluids), fullness from increased milk production, and/or engorgement
- Delay in milk production, baby underfed (weight loss ≥10%)
- Fast milk flow from overabundant milk production

BABY FACTORS include the following.

SLEEPY BABY   A difficult labor and delivery can leave baby exhausted. Some labor medications can sedate baby, decreasing alertness, and make the baby appear sleepy or uninterested in nursing. A severely jaundiced or ill baby may be less alert. If sleepiness begins on Day 2 through 5, baby may be unable to latch deeply enough to the firmer mammary tissue to trigger active sucking. Try reverse pressure softening (p. 333) before latch.

If a newborn sleeps so much that it is difficult to nurse at least 8 times each day:

- Make sure the baby is not too warm.
- Spend as much time as possible with parent and baby in full frontal contact, either skin to skin or lightly dressed.
- Cluster or bunch feeds together during baby's wakeful times.
- While baby is in a light sleep (eyes moving under eyelids) guide baby to latch.
- Make sure baby latches deeply to trigger more active sucking.

If baby quickly falls asleep after latching, this may be a sign of a shallow latch. In addition to latching deeper, adding breast compression (p. 309) may also speed milk flow and keep baby nursing.

Use weight as a gauge. The weight of a sleepy baby who is well fed will be in the expected range, and no interventions are needed. If baby's weight is borderline or low, eventually the baby will start sleeping more and become difficult to rouse. Rule out underfeeding as the cause of sleepiness via baby's weight gain. From Day 4 or 5 to about 3 months, expect babies to gain about 1 oz. (28 g) per day.

UNDERFED BABY Baby's weight gain can rule in or out nursing struggles caused by low milk intake. If a baby is not getting enough milk, this can lead to fussiness during feeds or even inability to latch. But low milk intake can also cause a loss of energy and alertness, and over time, babies begin to shut down. When underfed, some babies start sleeping more and more and become difficult to rouse. They may also fall asleep quickly during feeds.

With low milk intake, the first priority is to feed the baby with expressed mother's milk, donor milk, or a substitute recommended by the baby's healthcare provider. Second priority is to protect milk production by creating a milk-expression plan. Third priority is to get to the root cause of the baby's low milk intake, which may be due to baby not nursing often or long enough, low milk production, or ineffective nursing. Also, rule out any health problems or medications that may affect feeding.

PAIN DURING NURSING Possible causes of pain include birth injuries such as bruises, dislocated hip, hematoma, or broken bones. Circumcision may also cause babies to have trouble settling or shut down and become unresponsive. Pain medication may help. The following conditions may also affect nursing.

Torticollis, which means "twisted neck," is caused by a confined position in the womb in which baby's neck muscles are pulled to one side. This pulls the baby's lower jaw and affects jaw development in utero, giving the baby's jaw an asymmetrical look. Babies with torticollis may prefer to hold their head to one side and trying to turn it may be painful. Nipple pain, latching struggles, and ineffective feeding may be the first symptoms of undiagnosed torticollis. Suggest experimenting with different feeding positions to find the one most comfortable for them. Babies are more likely to achieve comfortable stable positions if placed prone on their semi-reclining parent. Some babies may nurse best when the same position is used on both sides by sliding baby's body over.

Hip dysplasia is caused by baby's hip socket not forming correctly. If the baby wears a brace or cast, finding a comfortable nursing position that does not stress the hips may be challenging. A straddle position, either upright or semi-reclined (p. 14), may make nursing more comfortable, as well as using a support pillow between baby's legs.

INCONSISTENT OR INEFFECTIVE NURSING often leads to slow weight gain or weight loss. Check for signs of effective nursing, such as wide jaw movements and ear wiggling during nursing, swallowing sounds, increasing relaxation, and baby coming off satisfied.

Signs of possible ineffective nursing:

- No swallowing heard. At milk ejection, most babies swallow after every one or two sucks, swallowing less and less often as feeds progress. Some babies swallow very quietly.
- Baby never seems satisfied. Families often say the ineffective baby nurses "all the time."
- Shallow latch. The baby's jaw angle appears narrow. This may cause slow milk flow, less milk intake, nipple pain, and/or difficulty staying latched.
- Coughing or sputtering during feeds can occur with very fast milk flow and uncoordinated sucking and swallowing or an airway abnormality.
- Low or high muscle tone. Low-tone babies include those with Down syndrome and other neurological impairments. Babies with high tone may be in the high-normal range or be neurologically impaired. High-tone babies may appear tense and arch away when nursing, especially in upright feeding positions.
- A clicking sound during nursing may be a sign suction is being broken. If baby is gaining weight well, this is not a problem.
- Cheek dimpling during feeds indicates the baby's mouth is empty and can occur with or without loss of suction. If the baby is gaining weight well, this is not a problem.
- Nipple pain or trauma can also be due to a shallow latch, unusual tongue movements, or anatomical variations, such as tongue-tie.
- Unrelieved mammary fullness or recurring mastitis can be a sign of ineffective milk removal.

If baby's swallowing cannot be heard, audible swallowing stops early in the feeds, or the baby falls asleep quickly, suggest increasing the time spent actively nursing by getting a deeper latch and using breast compression (p. 309) for a faster milk flow. If these strategies do not improve feeding effectiveness, see Box 4.2.

VARIATIONS IN BABY'S ORAL ANATOMY Some—but not all—babies with tongue-tie and other oral variations nurse ineffectively. The frenulum is the string-like membrane that attaches the tongue to the floor of the mouth. When the frenulum restricts normal tongue movement, this is called tongue-tie or ankyloglossia. Tongue-tie may run in families. For details on tongue-tie and other oral variations that may affect nursing, see p. 101. Whether a baby's oral variation affects nursing depends in part on the parent-child fit. A tongue-tied baby may have a much more difficult time feeding effectively when mammary tissue is taut and an easier time when it is looser.

AIRWAY ABNORMALITY   For effective nursing, a baby must coordinate sucking, swallowing and breathing. A baby with an airway malformation usually breathes more times per minute to get the oxygen needed. Faster breathing means less time to swallow, and breathing is always the priority. Coughing or sputtering during nursing may be a sign of an airway abnormality or it may occur when a young baby struggles with a fast milk flow. Baby's weight gain can help distinguish milk-flow issues from breathing issues, as babies with an airway abnormality often gain weight slowly. If a high-pitched squeaky sound known as **stridor** occurs, this may be a sign of an airway abnormality, such as laryngomalacia (narrowing of the upper airway), tracheomalacia (narrowing of the lower airway), vocal-cord paralysis, or other issues. When an airway abnormality compromises nursing, this can lead to ineffective feeding, coughing and gasping, and even a nursing aversion or "strike." For more details, see p. 111.

NEUROLOGICAL IMPAIRMENT   Babies with a neurological impairment often have either high or low muscle tone, which may cause nursing struggles. A neurological impairment may be caused by immaturity or obvious physical problems, such as a brain bleed, seizures, or Prader-Willi syndrome or others. When a baby's brain or nervous system is affected, it can compromise coordination and effective feeding. With practice, patience, and maturity, many can learn to nurse well. Babies with high tone may arch their bodies, over-respond to stimulation, and bite or clench during nursing. Babies with low muscle tone tend to under-respond to feeding triggers. Both may have trouble coordinating sucking, swallowing, and breathing. For details and strategies, see p. 126-130.

PARENT FACTORS include the following.

BIRTH-RELATED PAIN OR TRAUMA   A traumatic delivery can affect how birthing parents experience nursing. Some feel the need to stop nursing due to flashbacks of their trauma or the desire to go back to their "normal," pre-birth selves. Others find nursing comforting and healing. After a cesarean delivery, suggest comfortable feeding positions that do not put pressure on the surgical incision.

MAMMARY GLAND AND NIPPLE CHALLENGES include the following.

Taut Mammary Tissue Within the first day or two after birth—even before the milk increases—IV fluids received during labor can cause tissue swelling of the ankles and mammary glands that can make latching difficult. Swelling increases tissue tautness, which can flatten the nipple and make a deep latch more difficult. From the second to fifth days after birth, this is likely caused by normal fullness or engorgement. In this case, suggest starting with reverse pressure softening (p. 333) and/or mammary shaping (p. 321). To treat engorgement, see p. 28.

If severe engorgement occurs despite frequent nursing, this may be a sign the baby is not nursing effectively. If so, suggest the baby be checked for oral variations and other health issues. Also, suggest milk expression to relieve engorgement, safeguard milk production, and provide milk to feed the baby.

If mammary tissue is naturally taut, suggest the mammary shaping techniques on p. 321.

Nipple Shape and Size After birth, learning to nurse takes time and patience. If the parent's nipples are flat or inverted and baby has difficulty latching, review the suggestions in the checklist on p. 10 and those in the last section of this chapter.

Although flat and inverted nipples can make the early learning period more challenging for some, protruding (everted) nipples are not a requirement for effective nursing. Most babies are happy to suck on anything they can get into their mouth, including caregivers' arms, shoulders, and necks. But babies whose parents have flat or inverted nipples may be more at risk for nursing struggles after experiencing the "supernormal stimulus" of bottles and pacifiers/dummies. What is most important is the baby feeling the stimulation of the mammary tissue deeply in her mouth (protruding nipple or not) to trigger active sucking. Make the primary focus getting a deep latch.

In some cases, flat nipples may not be what they seem. IV fluids given during labor can cause mammary tissue swelling that causes protruding nipples to temporarily flatten.

Poor Fit If either nipple seems too large for the baby or their texture makes nursing challenging, this is called a poor nipple-baby fit (p. 56). This often occurs when the nipples are very wide and/or long and the baby has a very small mouth. Even with ideal latching dynamics, in some cases, the baby may fit only the nipple in her mouth, which can lead to nipple pain and/or slow milk flow. If long nipples trigger the baby's gag reflex, nursing struggles and even aversion may occur. The most reliable solution is the tincture of time. Newborns grow quickly, and it may take only a few weeks of growth before the baby's mouth is large enough to nurse well. If the nursing parent establishes full milk production with milk expression, the baby can begin nursing as soon as their fit issues are outgrown.

Mammary Gland Size and Nipple Placement Large glands do not always make it difficult to find a comfortable nursing position. But if they do, begin with a comfortable, well-supported semi-reclined position and place the baby tummy down on the parent's body, allowing her inborn feeding behaviors to be triggered before latching. Tissue support or shaping may be helpful for some babies, but encourage starting with the mammary gland at its natural height to see if the baby can latch well. The less lifting and supporting that is done, the easier nursing will be.

MILK FLOW Either fast or slow milk flow may contribute to nursing struggles.

Fast Milk Flow may occur with overabundant milk production, which may make managing flow during nursing difficult. At milk ejection, baby may gulp, cough, and sputter and latch on and off many times per feed to catch her breath. When a baby behaves this way, ask about weight gain. If she is gaining significantly more than 2 lb. (900 g) per month, overabundant milk production may be a factor (p. 200). The nursing parent may also have discomfort from fullness between feeds or recurring mastitis. If this is a likely cause, suggest slowing milk production (p. 203).

If the baby is not gaining more weight than average, suggest experimenting with feeding positions, beginning with the starter positions (p. 6), which give baby more control over milk flow. Nursing more often may also make the flow more manageable. If that doesn't help, suggest the baby's healthcare provider rule out any physical issues, such as oral variations (tongue-tie, unusually shaped palate), discomfort during feeds, airway abnormality, or neurological impairment (there would be an obvious physical cause). A nipple shield (p. 329) may also help.

Slow Milk Flow may be due to low milk production and can frustrate a hungry baby, causing nursing struggles. If milk production is low, see p. 193 for strategies to increase it, and if it is very low, see details on relactating on p. 271. When there is little milk, this can create frustration and feeding problems in some babies.

STRUGGLES AFTER THE EARLY WEEKS

When feeding struggles start after several weeks of uneventful nursing, anatomical variations and other conditions present at birth are less likely to be the cause but are still possible. The baby's age can provide clues to the cause of the nursing struggle. See possible causes in Box 4.3.

Box 4.3 Contributing Factors for Nursing Struggles After the Early Weeks

Baby Issues

- Use of artificial nipples (bottles, pacifiers), which can change sucking patterns. More likely ≤1 month
- Temperament. Some previously easygoing babies "wake up" at 2 to 3 weeks and become colicky
- Illness, such as ear infection, congestion, or others. Can happen at any age
- Gastroesophageal reflux disease (GERD). Symptoms usually first appear after about 4 weeks or so
- Hypersensitivity, intolerance, or allergy, causing discomfort, congestion, skin rash. Symptoms usually appear after about 3 or 4 weeks of age
- Pain when held. May be caused by injection, medical procedure, or injury. Can occur at any age.
- Candida (thrush). Can occur at any age
- Teething. Usually occurs after about 3 to 4 months of age
- Distractibility. Usually starts at around 3 months and increases over time
- Reaction to a new product the nursing parent uses, such as deodorant, detergents, etc.
- Nursing strike. Usually occurs after 2 months or so

Parent Issues

- Overabundant or low milk production, causing fast or slow milk flow
- Mastitis or other issues related to mammary health
- Stress, overstimulation, or upset, such as household move, holidays, anything that delays or decreases nursing, reducing milk production

Other factors that can provide clues to the cause of the struggles include physical symptoms, whether baby struggles to nurse on one or both sides, and when during the feed the struggle begins.

Nursing struggle starts before milk ejection. When an issue begins at the start of a feed, consider:

- Positioning causing discomfort or frustration. Was baby recently immunized or injured?
- Use of pacifiers/dummies or bottles contribute to nursing struggles in some babies.
- Mammary gland or milk-flow issues. Is the mammary tissue taut from missed feeds? Is the baby sleeping longer at night, causing milk production to slow? Has excess milk expression created an oversupply? Could the nursing parent have mastitis?

Nursing struggle starts at milk ejection. If the baby coughs or gasps, this may be a sign the baby is not coping well with milk flow. Suggest adjusting positioning, so baby's head is higher than the nipple (p. 6). Discuss possible overabundant milk production or health or anatomical issues in the baby.

Nursing struggle starts later in the feed. When baby starts fussing later, consider:

- The need to burp or pass a stool
- Low milk production, which is confirmed with slow weight gain
- Overabundant milk production, if weight gain is much above average (>2 lb. [900 g]/month)
- Gastroesophageal reflux disease (GERD), making feeds painful, usually after 4 weeks
- Hypersensitivity, intolerance, or allergy, usually accompanied by rash or wheezing/congestion

To rule out decreased milk intake, ask about their usual nursing pattern—feeds per day, time on each side. Overuse of bottles, pacifiers, and solid foods can cause a rapid decrease in the number of times each day baby nurses, which decreases milk production, resulting in an unhappy baby. If the exclusively nursing baby's weight gain is normal or high, consider other causes. Very fast weight gain may indicate overabundant milk production.

Nipple pain after a period of comfortable nursing can be caused by a shallow latch, candida (thrush), or teething (usually after 3 or 4 months). A history of nipple trauma increases the risk for a bacterial infection and/or thrush.

Mastitis, if recent, may cause temporarily slower milk flow or salty-tasting milk on the affected side, which may alter baby's response. After about a week of frequent nursing or milk expression, normal milk flow and taste will return.

BABY FACTORS include both physical and environmental causes.

PHYSICAL CAUSES may include the following.

Nasal Congestion can cause nursing struggles, because when a baby with a stuffy nose closes her mouth around the nipple, she may struggle to breathe. Congestion may also lead to an ear infection, which can cause pain during nursing. Persistent congestion may be a symptom of allergy or illness. For nursing strategies, see p. 238.

Colic is defined as crying at least 3 hours per day at least 3 days per week for at least 3 weeks. It often starts when a baby is about 2 to 3 weeks old. Parents may describe the baby as demanding or intense and find it difficult to help her settle and nurse. Holding, nursing, walking, and rocking may help, as well as the following strateigies.

Before nursing

- Be sure baby is not too warm or too cold and that her clothing is not binding.
- To help calm baby, if needed, offer a clean, trimmed finger to suck on, pad side up.

During nursing

- Keep sound and lights low.
- Begin nursing while baby is in a light sleep and not yet fully awake.
- Use a semi-reclined starter feeding position (p. 6) that allows the baby to self-attach.
- Let the baby finish feeding on one side before offering the other.

At other times

- Devote as much time as possible to holding baby either in skin-to-skin contact, lightly dressed, or in a soft baby carrier or sling.

Spend as much time as possible holding the colicky baby or wearing her in a soft baby carrier.

Allergy, Reflux, and Oversupply   Hypersensitivity, intolerance, or allergy usually involve physical symptoms (p. 118) and may also be associated with reflux disease (p. 116). A baby with reflux disease often nurses well for a few minutes then becomes increasingly agitated. Colic-like symptoms can also occur with overabundant milk production, which can often be confirmed with a well-above-average weight gain.

Teething usually occurs after about 3 to 4 months of age. A teething baby may nurse differently, bearing down on the mammary tissue, or even making chewing movements. Pressure helps ease gum discomfort. Some teething babies even go "on strike" when the pain is at its peak. For strategies, see p. 71.

Thrush symptoms include white patches on the inside of baby's cheeks that bleed or appear red when wiped off, a red, raised diaper rash, and nipple pain in the nursing parent. Thrush is an overgrowth of *Candida albicans,* a fungus that thrives in dark, moist places, such as the nipple, the baby's mouth, and diaper area. Because thrush can be painful, baby may latch eagerly, but pull away repeatedly from the pain. For strategies, see p. 227.

Infant Injury or Mouth Sores   If the baby bumped her mouth and has a sore area or developed cold sores, this could affect feeding comfort. Babies sometimes resist nursing if it involves touching a sensitive area, such as an injection site or a bruise. In this case, try a different feeding position until the sore area heals.

Developmental Distractibility usually starts after about 3 to 4 months and is a common cause of feeding struggles. Distractibility is part of baby's normal development and is not a sign baby is ready to wean. If the parent is concerned about short feeds, explain that older babies can get a lot of milk very quickly. Baby's weight gain will indicate whether or not the shorter nursing is a cause for concern. For strategies, see p. 203.

ENVIRONMENTAL CAUSES, such as the following, may affect nursing.

Unusual Stress or any major change in the baby's routine may affect nursing, especially in a sensitive baby. Examples include moving a household, family tensions, or the nursing parent's return to work. Even a positive stress, like holiday preparations, can sometimes affect a baby's willingness to feed.

Reaction to a New Product   Latching or nursing struggles sometimes start with the use of a new nipple cream or ointment, which may change the nipple's taste. A sensitive baby may register her dislike for a new product, like a new deodorant, body lotion, or even laundry detergent, by becoming unsettled while nursing or rejecting nursing altogether. If this is a possible cause, suggest rinsing the area with clear water before the next feed.

PARENT FACTORS may include the following.

Overabundant milk may cause a baby to have trouble coping with milk flow and gain weight faster than average. The baby struggling with milk flow may:

- Swallow a lot of air from gulping during feeds
- Spit up regularly
- Pass a lot of gas
- Wake soon after falling asleep and act hungry, even if she just nursed
- Have symptoms of colic
- Fuss during feeds, gasping, sputtering, or arching away when the milk ejects
- Have regular or occasional explosive green or watery stools

Similar symptoms may also occur in the baby with colic, reflux disease, and allergy. The baby may have a strong suck, strong muscle tone, and want to nurse often. Or she may refuse some feeds. This fussiness at feeds may continue as the baby gets older. The nursing parent may leak a lot of milk during and between feeds, and the milk ejection may feel painful. If fast milk flow continues to be an issue, some older babies:

- Become reluctant to nurse at all, even when obviously hungry
- Will not nurse to sleep, preferring instead to suck their fingers or thumb
- Use chewing or "biting" motions to avoid triggering fast milk flow
- Go on a nursing strike

When a baby has trouble managing milk flow, before taking steps to slow milk production, be sure that the baby is gaining much more than the average 2 lb. (900 g) per month. For strategies for coping with fast milk flow (p. 201) and slowing overabundant milk production, see p. 203.

If the baby sputters and coughs at milk ejection but weight gain is not above average, see p. 203 for other possible causes, such as airway abnormalities. If a baby's weight gain is borderline or low, nursing struggles may be due to low milk production. To increase it, see p. 193.

Menstruation Although unusual, some babies develop nursing struggles around the time of their nursing parent's menstrual cycle. Some families report that their baby rejects nursing for a day or so with each menstruation.

Mammary Health Mastitis (i.e., plugged duct, infection, abscess) is one cause of nursing struggles. One or both sides may be affected. Some babies are unsettled or reject the affected side. This may occur because milk flow from the affected side is slowed and/or because sodium and chloride levels increase, giving the milk a saltier taste.

Following the treatment recommendations for mastitis on p. 30 will cause milk production to rebound and its taste will return to normal, usually within a week or so. To help the baby accept the affected side again, use the strategies in the last section of this chapter and continue nursing on the other side.

NOT LATCHING TO ONE OR BOTH SIDES

When a baby seems unable or unwilling to latch to one or both sides, the first step is to rule out medical issues in the baby, such as torticollis, birth injury, oral anatomical variations, airway abnormalities, and illness. Nasal congestion, ear infection, allergy, reflux disease, and mouth injury are other health problems that can lead to nursing struggles. See Box 4.3 for a summary of possible causes after the newborn period.

NOT LATCHING TO ONE SIDE One-sided latching is not unusual. Many young babies latch and feed well on one side and not on the other. These are several possible reasons.

NIPPLE DIFFERENCES If one nipple is more everted (protruding) or less inverted than the other, the baby may latch to only one side. The same can be true in babies who respond better to the size or texture of one nipple over the other. If this happens, suggest using a semi-reclined starter position and first trigger the baby's inborn feeding behaviors so that she can self-attach (p. 6). Mammary support and shaping (p. 321) may also make it easier for the baby to latch deeper. In upright positions, helping the baby get a more asymmetrical latch (p. 319) may help.

MAMMARY FIRMNESS If one side is consistently firmer than the other, the baby may find it more difficult to latch deeply or latch at all. Suggest starting with reverse pressure softening (p. 333) to first soften the area around the areola before offering that side. Expressing just enough milk to soften the area around the areola may also help, as well as mammary support and shaping (p. 321).

DIFFERENCES IN MILK PRODUCTION OR FLOW Babies may prefer faster or slower milk flow.

- If baby nurses better with faster flow, suggest stimulating milk ejection before offering the unused side, so the baby won't have to wait.

- If baby nurses better with slower flow, suggest trying a semi-reclined starter position (p. 6) on the difficult side. In these positions, baby has more control over milk flow. See also p. 201.

NEWBORN FEEDING POSITIONS   Some newborns feel discomfort when held in certain positions and may latch to the difficult side if a more comfortable position is used. In the cradle or cross-cradle holds, typically the baby's head points in different directions on each side. If so, during latch attempts on the challenging side, suggest sliding the baby over in exactly the same body position (called the **slide-over position**) that worked on the easy side, so baby's head points in the same direction on both sides. Babies who struggle to latch when their position changes include those with:

- Torticollis (see p. 58), who may find it difficult or painful to turn their head
- A birth injury, which causes pain when pressure is applied in some positions
- A recent immunization or injury

In some cases, a nursing parent may be more coordinated on one side and nursing may go more smoothly when using the dominant hand to help the baby.

MAMMARY HEALTH   Mastitis may cause nursing struggles in a baby of any age. It can increase the saltiness of the milk and slow milk flow. If mastitis is a possibility (sore area or lump in one side), see p. 29.

Exclusive nursing is possible with one-sided feeding. It's possible to exclusively nurse twins, triplets, and even higher-order multiples, so most parents can produce enough milk on one side to fully nourish one baby. But depending on their storage capacity (p. 22), the baby doing one-sided nursing may feed more often than a baby taking both sides.

A common worry about one-sided nursing is whether the mammary glands will ever be the same size again, as the used side is often noticeably larger than the unused side. However, after weaning, the glands should return to their prepregnancy size. If they were the same size then, they will likely be the same size after weaning.

PERSUADING BABY TO TAKE THE UNUSED SIDE   If nursing parents want to help baby nurse on both sides, suggest during their normal waking hours they express milk from the unused side to establish or maintain good milk flow on that side. Strategies to make it easier for baby to latch and feed on the unused side include:

- Start nursing on the easier side, and after milk ejection, quickly slide the baby over to the other side without changing his body position.
- Offer the unused side after first stimulating milk ejection.
- Experiment with different positions, starting with semi-reclined starter positions (see p. 6).
- Use mammary shaping and support during latch attempts on the unused side (p. 321).
- Offer the unused side when baby is in a light sleep and less aware.
- Try nursing in a darkened room.
- Try the unused side while walking or rocking to distract baby.

If baby's milk intake is a concern, suggest monitoring baby's weight. Expected weight gain in the first 3 months is 1 oz. (28 g) per day and less after that. If the baby's weight gain is too low while nursing on one side and there is not enough expressed or donor milk available, ask the baby's healthcare provider about an appropriate supplement.

If a baby suddenly stops latching to one side without obvious cause, suggest parents see their healthcare provider to rule out mammary-related medical causes. Although unusual, this behavior is a possible indicator of mammary disease, such as abscess, infected galactocele (a milk-filled cyst), or even breast cancer.

THE NON-LATCHING BABY IN THE EARLY WEEKS If the baby has never nursed, suggest having the baby checked by her healthcare provider to rule out physical causes (Box 4.1). If the nursing struggles started between the second and fifth day, see Box 4.2. If nursing struggles started within the first month and the baby received artificial nipples, consider that as a possible contributing factor.

Some babies are suctioned at birth or shoved roughly during latch attempts without regard to their inborn feeding behaviors (Chapter 1). In some cases, parents are so motivated to nurse that they spend time at every feed trying to get their baby to latch while she gets more and more upset. Some babies will go on to nurse after these experiences, but some develop negative associations or aversions. In this case, suggest devoting some time to developing positive associations by making sure all the time spent on the nursing parent's body is happy time (see the last section).

Non-latching babies often struggle to nurse because they are looking for something they cannot find, such as:

- Full-frontal contact with the nursing parent to trigger their inborn feeding behaviors

- The chance to make their own way to the nipple in their own time
- The feeling of a deep latch, which stimulates active sucking
- A faster milk flow or a slower, more manageable milk flow
- A firm, protruding nipple (in babies who have been fed by bottle or given pacifiers)

In some cases, the best strategy is to allow baby to take an active role in latching. Suggest picking a time when the baby is not too hungry, getting into a comfortable, semi-reclined position with the nipple accessible to the baby, and putting the baby tummy down on their body near the nipple, triggering her inborn feeding behaviors, and letting her take the nipple in her own time.

A shallow latch may not trigger active sucking, and baby may become frustrated. In this case, try using mammary support or shaping (p. 321) to help the baby latch deeply. If using an upright position, it may also help to use an asymmetrical latch (p. 319). If engorgement interferes with a deep latch, see the earlier section "Taut Mammary Tissue." For more strategies, see the last section of this chapter.

If a baby received artificial nipples and is becoming frustrated with the soft nipple, suggest trying mammary shaping and support to help achieve a deep latch. Sometimes dripping milk on the nipple during latch attempts can help. In some cases, a thin, silicone nipple shield (p. 329) may be needed for the baby to transition to direct nursing.

NURSING STRIKE refers to the baby who was nursing well and suddenly rejects nursing. When babies go "on strike," some nursing parents wonder if this is their baby's way of weaning. But if the baby is younger than 1 year, this is unlikely, as before 12 months babies have a physical need for mother's milk. One way to tell a nursing strike from a natural weaning is that the baby is unhappy about it. Most often, a nursing strike lasts 2 to 4 days, but it may last as long as 10 days. It may require some ingenuity and careful analysis to find the cause and help the baby transition back to nursing. Sometimes the cause is never determined.

To determine the cause, all previous possible causes of nursing struggles should be considered. Individual babies respond to these factors differently, with some fussing at latch attempts, while others reject nursing completely. The causes of a nursing strike fall into two general categories:

Physical causes:

- Ear infection, cold, or other illness
- Reflux disease, which can make feedings painful
- Overabundant milk production, as a very fast milk flow can upset baby
- Hypersensitivity, intolerance, or allergy
- Pain when held, resulting from injury, medical procedure, or injection
- Mouth pain due to teething, thrush, or mouth injury or sores
- Reaction to a new product, such as deodorant, lotion, laundry detergent, etc.

Environmental causes:

- Stress, upset, overstimulation, or a chaotic home environment
- Feeding on a strict schedule, timed feeds, or frequent interruptions
- Baby left to cry for long periods
- Major changes in baby's routine, like traveling, a household move, or parent's return to work
- Arguments with others or yelling while nursing
- A strong reaction when the baby bites
- An unusually long separation

Finding a cause may influence which strategies to try. Even if the cause is unknown, suggest the strategies described in the next section.

While working to end the nursing strike, safeguard nursing by making sure the baby is well fed and express milk often enough to protect milk production.

STRATEGIES TO ACHIEVE SETTLED NURSING No matter what the cause, start with the basic strategies to help baby transition to direct nursing.

- Is baby calm?
- Are they looking into each other's eyes, touching, and talking?
- Is the baby in full frontal contact with the nursing parent and have foot contact?
- Is the baby's body stable and well supported?
- Is the baby relaxed with no muscle tension on either side of her body?

- Is baby's chin or cheek touching the parent's body?
- Can the baby's head tilt back slightly for easier swallowing?

Discuss the baby's alignment with the nipple. Make sure she can tilt her head back rather than tucking her chin. If needed, adjust their body positions. Also, avoid putting pressure on the back of baby's head.

Time-tested approaches to reduce stress at feeds can help the baby who's "on strike" nurse again.

- Keep the nursing parent's body a pleasant place, not a battleground. If nursing feels stressful, feed another way and instead give baby lots of cuddle time, letting baby nap with her head resting near the nipple.
- Spend time touching and in skin-to-skin contact. Between feeds, hold the baby as much as possible in skin-to-skin contact, with baby's bare torso resting against the nursing parent's bare chest. This is soothing and the oxytocin released makes them more open to one another.
- Attempt nursing while baby is in a light sleep or drowsy.
- Use feeding positions baby likes best, trying first the semi-reclined starter positions (p. 6).
- Trigger milk ejection before latch attempts for an instant reward, or try first expressing milk onto baby's lips.
- Try mammary shaping or support (p. 321), which may help the baby latch deeper to trigger active sucking.
- Try nursing in motion—walking or rocking.
- Spend as much time as possible nursing at those times the baby nurses well.
- Supplement if baby's weight gain slows to make sure she gets enough milk to be calm and open to nursing.

Tools and other strategies can help in some situations.

- Drip expressed milk on the nipple. If the baby attempts latching but won't stay there, ask a helper to use a spoon or eyedropper to drip expressed milk on the nipple or in the corner of baby's mouth. Swallowing triggers sucking, which can get baby started nursing. Give more milk if baby comes off.
- Feed a little milk first. Some babies are more willing to try nursing if they are not very hungry. Try giving the baby one-third to half a feed, and then offer to nurse. Another variation is **bait and switch**, which begins by bottle-feeding in a nursing position. After baby actively sucks and swallows for a minute or two, pull out the bottle teat and insert the nipple. Some babies just keep sucking.

- If using an upright position, try a pillow to support baby's weight. If baby finds close body contact too stimulating, she may be more willing to latch and feed if a firm pillow provides good body support.
- If flat or inverted nipples are an issue, draw them out with a suction device before nursing (p. 233).
- Try a thin, silicone nipple shield (p. 329).
- If slow milk flow is an issue, try a nursing supplementer.

CHAPTER 5 CONTRACEPTION

LACTATION, SEXUALITY, AND FERTILITY

NURSING AND SEXUALITY During the early months after birth, a change in sexual desire is common. Some parents report increased sexual desire, but the majority report less sexual desire. During lactation, milk leakage may occur during lovemaking. Skin-to-skin contact and orgasm release oxytocin, which triggers milk ejection. Milk flow can be stopped by applying gentle pressure to the nipples with palms or a cloth. The low estrogen levels occurring during early lactation may cause vaginal dryness, which can be easily remedied with lubricant.

THE EFFECTS OF NURSING ON FERTILITY For most parents, the hormones released during nursing delay the return of fertility after birth. A shorter time between birth and the first nursing session is associated with longer delay in the return to fertility.

BEFORE THE MENSES RESUME Baby's nursing pattern plays a major role in the timing of the return to fertility. Nursing exclusively and often day and night—with no long stretches between feeds—produces a longer period of infertility after birth than scheduled or supplemented nursing. A nursing parent's body chemistry also plays a major role in when fertility returns, which explains why return to fertility can vary so widely among nursing parents whose babies have similar feeding rhythms and sucking stimulation. It also explains why some parents who exclusively nurse day and night resume their menses within 8 weeks of giving birth while for others it takes 12 months, 24 months, or longer, even when their baby has long stretches of sleep or receives regular supplements.

The nursing parent's nutritional status has little effect on the return of fertility.

If menstruation returns during the first 6 months of nursing, it usually precedes ovulation (a "warning period"). Parents who nurse exclusively and intensively may have up to three menstrual cycles before they ovulate. The longer the menses are delayed by nursing and the less often parents nurse, the more likely it is that ovulation will occur before the first menstruation.

Milk expression has less of an effect on hormonal levels and fertility compared with nursing. It's important not to equate milk expression with nursing in terms of its effect on fertility.

How solid foods are started can affect nursing rhythms and therefore whether the nursing parent's menses return quickly or the period of natural infertility is prolonged. To delay the return of the menses as long as possible, nursing parents can:

- Nurse first before offering solid foods.
- Introduce solid foods gradually.
- Continue nursing often day and night, going no longer than 4 hours without nursing during the day and 6 hours at night.

As a growing baby nurses less often, the chances of ovulating before menstruating increase.

To increase the odds of ovulating before the first post-birth menstruation, parents can start solid foods or significantly increase their baby's consumption of other fluids, increase the length of time between nursing sessions at night, decrease overall nursing frequency, decrease total time nursing, and completely wean from nursing. Any changes that decrease nursing frequency increase the possibility of ovulation and pregnancy. If a nursing parent's goal is to become fertile before the menses return naturally, one option is to cut back on nursing.

In some rare cases, it may be impossible to become pregnant until the baby is completely weaned from nursing.

AFTER THE MENSES RESUME If more than 8 weeks after birth, vaginal bleeding lasts for 2 days or more or if bleeding occurs that is like a menstrual period, assume pregnancy is possible. Light bleeding or spotting is the first indication of the return to fertility. Ovulation is much more likely to precede regular or heavy bleeding, as opposed to spotting or light bleeding. Continuing to nurse after the menses resume reduces the chances of conceiving and maintaining a pregnancy.

After menstruation resumes, an increase in nursing or milk expression may suppress it again, but assume fertility has returned.

NURSING AND CONTRACEPTION

Cultural and religious values, as well as other factors, will affect the family planning choices each couple finds acceptable. Information that might rule in or out some contraceptive methods include:

- Their nursing rhythm and the baby's age (LAM and hormonal methods)
- The nursing parent's age (hormonal methods)
- The partner's opinion
- Their childbearing goals (temporary or permanent methods)

- Any health issues (temporary or permanent methods, hormonal methods)
- The family's financial resources, healthcare options, and locally available methods

NON-HORMONAL METHODS are the first choice for nursing families since they have no effect on nursing or milk production.

LACTATION AMENORRHEA METHOD (LAM) is a temporary family planning method that does not require sexual abstinence and is at least 98% reliable during the first 6 months after birth when certain conditions are met. Practicing optimal nursing provides a prolonged period of natural infertility, leads to better health outcomes in nursing parent and child, saves money that would otherwise be spent on supplements and contraception, and gives parents control over their fertility. LAM is also acceptable to virtually all religious groups.

For LAM to be effective, the answer to the following three questions must be "no."

- Have your menses returned? (Defined as 2 consecutive days of bleeding after 8 weeks post-delivery or a vaginal bleed considered to be a menses.)
- Are you supplementing regularly or allowing long periods without nursing either day or night?
- Is your baby more than 6 months old?

When using LAM, parents should ask themselves these questions regularly, and when the answer to any of them is "yes," to avoid pregnancy, the family needs to begin using another method of contraception. Parents can rely on LAM with confidence if their baby is exclusively nursing (only mother's milk and no other liquids or solids) or almost exclusively nursing (no more than two mouthfuls daily of other foods, drinks, medications, and/or vitamins/minerals).

LAM may continue to be effective after the first 6 months if the menses have not returned, solids are given after the baby nurses, and the gaps between nursing sessions are no longer than 4 hours during the day and 6 hours at night.

LAM appears to be slightly less effective in employed mothers expressing milk.

OTHER NATURAL FAMILY PLANNING METHODS involve abstaining from sex during fertile times. These include the Billings ovulation method (OM), Creighton model, Symptothermal method, and the Marquette method. Any of these natural family planning methods can be used by a nursing family even before the menses return. They all involve observing some combination of cervical mucus, temperature, and/or hormonal monitoring, which determines fertile times. Because no drugs or products are involved, they are safe for nursing couples and do not affect lactation. They may be as much as 98% effective when used correctly.

BARRIER METHODS WITH OR WITHOUT SPERMICIDES include condoms, diaphragms, contraceptive sponges, and cervical caps. Barrier methods do not affect nursing, are easily available in most places, are relatively inexpensive, can be used with other methods, and some provide protection from sexually transmitted diseases. When used correctly, condoms and diaphragms are relatively effective in preventing pregnancy.

Barrier methods also have some disadvantages. Unless lubricated condoms are used, they can cause irritation due to vaginal dryness from low estrogen levels during early nursing. Diaphragms and cervical caps require a physical exam for refitting after giving birth and whenever its user's weight varies by more than 10 lb. (4.5 kg). Allergic reactions can occur with contact with their materials. Some consider them inconvenient because they limit spontaneous sex.

Spermicides used alone or with a barrier method do not affect nursing.

NON-HORMONAL INTRAUTERINE DEVICES (IUDs) reliably prevent pregnancy and are compatible with nursing. They are inserted into the uterus and left in place long-term. They work by altering the user's hormonal state to prevent fertilization or implantation of a fertilized egg. Highly effective at preventing pregnancy, a non-hormonal IUD does not affect milk production, milk composition, or the nursing baby.

To reduce risk of expulsion, delay IUD insertion until at least 3 days after birth.

SURGICAL STERILIZATION includes vasectomy and tubal ligation. Both effectively prevent pregnancy by physically blocking the pathway between sperm and egg. These procedures should be considered permanent, as reversal cannot be guaranteed. Although neither affect lactation, with tubal ligation, there likely will be a temporary interruption of nursing during recovery, and the pain from the surgery may make nursing uncomfortable afterwards.

A full or partial hysterectomy will not affect nursing or milk production, which is regulated by hormones secreted from the hypothalamus and pituitary glands. But nursing parents undergoing any surgery will likely need help in maintaining nursing during the hospital stay. See p. 160.

HORMONAL METHODS are not the first choice for nursing families due to concerns about milk production and theoretical risks of exposure to the baby. Progestin, a synthetic form of the hormone progesterone, and estrogen, the hormone used in hormonal methods, are compatible with lactation, but the World Health Organization (WHO) and others consider these methods second and third choices for nursing parents.

Estrogen and progesterone have the potential to decrease milk production. The WHO recommends nursing families avoid using progestin-only contraception during the first 6 weeks after birth and combined hormonal contraceptives containing both progestin and estrogen during the first 6 months after birth. The U.S. Centers for Disease Control and Prevention (CDC) considers progestin-only methods acceptable during the early weeks after birth. The Academy of Breastfeeding Medicine (ABM) suggests avoiding hormonal contraceptives in cases of low milk production, a history of breast or chest surgery, multiple birth, preterm birth, and when the health of nursing parent or baby is compromised.

PROGESTIN-ONLY METHODS are considered the second choice for nursing families. They prevent pregnancy by thickening cervical mucus, making sperm penetration more difficult, blocking ovulation, and thinning the uterine lining. However, since the onset of copious lactation occurs with the rapid fall in natural progesterone levels after the delivery of the placenta, the use during the early weeks of methods that include progestin—a synthetic progesterone—has the potential to disrupt lactation. While studies have not yet identified any problems with these methods in large groups when initiated after 6 weeks post-birth, there are anecdotal reports of insufficient milk after these methods were started.

Differences among the following types of progestin-only methods may make one a better choice than another for nursing parents.

- **Progestin-only minipill** is most effective when taken at about the same time each day and is slightly less effective (and less forgiving of missed pills) than the combined pill with progesterone and estrogen. Irregular bleeding, a common side effect of the minipill, is less likely while nursing.

- **Progestin-only IUD** works like a non-hormonal IUD with small amounts of progestin released over time into its user's system. Depending on the model used, these devices may be effective for up to 12 years after insertion. They provide slightly better pregnancy prevention than non-hormonal IUDs (0.2% with hormonal IUDs become pregnant versus 0.8% with non-hormonal IUDs).

- **Progestin-releasing vaginal ring** is inserted in the vagina and removed for a week every 21 days.
- **Progestin-only injectable** (i.e. Depo-Provera or DPMA) is injected every 3 months and is used by about 6% worldwide. Since it is not reversible, be careful when using it during lactation.
- **Progestin-only implant** (i.e. Norplant or Implanon) is inserted under the skin and prevents pregnancy for up to 5 years. Used by only about 1% worldwide. Some implants, such as Nesterone or Elcometrine, deliver an orally inactive progesterone that baby cannot absorb, making it a better choice for nursing parents.

Timed-released methods (long-acting reversible contraception or LARC) are often recommended in low-income populations. They provide highly effective and continuous protection from pregnancy over a long period of time independent of human error.

The amount of hormone available to the baby through the milk is less with pills, implants and progestin-only IUDs and more with injectables, such as Depo-Provera (DPMA).

The WHO recommends nursing parents start progestin-only methods no earlier than 6 weeks after birth. The CDC and American College of Obstetricians and Gynecologists (ACOG) consider them acceptable immediately after birth, especially if providers consider parents at high risk of pregnancy before their first post-delivery checkup.

Effects of progestin on milk production is one concern when progestin-only methods are used early in lactation. In the first days after birth, the biological trigger for the rapid increase in milk production (lactogenesis II or secretory activation) is the sharp drop in progesterone that naturally occurs after the delivery of the placenta. If nursing parents receive an injection of progestin (a synthetic progesterone) right after delivery, this might alter their hormonal state enough to undermine milk production. Over the decades, most studies found little to no effect on lactation outcomes. However, there are anecdotal reports of nursing parents who experienced a drop in milk production after starting progestin-only methods.

When considering the timing of starting progestin-only methods, suggest families and healthcare providers take into account the period of natural infertility while the baby is fully nursing.

Effects of progestin on the baby is another concern when progestin-only methods are started early, because it may be difficult for the immature newborn to metabolize progestin.

But most experts consider these methods compatible with lactation. There were no clinically relevant effects on the baby, perhaps because progestin is not easily absorbed by the baby's gut. As of this writing, the children of nursing parents who used progestin-only methods were followed for up to 17 years, with no long-term effects found on growth or development, including sexual development.

METHODS CONTAINING ESTROGEN are considered the third and last choice for nursing parents, because the amount of estrogen in earlier versions of combined oral contraceptives decreased milk production and lactation duration. Estrogen is an effective lactation suppressant after birth.

Methods containing estrogen include:

- **The combined oral contraceptive pill** taken daily, containing estrogen and progestin.
- **Transdermal patch** (replaced weekly)
- **Combined vaginal ring** (replaced monthly)

The last two give continuous highly effective protection from pregnancy and as long as they stay in place are immune to human error.

Combined hormonal methods are not recommended for users over 35 who smoke and those with clotting problems, estrogen-dependent cancers, or severe migraine.

The CDC categorizes these methods differently depending on when they are started after birth:

- **Birth to 3 weeks:** Category 4, "an unacceptable health risk"
- **3 to 6 weeks:** Category 3, "the theoretical or proven risks usually outweigh the advantages"
- **After 6 weeks:** Category 2: "the advantages of using the method generally outweigh the theoretical or proven risks"

Concerns first arose about the use of combined oral contraceptives by nursing parents in the 1980s, when higher-dose estrogen pills taken during the first weeks post-delivery decreased milk production between 20% and 40%. When combined oral contraceptives with lower-dose estrogen were started after full milk production was established, they had less effect on both nursing duration and milk production. However, some studies found lower milk production among some parents using combined methods. More recent studies found that at 4 months after birth, those who used progestin-only methods were most likely to meet their nursing goals whereas those who used combined methods were least likely to meet their nursing goals. The WHO recommends nursing parents avoid combined methods until the baby is at least 6 months old, when the introduction of solid foods can offset any decrease in milk production.

Nursing babies whose parents use combined oral contraceptives receive no more estrogen than they would receive during nursing. Both estrogen and progesterone are considered compatible with lactation.

Previous concerns about changes in milk composition with combined contraceptives appear to be unfounded.

If a nursing parent uses a method containing estrogen, suggest continued nursing while monitoring the baby's weight gain.

EMERGENCY CONTRACEPTION The various types of emergency contraceptives, which are used to prevent pregnancy after unprotected sex, are compatible with lactation. These methods are most effective if used within 72 hours of intercourse but may be given up to 120 hours afterwards. Options include:

- Insertion of a copper IUD
- Combined oral contraceptives containing estrogen and progestin
- High doses of progestin, such as levonorgestrel (LNG), which is used in many of the previously described progestin-only contraceptive methods

As an emergency contraceptive, LNG is usually given in two 0.75 mg doses 12 hours apart. The ABM considers the amount of drug the nursing baby receives minimal and compatible with continued lactation. Download the ABM's Clinical Protocol #13 at **bfmed.org/protocols**.

CHAPTER 6   EMERGENCIES AND INFANT FEEDING

During emergencies, nursing is key to infant health and survival. In developed countries, even under normal circumstances, babies fed non-human milks are at greater risk of illness and death. But during war, famine, drought, flood, earthquake, hurricane, or other natural disasters, the risks of formula-feeding increase exponentially as conditions deteriorate and families face the following:

- Poor hygiene
- Limited or contaminated water supplies
- Less available food of all types, including infant formula
- Limited access to refrigeration and heat to sterilize containers
- Increased exposure to illness from crowds
- Decreased availability of medical treatment

RISKS OF NON-HUMAN MILKS

Babies fed non-human milks during an emergency are more likely to become ill from exposure to organisms in contaminated water and food. Risks of underfeeding increase when formula becomes scarce. Non-nursing babies are also more likely to become ill because they do not receive antibodies and other immunities from mother's milk. Formula and other foods also enhance infection in infants.

Nursing becomes vital during emergencies because it provides babies with unlimited safe food and fluids during their first 6 months, a safe partial food and fluids source after 6 months, and protection from illness. Along with all this, nursing also strengthens the close, loving parent-child bond and relieves stress in the nursing parent, which during emergencies can help prevent neglect and abandonment. Nursing also delays the return to fertility and enables families to nourish the baby during a time of more limited resources.

SUPPORT OPTIMAL NURSING PRACTICES

Following appropriate lactation practices is important to all families, but during an emergency, these actions may make the difference between life and death:

- Start nursing within an hour or so of birth.
- Maintain as much parent-baby skin-to-skin contact as possible after birth for increased infant stability.
- Nurse often and well day and night.

- Nurse exclusively for the first 6 months.
- Offer appropriate solid foods to baby at around 6 months of age.
- Continue nursing for at least the first 2 years.

MILK PRODUCTION IS RESILIENT The belief that stress or lack of food negatively affects milk quality or volume seems to be universal. But even when malnourished and stressed, nursing parents can produce good quality milk. Babies sometimes die unnecessarily because common misconceptions about nursing in emergencies lead to risky actions. For example, in Iraq during the Gulf War, the misconception that women could not produce adequate milk when malnourished and under great stress led some officials, journalists, and relief workers to discourage nursing. Although psychological stress can delay milk ejection, nursing is most definitely possible and milk will continue to be produced if nursing parents keep nursing. Stress, sleep difficulty, and fatigue do not necessarily affect milk volume. After a devastating 1978 earthquake in Guatemala, continued nursing by local mothers played a key role in infant survival.

As described in Chapter 14, nursing parents can produce ample milk even on very inadequate diets. A meta-analysis examining research from around the globe found that only when famine or near-famine conditions continue for several weeks does a parent's milk production or milk quality suffer. Even in famine conditions, milk production may be only slightly affected among previously well-nourished parents with good body stores. If famine occurs, providing nursing parents with food is less costly with better health outcomes than providing formula for babies.

Fluid intake appears to be unrelated to milk production. Increasing nursing parents' fluids by 25% was not found to affect milk production (p. 237).

PROVIDE LACTATION SUPPORT In every culture, lactation support during a crisis is critical. In countries where nursing is the norm, nursing parents often worry about not making enough milk, even when their milk production is ample. "Perceived insufficient milk" does not necessarily mean milk production is low. It may be a misinterpretation of normal infant behaviors or unrealistic expectations of how often a newborn should nurse. For this reason, health workers in emergencies need to understand nursing norms, so they can help families learn to gauge adequate milk production and encourage feeding more often if milk production needs a boost.

In emergencies, trained relief workers and experienced nursing parents can provide the necessary lactation support.

Part of any relief effort should be establishing policies that make nursing information and support a priority. An effective way to support nursing is to find parents who are currently nursing in the affected areas or those who have previously nursed and have the knowledge and skills to help others. Experienced nursing parents can counsel others on overcoming common challenges, such as nipple pain, worries about milk production, and mastitis. They can also provide information on boosting milk production for those mostly nursing; and explain relactation or induced lactation for those who never nursed or weaned before the emergency.

ENCOURAGE EXCLUSIVE NURSING AND RELACTATION
In emergencies, encourage exclusive nursing, wet nursing, induced lactation, and relactation, as even partial milk production can save babies' lives. To prevent infant deaths in an emergency, birthing parents who previously weaned or never nursed can relactate. Adoptive parents can induce lactation. Even partial milk production provides a source of safe, uncontaminated food and protection from illness. See Chapter 17 for details.

The main focus in an emergency should be on basic approaches, such as nursing for food and comfort and when baby is not nursing, using hand expression to stimulate milk production, as well as frequent parent-baby skin-to-skin contact day and night.

GIVE FORMULA ONLY TO THOSE NOT FULLY NURSING

During emergencies, infant formula and other foods that replace nursing should only be given to those caring for babies who cannot fully nurse, along with intensive support to improve survival rates. When a war or natural disaster occurs, the first impulse among many in developed nations is to offer aid in the form of infant formula. But this can cause more problems than it solves. Because exclusive nursing is not common anywhere in the world, making formula available puts nursing babies at risk. Providing formula to the affected areas can increase formula-related deaths, undermine families' confidence in nursing, and create an unnecessary dependence on commercial products. Nursing parents may decide to start giving their babies formula. The following are common reasons nursing parents request formula in emergencies:

- **The misconception that they can't fully nurse** due to stress, food shortages, or their misinterpretation of their baby's behavior.
- **Cultural beliefs**, for example that trauma will make their milk "bad."

- **An aspiration to bottle-feed.** In developing countries, formula-feeding is associated with higher socioeconomic status, which makes it appealing to some families.
- **Formula is expensive**. Some nursing parents may not feed their babies donated formula but request formula so they can sell it. A month's supply of formula in the Philippines may cost those in the lowest income group 75% of their monthly household income.

In 1991, during relief efforts in Iraq, Kurdish parents were told by British health personnel about the health risks of infant formula, but many were skeptical because formula-feeding originated in the West. In conflict situations, many families stop nursing, which makes nutritional challenges worse. Relief workers need to know that when nursing babies are fed formula, it will decrease the nursing parent's milk production and increase babies' risk for formula-related illness and death. Use of infant formula actively and passively harms babies' immune systems, making them vulnerable to infection and death from diarrhea and pneumonia.

When an emergency occurs in areas where nursing is not yet the norm, health risks to babies increase when formula is no longer easily available and hygiene deteriorates. In these areas, relief workers wanting to support nursing may encounter the extra challenge of dealing with traditional practices that undermine nursing. During the war in Bosnia, for example, many formula-fed babies died when formula became scarce and safe preparation became difficult. However, traditional practices, such as scheduling feeds and early and regular use of formula undermined milk production. Lack of access to infant formula can kill within a few days. After Hurricane Katrina in New Orleans, formula-fed infants died because they did not have access to formula or human milk.

FOLLOW INTERNATIONAL FORMULA GUIDELINES

If formula is provided in a crisis area, this should be done only under existing international guidelines, which include:

- Limit formula distribution to specifically defined situations
- Guarantee its availability as long as the baby requires it (until at least 6 months)
- Provide formula only in unbranded, generic packaging so sales are not promoted
- Distribute the formula only to babies younger than 12 months who are partially weaned along with making available clean water, fuel and containers for heating and sterilization, instructions and measuring tools, and

extra medical support for formula-related illness, such as treatments for diarrhea, and specific plans for lactation promotion to offset the availability of formula
- Adjust practices as needed to better reflect cultural values

Easily cleaned feeding cups may need to be provided in areas with poor hygiene to avoid the use of feeding bottles and nipples/teats, which are easily contaminated. Extra food allowances may be offered to nursing parents as an incentive to keep nursing.

Infant formula is not the only cause for concern. During the 2016 European refugee crisis, commercial infant foods were distributed in the refugee camps. Their packages recommended giving them to babies at 4 months, which is not best practice and if followed, could increase health problems.

Promoting the survival of babies in emergencies involves promoting exclusive nursing and measures that help families achieve this, such as:

- Give nursing parents priority access to food and other resources.
- Provide "safe spaces" where nursing parents can care for their baby and get lactation help.
- Prevent the uncontrolled distribution of infant formula or other milk products.

Yet despite these guidelines, infant formula continues to be distributed inappropriately in emergencies.

DIGITAL RESOURCES

bit.ly/BA2-CDCDisasters—U.S. Centers for Disease Control and Prevention's (CDC) 2018 webpage "Disaster Planning: Infant and Child Feeding."

bit.ly/BA2-WHOEmergencies—2017 publication "Infant and Young Child Feeding in Emergencies" distributed by WHO and created jointly by many international organizations. Free and downloadable.

bit.ly/BA2-WHORelactation—World Health Organization's (WHO) free, downloadable booklet, "Relactation: Review of Experience and Recommendations for Practice."

ennonline.net—U.K.'s Emergency Nutrition Network, whose Infant and Young Child Feeding in Emergencies (IFE) Core Group offers downloadable information for the public and relief workers on protecting nursing during emergencies.

CHAPTER 7 EMPLOYMENT

LENGTH OF PARENTAL LEAVE AND NURSING

How should nursing parents plan for their return to work? This depends on whether they work full time or part time (working fewer hours makes continued nursing easier) and whether they can nurse during work hours. Baby's age is a major factor, too. In general, the older the baby when the parent returns to work, the easier it is to meet long-term nursing goals. Here are some factors that affect nursing when parents' return to work occurs during these six time windows.

- **Birth to 5 weeks** is most challenging, because both parent and baby are physically vulnerable after childbirth and milk production is still ramping up. To reach full milk production, plan for 10 or more milk removals per day. The newborn's feeding volumes increase rapidly during this time. See Table 20.1 on p. 305 for realistic expectations.

- **6 weeks to 3 months** is easier because maintaining full milk production requires fewer milk removals per day (usually 6 to 8) than boosting it. Many parents still have childbirth-related physical symptoms, and babies this age are often fussy for parts of each day.

- **4 to 5 months** is a time when both baby's daily fussiness and physical symptoms from childbirth have resolved. According to studies, parents who start work now nurse longer.

- **6 to 8 months** is a period when the baby's need for milk decreases as solid foods are started. Babies this age can learn to drink from a cup, which eliminates the need to bottle-feed.

- **9 to 11 months** is a time when baby's need for milk further decreases, while his skill with a cup increases.

- **1 year or older** is the easiest time for nursing parents to return to work, because regular milk expression is not usually required, since baby can drink other beverages, including cow's milk or non-dairy beverages from the store. Parent and baby can continue nursing whenever they are together.

PRIORITIES DURING PARENTAL LEAVE

BABY TIME Think of the time at home during the early weeks after birth as a welcome period of closeness and togetherness. While on leave, a top priority is to nurse long and often to help set milk production at the level needed to meet long-term feeding goals. Support for nursing and lactation help are critical during this often overwhelming time.

If nursing is going well, milk production is best set by the baby, so suggest parents wait until returning to work before adopting their work schedule. Limiting nursing to certain times or feeding at set intervals is likely to slow milk production and undermine their long-term feeding goals. A baby's ability to adapt to change increases with age.

In the week or two before going back to work, suggest parents note how many times in 24 hours the baby nurses to get an idea of their magic number (p. 98), the number of milk removals (nursing plus pumping sessions) needed each day to keep milk production steady over time. Differences in storage capacity (p. 18) account for the variations in this number from parent to parent.

MILK EXPRESSION OPTIONS AND LOGISTICS When considering how to express milk, know that hand expression and breast pumps are often more effective when used together.

CHOOSING A BREAST PUMP If a family wants help in choosing a breast pump, ask how many hours per week others will feed the baby. When a pump plays a major role in maintaining milk production, choosing an effective pump may make a significant difference in parents' ability to meet their feeding goals. The best choice will depend in part on the family's means and situation.

Pump Plays a Major Role in Maintaining Milk Production If others will feed the baby for 32 hours or more per week, baby is younger than 6 months, and the family plans to feed only expressed milk for missed feeds, suggest looking for a pump with a motor warranty of at least 1 year that has a double-pumping option, and if its nipple tunnels are hard plastic, there are at least three different size options available. Separate vacuum and cycles controls have advantages over a single control dial, because separate controls allow users to customize the pump's settings to their body's response.

Pump Plays a Minor Role in Maintaining Milk Production If others will feed the baby less than 32 hours per week or the baby will receive foods other than expressed milk for missed feeds, a pump designed for occasional use (single pumps and muscle-powered manual pumps) may suffice.

WHEN TO EXPRESS AT HOME AND HOW MUCH TO STORE If the baby is younger than 1 year and the goal is to provide only expressed milk for missed feeds, before going back to work, allow 3 or 4 weeks to practice milk expression and store milk. This practice time allows parents to get comfortable with their expression method, so they can go through the "conditioning phase" at home rather than at work, where there will be a greater need to express quickly and effectively.

How Much Milk to Store Unless parental leave is shorter than 8 weeks, it may not be a good time investment to do much pumping and storing during the first month after birth, when milk production and therefore pumping yields are naturally lower. When parental leave is at least 8 weeks, suggest expressing milk for storage after milk production reaches its peak, around 4 to 5 weeks. At first, most parents express very little milk. With some practice, an expression session in the morning about 30 to 60 minutes after nursing usually yields about half a feed (1.5 to 2 oz. [45 to 58 mL]). Expressing once daily for 4 weeks should reasonably yield about 14 feeds (half a feed each day for 28 days) as a back-up. A reserve of frozen milk is helpful for parents working full-time planning for expressed milk only for a young baby. Once at work, they can usually express enough milk at work for the next day. A freezer stash serves as a hedge against the unexpected, such as spilled milk.

When to Express Milk at Home To store milk at home without affecting nursing, parents can:

- Store whatever milk they express to stay comfortable during the early weeks
- Express milk from one side while baby nurses on the other side
- Plan to express in the morning (when milk levels tend to be higher) about 30 to 60 minutes after a feed and at least an hour before a feed

If the baby wants to nurse right after a milk expression, go ahead. Most babies do not mind feeding longer to get the milk they need or nursing again sooner.

To avoid waste, suggest storing no more milk in a container than the baby will consume at one feed. (See Table 20.1 on p. 305 for average feeding volumes by age.)

PLANNING AHEAD FOR WORK A key aspect of any planning is deciding whether or not to express milk at work. If not, discuss other options. Those with a very large storage capacity (p. 18) may comfortably go for a long workday without expressing milk. But over time, without milk expression, most exclusively nursing parents of young babies will risk mastitis and/or reduced milk production.

When formulating a plan, ask if the workday will be longer than the baby's current longest stretch between feeds at home (usually at night). If the parent is already going this length of time without a problem, it may not be necessary to pump at work.

Partial Weaning is an option if the workday is much longer than the current longest stretch between milk removals at home and the parent does not plan to pump at work. This involves gradually reducing milk production so the parent can be away from the baby for long stretches without uncomfortable fullness yet still nurse at home.

Here are two approaches to partial weaning:

- Note the usual feeding times during the workday hours. A week or two before returning to work, pick one nursing session during that time and instead feed a substitute. (Avoid the first morning feed, when most nursing parents feel full already.) Feed this substitute at about the same time every day. After eliminating one nursing session, wait at least 2 to 3 days before dropping another. If uncomfortable, pump to comfort to prevent mastitis. The partial weaning is complete when the parent feels comfortable without nursing for the entire workday.

- Continue nursing at all feeds while at home and offer the supplements in between. When the baby regularly takes as much supplement as he would take during the workday, the partial weaning is complete.

Expressing Milk at Work takes planning. Discuss finding a private place to pump and where to store milk (insulated tote bag with cooling elements, communal refrigerator). Available break time for pumping may influence whether to double-pump to save time.

The number of pump sessions needed during the workday to maintain milk production depends on whether the baby is exclusively human-milk fed, the number of hours per day others feed the baby, and the parent's storage capacity. For an exclusively human-milk-fed baby younger than 6 months, as a starting point, divide by three the number of hours others will feed the baby, including travel time:. For example: 12 hours, 4 expressions ($12 \div 3 = 4$) or 9 hours, 3 expressions ($9 \div 3 = 3$).

After following this routine at work for a week or two, adjust as needed. Most parents of exclusively nursing babies younger than 6 months express milk 2 to 3 times per workday and spend less than 1 hour per day expressing milk. On average, parents stop pumping at work by their baby's first birthday.

MILK VOLUMES NEEDED during the workday can be calculated based on how many hours others feed the baby. Before the family learns how much milk baby actually consumes once back at work, keep in mind that on average, nursing babies take about 25 oz. (750 mL) of milk each day (24-hour period), but babies differ. To calculate the volume of milk needed during work hours, add a little extra milk to account for big eaters and use 30 oz. (887 mL) per 24 hours as a benchmark. Then divide this volume by the portion of the day that others feed the baby:

- **6 hours** (one-quarter of a 24-hour day) one-quarter of 30 oz. (887 mL) is 7.5 oz. (252 mL)
- **8 hours** (one-third of a 24-hour day) one-third of 30 oz. (887 mL) is 10 oz. (296 mL)
- **12 hours** (half of a 24-hour day) half of 30 oz. (887 mL) is 15 oz. (444 mL)

Most parents working full time are away from their babies for 8 to 12 hours per day, so most of these babies will need between 10 and 15 oz. (296 to 444 mL) of milk. This assumes that the baby nurses often at home. If the baby feeds very little at home or the baby sleeps for very long stretches at night without feeding, the baby will need more milk during work hours. For example, a baby who sleeps 8 hours at night will need the full 30 oz. (887 mL) during the remaining 16 hours left in the day.

Between 1 and 6 months, nursing babies need about the same volume of milk per day. After solids are started, the volume of milk needed gradually decreases.

INTRODUCING A FEEDING BOTTLE is best delayed until baby is at least 3 to 4 weeks old to allow him to first master nursing. If the nursing parent returns to work within the first month after birth, it may be necessary to start bottles earlier. If the nursing parent returns to work after 6 months, learning to feed from a bottle may be unnecessary, as many babies this age can transition directly to a cup.

Some families delay bottles until the return to work and arrange for the caregiver to introduce bottles then. But most parents prefer to introduce the bottle earlier, so they know their baby will accept it.

Suggest the parents try different types of bottle nipples/teats and choose the slowest-flow teat the baby accepts. A fast-flow teat can lead to overfeeding. A baby using a slow-flow teat is more likely to feel full after less milk, minimizing the volume of milk needed during the workday.

Because babies' mouths are different shapes, one type of bottle and nipple will not be the best choice for all babies. Suggest trying several types and styles of teats and see which the baby accepts.

In many cases, the best person to introduce a bottle is the baby's caregiver, since the bottle will be a part of their relationship. Bottle-feeding may go more smoothly if the caregiver has the chance to have a few visits and get to know the baby first. But some believe it's easiest for nursing parents to introduce the bottle, since they are the person baby knows best.

If a baby is reluctant to take a bottle, try these strategies:

- Have someone other than nursing parent offer the bottle while the parent is out of the building.
- Offer the bottle before baby is very hungry.
- Offer short trials with the bottle at first. If baby resists, stop and put it away.
- Try different feeding positions. If baby won't take it in a nursing position, try with baby facing forward, back against caregiver's chest, propped on raised legs, or in a baby seat.
- Wrap the baby in an item of the nursing parent's clothing with their scent on it.
- Warm the bottle teat to body temperature by running warm water over it first. Try dipping it in warm milk. If baby is teething, try chilling it.
- Tap baby's lips with the bottle teat, wait until baby opens, and allow baby to draw the teat into his mouth rather than pushing it in.
- Move rhythmically (walking, rocking, swaying) when offering the bottle to calm baby.
- Experiment with different types of bottles and teats.
- Try offering the bottle while baby is drowsy or in a light sleep.
- If baby is older, give him a bottle to play with for a few days before using it for feeding.
- Give some milk by spoon first and then offer the bottle or let baby suck on a finger and slip in the bottle along the side as he sucks.

If none of these strategies work, try feeding baby with a cup, spoon, or eyedropper. Try giving a partly frozen human-milk "slushie" by spoon.

Taking more milk from a bottle than the volume expressed for a missed feed is not necessarily a sign of low milk production. Unless paced-feeding techniques are used (p. 312), this difference may be caused by overfeeding from the fast, consistent flow of the bottle and so is more of a reflection of differences in feeding methods.

JOB OPTIONS AND CHILD CARE may significantly affect feeding outcomes.

WORK SCHEDULES AND SETTINGS may or may not provide the flexibility that makes nursing easier. When possible, suggest parents explore these options:

- Part time—Working fewer hours per week
- Job-sharing—Sharing one position with another person
- Phase back—Gradually increasing work hours from part time to full time
- Flex-time—Adjusting work hours to baby's routine
- Compressed work week—Working the same hours in fewer days
- Telecommuting—Working from home some or all workdays
- On-site day care—Going to baby for feeds as needed

Professional or management positions are more likely to provide flexibility and worksite lactation support. Lactation support is much less likely in the service, production, and transportation industries.

If the work schedule or setting is inflexible, explore the possibility of **reverse cycle nursing**, when most feeds occur while the nursing parent is home with the baby and the baby takes his longest sleep stretch during the workday. Parents can schedule their work hours during the baby's naturally occurring longest sleep period. Or after the return to work, the baby may change his feeding pattern so he is awake and feeding more often when the nursing parent is home. Reverse cycle nursing often requires less milk expression, but nursing often all night may be exhausting for the nursing parent.

WORKSITE LACTATION SUPPORT increases initiation, duration, and exclusivity of nursing.

When nursing parents talk to their boss about their needs, suggest they focus on the benefits to the employer of providing worksite lactation support. In companies when families do not nurse their babies, they experience:

- Significantly higher healthcare expenses
- Twice as many 1-day absences due to illness
- Lower employee retention rates after birth (national average: 59%, in companies with worksite lactation support: 94%)

In some parts of the world, employers are required by law to provide a time and place for nursing or milk expression. However, when discussing lactation laws, bring up this subject carefully so the employer does not see it as a veiled threat. Most U.S. worksite breastfeeding laws carry no penalty if not followed.

Many common barriers to worksite lactation support, such as the following, can often be overcome with creative thinking and an open mind.

- **Time away from work duties.** Many parents can express their milk during regular breaks and mealtimes. If not, they may arrange to make up time by coming in early or leaving later. Stress that the need to express at work is temporary and most stop expressing by 1 year.
- **Discomfort with breastfeeding.** Try using the word "lactation." Avoid promotional materials with nursing photos. Suggest coworkers share their stories to show the need.
- **Resistance from other employees** can be avoided by including others in the planning and with staff training. For greater fairness, some companies offer lactation education and equipment to the partners of employees, too. Discuss the financial benefits to the company.
- **Lack of available space,** such as a private office. The needed space may be as small as 4 by 5 feet (1.5 by 2 meters), such as a modified storage room. Alternatively, rather than a separate room, screen off an area.

Even if employers do not offer an official lactation program at work, they can support nursing by offering longer parental leave after birth, flexible work hours, break times for nursing or expressing, and a place to express and store milk.

ACCESS TO BABY DURING THE WORKDAY by either bringing baby to work or going to the baby for feeds, can make it easier to meet feeding goals.

Bringing baby to work may involve caring for the baby in the work area or the employer may provide on-site child care.

If bringing baby to work is not possible, ask if the nursing parent can go to the baby for some or all feeds. Even one nursing session during the workday reduces the time spent expressing milk and the volume of expressed milk the baby needs. Choosing a caregiver near work also reduces travel time from the baby, further reducing the expressed milk needed.

RETURNING TO WORK

In most families, the nursing parent's return to work is a major transition that can be made easier with good planning.

EASING THE TRANSITION Start back to work near the end of the work week, such as on a Thursday or Friday or start back part time, working shorter hours.

Plan the work wardrobe with nursing and expressing milk in mind. Have breast pads on hand and an extra top available in case of milk leakage. Wear two-piece outfits so nursing and milk expression are possible without fully undressing. Wear patterned tops rather than solid colors to better camouflage leaks or spilled milk. Have a jacket or sweater handy for use as a cover-up if needed.

Returning to work can be an emotional and overwhelming time. Suggest getting support from other employed nursing parents. If there are none at work, look into online peer support groups.

STRATEGIES TO MINIMIZE MILK NEEDED AND AVOID WASTE When baby is younger than 1 year, parents' daily routine can affect how often they need to express milk at work. To keep milk expression to a minimum:

- Nurse at least twice in the morning before leaving the baby with the caregiver. Nurse once upon awakening and again just before leaving baby.
- Nurse as soon as the nursing couple are reunited after work. If the baby seems hungry just before the parent arrives, suggest the caregiver feed a little milk so baby is still hungry when the parent gets there.
- Nurse often at home, day and night. The baby needs a fixed amount of milk per 24 hours. The fewer times baby nurses while at home, the more milk needed during the workday.
- Choose a caregiver close to work rather than home to reduce travel time and time apart.
- If possible, plan to nurse baby at least once during the workday. If the caregiver is nearby, the parent may be able to go to baby or have baby brought to the workplace for a feed.

Depending on workday length, these strategies can reduce the volume of expressed milk needed significantly.

To minimize the volume of expressed milk the baby needs during the workday, suggest the family:

- Store expressed milk in the smallest volumes baby may take. After 1 month, the average volume consumed during a nursing is 3 to 4 oz. (88 to 118 mL), but provide some 1- to 2-oz. (30 to 59 mL) snacks to avoid waste when the baby wants just a little more.
- If bottle-feeding, choose a slow-flow teat and use paced bottle-feeding techniques (p. 312) so baby feels full with less milk.

KEEPING MILK PRODUCTION STABLE LONG TERM hinges on several factors.

THE MAGIC NUMBER refers to the number of daily milk removals (nursing plus pumping sessions) needed to keep milk production steady long term. The specific number of milk removals varies by nursing parent due to differences in storage capacity (p. 18), but usually falls between 4 and 8.

In parents with a large storage capacity, it takes longer for enough milk to accumulate to slow milk production. Large-capacity parents can maintain milk production with fewer milk removals per day and express more milk at each session compared with smaller-capacity parents. Small-capacity parents feel full faster and must remove the milk more times per day to express the same volume of milk. Both can make plenty of milk overall, but the number of milk removals needed to keep milk production stable may vary greatly.

Once back at work, at least once per week suggest noting the number of daily milk removals. Over time, many parents keep their number of milk expressions at work steady but nurse less at home. When baby begins sleeping longer at night, for example, the number of daily milk removals may drop below the magic number. If milk production decreases, ask about the number of daily milk removals now and how that compares with their total during parental leave. Increasing the number of daily milk removals is often all that's needed to boost decreasing milk production.

Parents who travel for work without baby can use their magic number as a guide.

THE LONGEST STRETCH between milk removals (usually at night) is another key variable. Because "full glands make milk slower," when the longest stretch is too long, it can slow milk production. Suggest limiting the longest stretch to 8 hours or less.

When the baby starts eating solid foods, expect milk production to gradually decrease, because solids take the place of human milk in baby's diet.

PROBLEM-SOLVNG During the workday, if the baby takes more milk than parent expresses, gather more information before offering suggestions. Ask the baby's age and how many hours they are apart during the workday, including travel time. If the baby is younger than 1 year and the workday is 8 to 12 hours long, average milk intake is between 10 and 15 oz. (296 to 444 mL).

IF BABY IS TAKING MUCH MORE MILK THAN AVERAGE, baby may be overfed during the workday, either due to bottle-feeding that is not paced (p. 312), the caregiver overfeeding to keep baby content, or wasted milk discarded from too-full bottles.

IF PARENTS EXPRESS TOO LITTLE MILK AT WORK, look for the root cause. Consider too few daily milk removals (dropping below the magic number), a longest stretch so long that milk production drops, and issues with milk expression. (Are parents using hands-on pumping? Has their pump fit changed? Does the pump need new parts or is it malfunctioning?).

INCREASING MILK PRODUCTION   Because nursing parents differ, be prepared to offer different options for boosting milk production (p. 193). The sooner action is taken to increase flagging milk production, the more quickly improvement is likely to occur. The longer parents wait to take action, the more difficult it can be to boost milk production and the longer it takes.

CHAPTER 8 HEALTH AND ANATOMY ISSUES: BABY

ORAL ANATOMY OF THE NURSING BABY

The baby's tongue, lips, cheeks, palate, and jaws all play important roles in nursing effectiveness. Their characteristics are determined by genetics and environment.

BABY'S TONGUE For effective nursing, a baby's tongue needs the freedom of movement to extend, lift, lower, and form a groove.

TONGUE-TIE (ankyloglossia) refers to a condition in which the membrane under the tongue that attaches it to the floor of the mouth (***lingual frenulum***) is tight, fibrous, or thick enough to restrict normal tongue movement. At this writing, there are no agreed-upon definitions of a normal frenulum. If a tongue-tie is suspected, the International Association of Tongue Tie Professionals uses the term ***asymptomatic tongue-tie*** to describe tongue-tied babies who nurse comfortably and effectively and the term ***symptomatic tongue-tie*** to describe tongue-tied babies who have nursing problems after receiving skilled lactation help.

Incidence of Tongue-Tie Between 3% and 13% of all babies are tongue-tied, and tongue-tie runs in families. No more than 50% of tongue-tied babies develop feeding problems, so when a tongue-tied baby has nursing problems, it is important to consider other causes and first try basic strategies to improve nursing dynamics.

Nursing problems common among symptomatic tongue-tied babies are difficulty latching, parental nipple pain, and poor milk transfer. These symptoms can lead to continuous feeding and slow weight gain. Other possible signs of tongue-tie include a clicking sound during nursing, long rest periods during feeds, slipping off the nipple while nursing, and frequent coughing during feeds. Not all tongue-tied babies have all of these symptoms.

It is unclear from the research to what extent untreated tongue-tie is associated with later issues, such as speech problems, reflux, difficulty eating solid foods, tooth decay, and sleep apnea.

Coryllos Tongue-Tie Classification System categorizes tongue-ties into one of four or five different types. These types are unrelated to whether the tongue-tie is symptomatic or asymptomatic. A tongue-tie's type is determined by where one end of the frenulum attaches to the baby's tongue and where the other end attaches to the floor of the baby's mouth. Types 1 and 2 are considered anterior, or near the front of baby's mouth (which may give the tongue a heart-shaped appearance). Types 3 and 4 are considered posterior, or near the back of baby's mouth. A posterior tongue-tie may cause the tongue tip to curl down or impair baby's ability to lift her tongue. A possible Type 5 tongue-tie is the submucosal type, a posterior tongue-tie in which the frenulum attaches to the floor of the baby's mouth underneath its mucous membrane.

Identifying the type of a tongue-tie is unrelated to whether it is symptomatic or asymptomatic. Other factors may affect nursing in tongue-tied babies, such as the consistency of the mammary tissue and the floor of baby's mouth, as well as the elasticity and consistency of the frenulum. The baby's tongue function is more important to nursing than its appearance.

Tongue-Tie Assessment Tools Several validated tongue-tie assessment tools were created to help gauge tongue function as well as appearance. These include Alison Hazelbaker's Assessment Tool for Lingual Frenulum Function (ATLFF) and the Bristol Tongue Assessment Tool (BTAT), along with the picture-based Neonatal Tongue Screening Test (NTST) from Brazil and the Tongue-tie and Breastfed Baby (TABBY) assessment tool from the U.K.

Nursing Strategies for Symptomatic Tongue-Tied Babies If a tongue-tied baby has nursing problems, a good first strategy is to begin by seeing if adjusting positioning and latch, mammary shaping, and other basic strategies make a difference. In many cases, improving nursing dynamics can help increase comfort and feeding effectiveness.

In some cases, using a nipple shield may help, because it can reduce the sensation of painful nursing enough to make it bearable.

If nursing parents of symptomatic tongue-tied babies can handle some nursing but not exclusive nursing, expressing milk for some feeds is an option.

If after trying basic strategies, feedings are still painful or the baby is unable to nurse effectively, it's important to rule out other possible causes, such as poor positioning dynamics, aversion from negative experiences (deep suctioning, forceful latching attempts, family mental-health issues), structural issues (asymmetry or torticollis, unusually shaped palate), pain from an undiagnosed birth injury, hip dysplasia, or medical conditions (prematurity, neurological issues, congenital, respiratory, or cardiac abnormalities).

After other causes are ruled out, discuss having the baby evaluated for diagnosis of tongue-tie and possible tongue-tie release (frenotomy). A frenotomy is usually a simple procedure that can be done in a provider's office. In most places, it is performed by a doctor or dentist and involves releasing the baby's frenulum with scissors or a laser to improve the tongue's range of movement. It involves no stitches and is usually done without anesthesia. The evidence on the effectiveness of frenotomy indicates it usually improves the nursing parent's comfort. Symptomatic tongue-tie is less likely to lead to premature weaning if it is done earlier rather than later. After a frenotomy, if improvement occurs, it may be obvious immediately, or it may take some time.

Post-frenotomy care is recommended by some expert clinicians. Some say nursing alone provides enough "tongue exercise" after a frenotomy to prevent scarring or reattachment of the frenulum. Others believe that some gentle stretching exercises provide better results. Still others express concern that painful practices may cause nursing aversion.

TONGUE SIZE AND TONE can affect nursing. If the baby has a large or low-tone tongue, it may stick out of baby's mouth when she is at rest. If so, try triggering the baby's inborn feeding behaviors and allow her to self-attach. If the baby has Down syndrome, see the later section on p. 127.

BABY'S LIPS AND CHEEKS may affect nursing in some situations.

BABY'S LIPS play a vital role in allowing baby to form a seal during nursing.

Lip Flanging Despite common misconceptions, the baby's upper lip does not need to be flanged out for comfortable nursing. While the lower lip is usually completely flanged out, the upper lip may have a neutral position or be slightly flanged. There's no benefit to parents pulling out baby's lips after latch. In fact, this action may inadvertently cause a deep latch to become a shallower latch. What's most important after latch is that the nursing parent is comfortable and the baby is sucking actively. If both of these occur, there is no need to worry about or adjust the position of baby's lips.

Upper Lip-Ties The superior or maxillary labial frenulum (or frenum) is the membrane that connects the upper lip with the upper gumline. As a child grows, a very thick upper lip-tie may create excess space between the two upper front teeth, which in some cases, contributes to gum disease.

This membrane is not part of the normal newborn exam, so no one knows what characteristics are typical or atypical. Even its function is unknown. Much like tongue-tie, even without agreed-upon definitions, lip-ties are being identified and surgically released.

What problems are attributed to lip-tie? Some think lip-tie may reduce nursing effectiveness by preventing upper lip flanging, complicate latch by preventing baby from forming a seal on the mammary tissue, and contribute to poor milk transfer, nipple pain, and tooth decay from milk pooling around upper front teeth. But because lip-tie release is usually done at the same time as tongue-tie release, at this writing, it is impossible to separate the effects of lip-tie release from tongue-tie release.

Neither of the two proposed lip-tie classification systems (Kotlow and Stanford) are considered reliable.

BABY'S CHEEKS contain muscles and fat pads to help stabilize baby's tongue during nursing and play a role in the baby's ability to generate suction. Term babies have rounded cheeks because in utero they laid down fat pads in their cheek muscles. Their cheeks support the grooving of baby's tongue during nursing and make it easier to generate the suction needed to nurse effectively. Depending on gestational age, babies born preterm may lack these fat pads, which can cause their cheeks to dimple during nursing, reducing suction, which may reduce feeding effectiveness.

Some suggest that in rare cases, abnormal membranes known as **buccal-ties** may extend between the baby's gum and cheeks and cause nursing problems. As with lip-ties, data on normal membranes in the cheeks (such as those that create dimples) is scarce. Little is known about this possibility, so it is safe to say that when nursing problems arise, the first priority is to first go back to basics and try other strategies to improve nursing before a buccal-tie release is considered.

BABY'S PALATE, otherwise known as the roof of baby's mouth, can affect nursing.

PALATE SHAPES can vary greatly among babies. Possible palate shapes include:

- Reference (average) palate, the most common, is smooth and sloping. When given a finger pad side up to suck, the baby will draw it back about 1.5 inches (3.75 cm)—near where her soft and hard palates meet—and the entire length of the finger will stay in contact with the palate. An average palate slopes upward about 0.25 inches (0.5 cm).

- Grooved palate is unusual and features a thin groove along its length, which may make it more difficult for a baby to maintain suction during nursing.

- High or bubble palate may cause broken suction and a clicking sound during nursing. Its slope is more angled than a reference palate. With a bubble palate, a finger cannot feel the whole palate. Instead, a gap (bubble) is felt above the finger, which may be round or oval, shallow or deep.

In some cases, a baby with a high or bubble palate may resist drawing in the nipple deeply because she is not used to having the highest part of her palate touched. This touch may stimulate the gag reflex. If this happens, over several days, gradually help the baby adjust to normal touch on her palate by making it a pleasant game to first touch her lips, wait for an open mouth, and then gently slide a clean finger with a closely trimmed nail back—pad side up— along her hard palate, stopping just before the gag reflex is triggered. By making this a happy time and gradually moving the finger further back, it can help a baby get used to this feel and overcome this sensitivity.

Because the palate can be molded by tongue movements, pacifier/dummy, bottle use, and anything else that comes in regular contact with it, when a baby has an unusually shaped palate, suggest parents have their baby evaluated for tongue-tie.

CLEFT LIP AND PALATE, one of the most common birth defects, involves an opening (cleft) in the lip or palate. The cleft is correctable by surgery, and its type, location, and severity will determine its effect on nursing.

Cleft Lip Only A cleft lip may be either incomplete or complete (all the way up into the baby's nasal cavity), on one side (unilateral), or both (bilateral) and may involve the gum (alveolus). Babies with only a cleft lip have far fewer feeding problems than those with a cleft palate. An intact palate allows them to generate suction inside their mouth and therefore nurse more effectively.

Nursing strategies. With a cleft lip only, depending on its size and type, some babies need help forming a complete seal around the mammary tissue. If so, the following strategies may help.

- Experiment with different feeding positions.
- After baby latches, try using thumb or mammary tissue to fill in the lip opening to help the baby form a complete seal, which is needed to generate suction.
- Try pulling up mammary tissue between two fingers and press it into the cleft
- If the cleft is on one side only (unilateral), position the nipple to one side of the baby's cleft and use the thumb or a finger to fill the opening.

If these strategies don't solve the problem, have the baby checked for tongue-tie and a submucous cleft (p. 106), which is much more likely among babies with a cleft lip.

Because mammary tissue is flexible and can be molded to fill gaps more easily than an artificial teat, nursing may be easier than bottle-feeding for babies with a cleft lip. For nursing families who also plan to use feeding bottles, if the baby has a wide cleft, a wide-base teat may be easier for baby to manage.

Corrective surgery for a cleft lip may be performed as early as the first week or two after birth or as late as months later. Nursing rates among babies who have the early surgery are comparable to those in the general population.

After cleft lip repair, nursing may be interrupted for a few hours. No increased risk of wound separation was found when babies nurse or bottle-feed immediately after cleft lip repair. But nursing shortly after surgery needs to be arranged in advance with the baby's surgeon. If the surgeon has no personal experience with early nursing after surgery and is reluctant to allow it, ask if a nurse could observe the baby for signs of damage to the stitches. If the family is not happy with the surgeon's response, a second opinion is an option. If the surgeon requires a longer interruption, suggest expressing milk to stay comfortable and maintain milk production.

Some babies happily nurse after surgery and some do not. If the baby will not nurse, see p. 72 for strategies to help the baby return to nursing.

CLEFT PALATE WITH OR WITHOUT CLEFT LIP A cleft palate occurs when parts of the baby's palate do not fuse in utero, leaving an opening in the roof of her mouth. A cleft may occur in the hard palate, the soft palate, or both, and its location and size will affect the baby's ability to feed effectively. As with a cleft lip, a cleft palate can occur in one side (unilateral) or both (bilateral).

Another type is called a **submucous cleft**, which is an opening of muscle or bone beneath intact skin that may be invisible to the eye or may appear as a depression in the roof of baby's mouth. A cleft palate may be one feature of a genetic syndrome, such as Pierre-Robin sequence. It is not uncommon for cleft palates to be missed during newborn exams.

Hard and Soft Palate Clefts A cleft palate makes feeding challenging for several reasons.

- It may make it impossible for the baby to generate suction in her mouth, which is needed to keep the nipple in place and draw milk from the mammary gland or bottle.
- It allows milk in the baby's mouth to flow into her nasal cavity, where it can enter the airway.
- Depending on the cleft's size and location, there may be no firm surface against which the baby can compress a nipple or teat.

- The baby may keep her tongue mostly in the cleft and when she does move it forward, its movements may be uncoordinated rather than smooth.

For these reasons, a baby with a cleft palate may take up to two or three times longer to feed (while nursing, bottle-feeding, or both) than other babies.

Nursing options and influencing factors. Some babies with a cleft palate exclusively nurse, either early or later, but may need extra help transferring milk or supplements by another feeding method. Factors that affect how feeding goes include the birth facility's approach to nursing, available lactation options (help, support, tools, techniques), and the following physical factors that can influence nursing effectiveness:

- Whether or not the mammary tissue is malleable
- Whether milk production is low or abundant
- The location and size of the baby's cleft

If the cleft is small and it can be plugged with mammary tissue during nursing, the baby may be able to form an air seal and generate the suction needed to keep the nipple in place and the milk flowing in the right direction. The Academy of Breastfeeding Medicine (ABM) recommends in its Clinical Protocol #17 evaluating each cleft-affected baby individually for nursing. This protocol can be downloaded at: **bfmed.org/protocols**.

Milk expression from birth will likely be needed to establish and maintain adequate milk production for the baby with a cleft palate. Learning and practicing hand expression soon after birth stimulates milk production and provides colostrum to supplement the baby. Hand expression and breast compression during direct nursing may help compensate for a baby's lack of suction.

Discuss the family's goals. If exclusive human-milk feeding is important to them, do they prefer pumping and bottle-feeding? Would they rather express milk into the baby's mouth during direct nursing with compression? Both methods are time consuming in different ways. Some parents settle on a combination of methods. Even without much milk intake, the act of nursing can be soothing to parent and child and promote healthy development of baby's mouth, tongue, and facial muscles.

Feeding positions. When choosing a nursing position, try first the starter positions described on p. 6. In these positions:

- Gravity helps maintain latch in a baby who can't generate suction.

- Baby's tongue is drawn forward and down by gravity, which is helpful if the baby rests her tongue in the cleft.
- Baby's head is positioned higher than the nipple, reducing milk flow into the nose and ear tubes.
- There is less muscle strain during long feeds, since baby's weight rests on the parent's body.
- It is easier for the baby to use her instinctive feeding behaviors to self-attach.

Suggest beginning with the slightly more upright versions of the starter positions, with parent's body slope between 55 and 65 degrees (Figure 8.1).

If sitting-up-straight positions are used, the ABM protocol suggests starting with a football/rugby hold rather than cross-cradle position. The ABM also suggests positioning the nipple toward the side of the palate that has the most intact bone to prevent the nipple being pushed into the cleft.

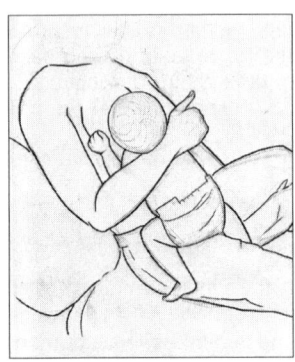

Figure 8.1 Semi-reclined straddle position
©2021 Nancy Mohrbacher Solutions, Inc.

Other strategies to improve milk intake in babies with a cleft palate include:

- *Provide mammary support* to help keep the nipple in back of the baby's mouth during feeds.
- *Hand express milk into baby's mouth* during nursing. To coordinate milk flow with baby's suck/swallow/breathe rhythm, compress firmly with thumb and forefinger when baby starts moving her tongue. Stop compressing while baby swallows and takes a breath.
- *Experiment with firm and soft mammary tissue*. Some babies nurse more effectively when the glands are firm, others when they are soft.
- *Provide jaw and chin support*. Some babies with a cleft palate need support to hold their jaw and chin steady while nursing. If the baby's cheeks dimple inward as the baby nurses, try the Dancer Hand position (Figure 8.2). As baby grows and gets more nursing practice, her muscle tone will improve and she may need chin support with only an index finger.

- *Try a nursing supplementer*, which can provide the cleft-affected baby with an experience similar to that of other babies. At this writing, all commercial nursing supplementers provide milk flow only when a baby generates suction, which many of these babies cannot. But gravity can speed milk flow by attaching the supplementer to an object much higher than the baby or making a hole near the top of the supplementer container to equalize the internal and external pressure for a faster milk flow. Alternatively, create a makeshift nursing supplementer that allows the feeder to actively deliver milk to the baby (p. 316), using either a #5 French feeding tube or a butterfly catheter, a port, and a syringe full of milk with the needle removed.

- *Nurse two babies together*. When the cleft-affected baby is a twin or the parent is tandem nursing, if the other sibling has an intact palate and can nurse effectively, by nursing them together, the more effective feeder can stimulate milk flow for the cleft-affected baby.

- *Be patient*. Finding ways to make nursing work with cleft-affected babies takes time. Until then, take advantage of all available help.

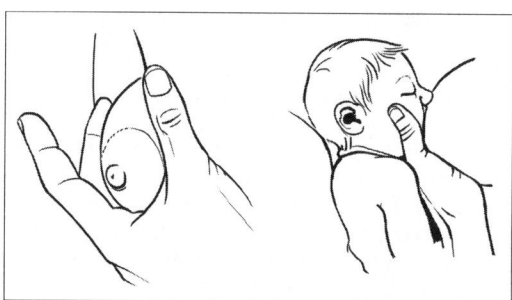

Figure 8.2 Dancer hand position to provide extra jaw support during nursing
©2021 Nancy Mohrbacher Solutions, Inc.

Slow weight gain is a common issue among babies with a cleft palate, but these interventions used in combination may enhance weight gain and make feeds easier.

- *Education and support* in combination with other interventions improve weight gain and growth. When counseling is started at birth by trained health professionals, these babies grow at the same rate as those without clefts.

- *Specialized feeding bottles* and nipples/teats. With today's online marketplace, families have greater access to squeezable bottles and teats and others designed for cleft-affected babies. Products like the Haberman and Pigeon Feeders are not always necessary or helpful. Many parents of cleft-affected babies report that regular feeding bottles work as well or better.

- *Palatal obturators* are plastic plates fitted to the baby's mouth. Some types are used before corrective surgery to keep the cleft in the baby's hard palate from closing improperly. Their use does not enable the baby to generate suction, but they provide a firm surface for baby to compress mammary tissue or a bottle teat with her tongue during feeds. The use of these devices does not always improve infant growth. If used, suggest requesting one with a smooth surface to reduce friction on the nipple.
- *Nasogastric (NG) tube*, which goes through the baby's nose into her stomach. It may be used when a cleft palate makes feeding profoundly challenging.

Cleft palate repair may be done as early as 3 months and as late as 32 months. Its timing and approach will vary by the surgeon and center. Cleft-palate repair may be done in stages during the baby's first or second year, after the face and mouth have matured, but before baby begins doing much talking.

After cleft palate repair, nursing may be uncomfortable for baby at first. With a newly structured palate, sucking will feel different to baby, and this new sensation may be unsettling. But within a few weeks, as nursing becomes easier, baby may begin nursing with more enthusiasm than before.

Submucous Cleft is an opening of muscle or bone beneath intact skin that may appear as a depression in the roof of baby's mouth. Depending on which muscles are missing, some babies can generate suction, but because the muscles of the soft palate are affected, it may make swallowing difficult and/or prevent the muscles of the soft palate from closing off the passage to the nose during feeds. Symptoms of submucous cleft include prolonged /ineffective nursing and milk flow through the nose.

Many babies with submucous clefts feed better during nursing than from the bottle, even specialty bottles. Using the semi-reclined and other feeding positions described in the previous section can make nursing easier if the baby has difficulty swallowing by providing more control over milk flow, which reduces milk flow through the nose.

BABY'S LOWER JAW AND AIRWAY A wide-open mouth at latch helps ensure the baby draws in enough mammary tissue for good milk transfer. After latch, the effectively nursing baby uses smooth jaw movements with a slight pause as her jaw lowers. But if baby's lower jaw is small or recessed or the baby has an airway abnormality, this can decrease nursing effectiveness.

SMALL OR RECESSED LOWER JAW All babies are born with receding chins, due in part to their chin-to-chest-position in utero. Although there is no agreed-upon objective definition for an unusually small lower jaw (**micrognathia**), if the baby's lower jaw seems obviously small in relation to the upper jaw, the baby may be more likely to have problems nursing.

A short or recessed jaw (**retrognathia**) may be problematic because of its effect on tongue placement. If both jaw and tongue are recessed, this may restrict the baby's ability to lift her tongue during nursing. Micrognathia is also associated with a narrower upper airway. To keep their airway open, these babies may tilt back their head and position their tongue on the palate, which can interfere with nursing.

These positioning strategies may help babies with a short or recessed jaw nurse more effectively:

- A very asymmetrical latch (p. 319) with head tilted back and baby's body pulled in close to the nursing parent's opposite nipple.
- Side-lying positions or semi-reclined starter positions, (p. 6) may help increase the baby's head extension for easier breathing.

If these strategies aren't enough, other options include the use of a nipple shield (p. 329) or finger-feeding (p. 314) as a way to help the baby learn to coordinate sucking, swallowing and breathing and improve her muscle strength.

AIRWAY ABNORMALITIES that cause a narrowed airway may contribute to slow weight gain, fast and noisy breathing, frequent coughing during nursing, and/or a high-pitched squeaky sound called **stridor**. The most common airway abnormalities are laryngomalacia (narrowing of the upper airway), tracheomalacia (narrowing of the lower airway), and vocal cord paralysis.

For effective nursing, a baby needs to coordinate sucking, swallowing, and breathing. A baby with an airway malformation or instability usually breathes more times per minute than other babies to get the oxygen needed. Faster breathing allows less time to swallow. When choosing between breathing and eating, breathing always wins.

A baby with laryngomalacia often nurses in bursts of three to five sucks with longer breathing pauses and may sometimes look bluish during feeds. Mild or severe symptoms may appear at birth or during the first few weeks and usually worsen until 6 months and then improve until 18 to 24 months.

Baby's weight gain can help distinguish simple milk-flow issues from breathing issues. When babies have trouble coping with milk flow, some assume this indicates oversupply (p. 200). Not so in a baby with an airway abnormality, who gains weight slowly because their faster breathing requires more energy and therefore more calories. Babies struggling with oversupply, on the other hand, usually gain weight faster than average, well above 2 pounds (900 grams) per month.

The increased airway pressure babies with airway abnormalities generate puts them at increased risk of reflux disease, which can cause painful feeds. Suggest they be evaluated for GERD (p. 116).

Babies with respiratory issues may nurse more effectively when the following basic strategies are used:

- Slow the milk flow (nurse after expressing some milk, paced bottle feeds)
- Relax baby before feeds to slow breathing (rock, walk, massage, eye contact, babywearing)
- Treat reflux disease, if present
- Use positioning to keep the airway as open as possible

Most babies find nursing easiest in starter positions (p. 6). Lying tummy down on the parent's body is especially helpful to these babies because milk flowing "uphill" gives them more control over milk flow. Whatever position is used, allow baby's head to tilt back while nursing. Head extension opens their upper airway and reduces respiratory distress. Head extension is possible in any feeding position by sliding the baby's body in the direction of her feet. Whatever the position, make sure the baby can release the nipple whenever needed for breathing breaks, as opposed to holding baby's head in place.

Some babies with an airway abnormality are more comfortable feeding for long periods at a leisurely pace, while others prefer to feed often for a short time.

If needed, suggest expressing milk as a supplement and to safeguard the milk production. If baby has difficulty bottle-feeding, consider supplementing with a specialized feeding device, such as a Haberman Feeder set to the slowest flow setting to make milk flow easier to manage.

ILLNESS IN THE NURSING BABY

When a child is ill, continued nursing is almost always the best option, because it comforts a sick baby and speeds recovery by providing antibodies specific to that illness.

COLDS, FLU, CONGESTION, AND EAR INFECTIONS When a nursing baby with nasal congestion struggles to breathe during feeds, some basic strategies can make nursing easier.

- Before nursing, keep the baby mostly upright so her sinuses can drain.
- If recommended, use a soft nasal aspirator to gently clear her nose of mucus.
- Nurse in a position upright enough so that baby's sinuses can drain.
- Nurse more often, as frequent feeds are often easier to manage.
- Nurse where the air is moist; use a cool-mist vaporizer or nurse in the bathroom with the shower running.
- For symptom relief, contact the baby's healthcare provider.

During a cold or ear infection, if the baby won't nurse, express milk and feed it by spoon or cup.

A baby with chronic congestion or trouble breathing should be evaluated by a healthcare provider. Chronic congestion can be a sign of allergy, GERD, or other physical problems. Struggles with breathing during feeds may be due to mouth or throat inflammation from rough suctioning or intubation after birth, spasms, or physical abnormalities (p. 111).

GASTROINTESTINAL ILLNESS nearly always resolves faster if baby keeps nursing.

Even during vomiting, human milk is absorbed quickly, so some fluids and nutrients will be retained.

When a gastrointestinal illness causes diarrhea and/or vomiting, be alert to the following signs of dehydration, and if they occur, contact baby's healthcare provider right away.

- Listlessness, lethargy, and/or sleeping through feeds
- Weak cry
- Baby's skin loses its resiliency (when pinched, it no longer bounces back)
- Dry mouth and eyes
- Fewer tears
- Fewer wet diapers (≤2 in 24 hours)
- Baby's fontanel (soft spot) appears sunken or depressed
- Fever

Dehydration can be prevented by feeding the baby frequently to improve fluid intake.

DIARRHEA differs from normal nursing stools in frequency, consistency, and/or smell.

The difference between normal nursing stools and diarrhea include:

- More stools, as many as 12 to 16 per day
- Watery stools, often with few "curds"
- A stronger, more offensive smell

Diarrhea occurs less often among nursing babies, but when it occurs, it may be caused by gastrointestinal (GI) illness or as a side effect of a food or medication either consumed directly by the baby or passed to the baby via mother's milk.

Diarrhea that lasts for weeks after an illness is often due to temporary lactose intolerance, and continued nursing is recommended. Many babies switched to lactose-free formulas do not improve.

Lactose Intolerance refers to the bloating, gas, abdominal pain, diarrhea, and nausea that occur when a lack of the enzyme lactase leaves lactose unprocessed in the gut. Most cases of lactose intolerance occur only in older children and adults. These are the four main types.

- *Primary lactase deficiency*, the most common type, does not affect young babies. It occurs later in life in about 70% of the world's population. Lactase production gradually decreases as early as age three and as late as adulthood. If a nursing parent has this type, the baby will not become lactose intolerant until she is older. It does not cause diarrhea in babies.
- *Congenital lactase deficiency* is a very rare genetic disorder that becomes obvious shortly after birth, causing dehydration, illness, and lack of weight gain. Like babies with classic galactosemia, the few babies with this condition cannot be safely nursed.
- *Developmental lactase deficiency* is a temporarily lower level of lactase production common in preterm babies younger than 34 weeks gestation.
- *Secondary lactase deficiency* is the most common type in babies and young children. This temporary condition is caused by damage to the lining of the small intestine from an infection, medication, celiac disease, or other illness.

This last, temporary type usually occurs in a baby or toddler after gut damage from a GI infection temporarily slows or stops lactase production. Other causes of "nuisance diarrhea" from intestinal damage include treatment with antibiotics, solid foods that irritate the lining of the gut, and excess fruit juice consumption. While the damage heals, diarrhea continues for on average 2 to 4 weeks and then resolves on its own. When the diarrhea does not immediately resolve, some recommend weaning the nursing babies to formula. But the American Academy of Pediatrics (AAP) suggests continued nursing during infectious illness with diarrhea and after in babies with no more than mild dehydration.

Green, Watery Stools without symptoms of illness may indicate the baby is sensitive to a food or drug either given directly or via mother's milk. Based on a 1988 article, a foremilk-hindmilk imbalance was suggested as a possible cause of green, watery stools, along with irritability, gas, and slow weight gain. In parents with oversupply who feed by the clock, switching sides before baby reaches the fatty hindmilk could overload the baby's small intestine with more lactose from the low-fat foremilk than it could absorb, causing these symptoms. But nursing babies using a wide variety of feeding patterns receive the same balance of foremilk and hindmilk.

A temporary or permanent weaning during a bout of diarrhea is not usually beneficial and may even lead to more problems. Babies return to health faster when they continue to nurse, with exclusively nursing babies recovering faster than mixed-fed or formula-fed babies.

VOMITING   When baby is vomiting, rule out the possibility that the baby is not ill but "spitting up" after feeds, which is common in young babies. If vomiting starts after weeks of uneventful nursing without other signs of illness, this may be a sign of a sensitivity to a food or drug baby receives directly or through mother's milk. When due to a reaction, spitting up could occur as soon as right after the exposure or as long as 48 hours later. See p. 238.

Pyloric Stenosis   If a baby projectile vomits once a day or more, suggest an evaluation for pyloric stenosis, whose symptoms usually appear between 2 and 6 weeks of age. At first, projectile vomiting happens only occasionally, but with pyloric stenosis, it happens more and more over time until the baby projectile vomits after every feed, which can lead to weight loss and dehydration.

The treatment for pyloric stenosis is to first evaluate the baby for dehydration and, if needed, restore her electrolyte balance before performing a simple surgery. During the surgery, the nursing parent may need to express milk, but if the surgery is uncomplicated, the baby can likely nurse after she recovers from the anesthesia. Early feeding post-surgery is associated with decreased length of hospital stay.

Keeping a Vomiting Nursing Baby Hydrated   If an obviously sick baby vomits after every nursing session, these strategies may help keep the baby hydrated and decrease the vomiting.

- Express most of the milk before the baby nurses, and offer a less-full gland.
- In babies 6 months or older, offer ice chips or water from a spoon.

REFLUX DISEASE (GERD) In a baby's first months, several times each day her stomach contents typically wash back into her esophagus, known as gastroesophageal reflux (GER). Spitting up occurs when the stomach contents make it up the esophagus and out the mouth. Spitting up occurs in up to 70% of babies and peaks around 4 to 5 months, occurring less and less often as the digestive system matures. By 12 months, only about 4% of babies still spit up.

When a thriving baby is feeding normally, spitting up is a temporary inconvenience. But when GER causes damage to the lining of the esophagus, normal GER becomes gastroesophageal reflux disease (GERD). A baby with GERD may spit up or she may not, because damage to the esophagus can occur even if the stomach contents don't reach baby's mouth. GERD may cause congestion, coughing, wheezing, bronchitis, pneumonia, apnea, esophageal narrowing, anemia, failure to thrive, and inflammation of the esophagus, which may cause pain during and after feeds. GERD also may cause:

- Crying and irritability
- Poor weight gain
- Sleep problems day and night
- Back arching and head turning
- Feeding aversion, which sometimes leads to feeding refusal

GERD may be an underlying cause of colic. GERD in babies is usually diagnosed by symptoms alone, because there is no diagnostic test that is reliable.

When a baby is unhappy during nursing sessions, parents may wonder if weaning will help. But formula can actually make the discomfort worse. Episodes of reflux are shorter among nursing babies compared with those fed formula. Nursing babies also stop spitting up earlier than babies formula-fed.

The following basic strategies can reduce GERD symptoms by 50%.

Use positioning therapy to minimize reflux. Keep baby's "head above bottom" so stomach contents stay in place.

- After feeds, keep baby upright for 20 to 30 minutes, in arms or in an upright baby carrier.

- At diaper changes, avoid lifting baby's legs; instead roll her on her left side to wipe.
- Nurse with baby's head higher than bottom in the starter positions (p. 6) or hold baby's bottom in parent's lap or on a pillow.
- When baby is awake and horizontal, lay her on her left side or on her tummy. Lying prone triggers less reflux than back-lying (supine).
- Avoid putting baby in a car seat except when in the car, as this position increases reflux.

Eliminate dairy from the nursing parent's diet, as cow-milk protein allergy produces similar symptoms. Avoid all forms of cow's milk protein, including all sources of dairy, casein, and whey for 4 weeks to see if baby's symptoms improve (p. 238). During the elimination diet, if formula is given, use a type in which the protein is at least partially broken down, such as Nutramigen.

Feed often. A baby needs on average 25 oz. (750 mL) every 24 hours to thrive. Taking smaller volumes of milk more often means less milk in the stomach to wash back into the esophagus and less time with an empty high-acid-content stomach. As in adults, an overly full stomach worsens GERD symptoms.

Thickening milk is recommended to reduce reflux in formula-fed babies but not in nursing babies with GERD. No evidence supports this practice. When starch-based thickening agents are added to expressed human milk, the enzymes in human milk digest the thickener.

Direct nursing alone reduces reflux. Feeding solids is not protective of reflux in nursing babies, and the addition of formula and bottle-feeding increases reflux.

Most babies outgrow reflux, but lack of treatment can contribute to slowed weight gain and later health problems, such as adult GERD and esophageal strictures. The first step in treating suspected GERD is to try the basic strategies beginning on the previous page for at least 2 to 4 weeks. If no improvement, see baby's healthcare provider to discuss prescription medication. If the medication reduces symptoms, keep in mind the drug's dose may need to be adjusted as baby's weight increases.

CHRONIC CONDITIONS IN THE NURSING BABY

When a baby is born with special needs, the parents may grieve the healthy baby they expected before they can accept the baby in their arms. Even if the diagnosis comes later, they may be wrestling with strong feelings and find it difficult to remember information given verbally, so provide it in writing and be prepared to go over it with them several times. When talking with parents:

- Acknowledge their feelings, which makes it easier for them to think through their situation.
- Suggest taking one day at a time and determine what works best for them by watching their baby's response.
- Ask normal questions like who the baby looks like and how she responds to others.
- If support organizations exist, discuss ways to connect with others in the same situation.

ALLERGY in children is increasing. It is less common in exclusively nursing babies, but this is not a guarantee, especially in those with a family history of allergy.

DEFINITIONS The terms allergy, hypersensitivity, and intolerance are often confused. An ***allergy*** or ***hypersensitivity*** is an immune response, often severe, and its symptoms usually affect many organs and occur predictably with each exposure. The most common U.S. food allergy is to peanut, followed by dairy, shellfish, tree nuts, egg, fin fish, and strawberry. With a food ***intolerance***, there is no immune response and the symptoms are usually not severe and limited to the digestive tract. People with a food intolerance can often eat small amounts of the food without a reaction.

Allergy occurs more often in children with a family history of allergy. If one parent has an allergy, the baby has a 20% to 40% increased risk of being allergic, and if both parents have an allergy, the baby's risk increases to 50% to 80%.

ALLERGY SYMPTOMS include fussiness (especially during feeds), but most allergic children also have physical symptoms, such as:

- Skin reactions: eczema, dermatitis, hives, rash, dry skin
- Gastrointestinal issues: vomiting, diarrhea, pain, blood or mucus in stools
- Respiratory problems: congestion, runny nose, wheezing, coughing

For strategies, see p. 238.

CARDIAC ISSUES at birth, known as congenital heart disease (CHD), include defects of the heart and major blood vessels and may occur alone or with Down syndrome or other syndromes. About 20% of babies with CHD gain weight slowly no matter how they are fed, because they take more breaths each minute and their hearts beat faster, using more energy.

Nursing challenges common when nursing a baby with cardiac issues include:

- Delayed first feed
- Separation from the baby during the hospital stay
- The need for the baby to fast before some medical procedures
- Inconsistent feeding support from healthcare providers
- Anxiety about feeding

One common concern in special-care nurseries is the ability to measure baby's milk intake. Weighing babies before and after nursing with a scale accurate to 2 g allows parents and providers to accurately measure baby's milk intake during nursing, even when baby is wearing leads.

FACTORS THAT SUPPORT NURSING SUCCESS Direct nursing is easier than bottle-feeding for babies with CHD and results in better health outcomes. Some babies with cardiac issues have difficulty nursing and bottle-feeding. Factors important to nursing success include:

- Encouragement and support from healthcare providers
- Consistent and careful lactation management
- Help from lactation specialists
- Parental motivation

NURSING STRATEGIES WITH CARDIAC ISSUES Unrelated to the severity of the baby's condition, families often worry about inadequate weight gain and breathlessness and fatigue during nursing. Suggest parents try these strategies:

- If surgery is imminent, spend as much time as possible nursing to ease baby's transition back to nursing afterward.
- Try the starter positions (p. 6) or side-lying (p. 12), which allow the baby's head to extend for easier swallowing and breathing.
- If the baby fatigues easily and only nurses well from one side, use breast compression (p. 309) or the "milk shake" (p. 201) to give baby access to more hindmilk more quickly.
- Feed often, as a baby with less stamina may do better with smaller, frequent feeds.
- Stop nursing if the baby is short of breath, her lips turn blue, or she looks pale or tired.
- If the baby nurses ineffectively, express milk after feeds to safeguard milk production and try the Dancer Hand position (p. 109) for more support or a nipple shield (p. 329).

- During medical procedures, as needed, request a place to express milk and arrange for food and drink, a place to rest, a breast pump, refrigerator, and/or cleaning supplies.

TIPS FOR BOOSTING WEIGHT GAIN Exclusive direct nursing is possible for many babies with cardiac issues, but some need extra help to gain weight adequately, for example

- Consistent use of breast compression (p. 309) during nursing to increase milk fat content.
- Adding a calorie-rich supplement to expressed milk.
- Nursing during the day and feeding baby with a continuous feeding pump at night.
- Following nursing with a high-calorie supplement via a nasogastric tube.
- Using a nursing supplementer or other method to supplement the baby with high-calorie hindmilk.
- If baby's fluids are restricted, feeding only high-calorie hindmilk (28-30 calories/oz. [30 mL]) or high-calorie preterm formula.

To provide hindmilk, express milk after nursing. If exclusively expressing, suggest storing the milk expressed during the first few minutes for later (or maybe the first half of the pump session to get even higher-calorie milk), and then collecting the later milk expressed for supplementing. A device called a creamatocrit can measure the fat content of human milk. Expressed milk can also be **fractionated,** meaning the fattier milk is separated from the lower-fat-milk in a centrifuge and fed to the baby.

Whatever supplement is used, discuss with the baby's healthcare provider how often and how much to give. Depending on the baby's weight gain and feeding effectiveness, the baby may be supplemented after every feed, after every other feed, or less often. Emphasize the value of expressed milk and explain that with cardiac issues, simply increasing milk intake may not be enough

If parents are discouraged, stress that the baby's nursing effectiveness will likely improve with practice, the right medication, or if the problem is severe, with surgery.

CYSTIC FIBROSIS is a genetic disease that causes a thick, gluey mucus to be secreted that clogs the bronchial tubes, interfering with breathing and blocking the digestive enzymes from leaving the pancreas, which causes incomplete digestion. The sweat glands reabsorb chloride normally, which causes baby's skin to taste salty when kissed.

The disease can range from mild to severe. Some cases are detectable only by lab tests while others are life-threatening. The baby may have breathing problems and regular respiratory infections and may look thin, pale, and undernourished.

The first clue that a baby has cystic fibrosis may be a puzzling slow weight gain in a baby who vigorously nurses and has many wet diapers and stools. In this case, slow weight gain is due to incomplete digestion and is unrelated to the baby's milk intake.

Babies with cystic fibrosis who do not nurse have poorer health outcomes and earlier onset of symptoms. Several downsides to less-than-exclusive nursing in the baby with cystic fibrosis are a slower weight gain and shorter height, more severe disease, earlier onset of symptoms, more infections, and greater decline in lung function.

At this writing, only about 50% of these families do any nursing. While babies were once not diagnosed with cystic fibrosis until they were at least several months old, now, newborn blood screening makes it possible to diagnose cystic fibrosis soon after birth. As a result, concerns about boosting weight gain and a lack of confidence in nursing convinces many families to formula-feed. One way to counter this trend is to include an IBCLC at the visit where cystic fibrosis is diagnosed and provide a lactation plan and access to IBCLC support, which can significantly increase nursing rates.

In about half of the babies with cystic fibrosis, the flow of digestive enzymes from the pancreas is reduced and replacement enzymes are needed to grow and gain weight appropriately. These enzymes can be dissolved in soft foods and given by spoon before nursing. Some of these babies also need extra vitamins, minerals, and salt, especially in hot weather. To prevent respiratory infections, the family may be advised to keep the baby upright when possible and to use aerosols, antibiotics, and/or expectorants.

DIABETES Type 1 diabetes occurs when the insulin-producing beta cells in the pancreas are destroyed, leaving the body unable to produce insulin, a hormone needed to convert sugar, starches, and other foods into fuel for the body. Without insulin, blood sugar can rise to dangerous levels and cause health complications and even death.

When Type 1 diabetes is diagnosed in babies younger than 9 months, it is likely a genetic form of the disease. Insulin may be used to treat it, or after the baby is stabilized, it may be treated with an oral medication. Babies diagnosed with Type 1 diabetes may also have other neurological issues that sometimes make early nursing more challenging, but nursing is recommended.

Caregivers need to check the diabetic child's blood-sugar levels regularly and provide daily medication or insulin replacement therapy via injections or subcutaneous pump, so their blood sugar doesn't become dangerously low or high. During infancy and childhood, keeping blood-sugar levels within the normal range is important to healthy brain growth and cognitive development.

Some parents report their healthcare providers seem frustrated because they cannot say exactly how much milk the nursing baby consumes. This can add to the family's stress after diagnosis and may leave the impression that continuing to nurse is bad for their child's health. There is no evidence to support this point of view. But there is evidence that nursing children in general have better brain development and cognitive outcomes independent of the family's means. The infection-fighting aspect of nursing is also important, as diabetics are more prone to infections than those with normal insulin levels.

CARBOHYDRATE CONTENT OF HUMAN MILK   Parents need to track the child's carbohydrate intake to calculate the dose of insulin needed to keep blood-sugar levels within the normal range. The ABM Clinical Protocol #27 (at **bfmed.org/protocols**) noted that human milk contains 70 g of carbohydrates per liter, the same carbohydrate content as infant formula. Formula's fat content is about 10 g/L lower than human milk, but this difference in fat content makes it likely that babies fed human milk have less blood-sugar variability than babies fed formula.

CALCULATING VOLUME OF MILK CONSUMED DURING NURSING   When nursing directly, the ABM protocol provides different ways to calculate milk intake during nursing.

- Test weights, using baby scales accurate to 2 g (available for rent in some areas) provides an accurate measure. Weigh the baby before and after every nursing session around the clock for several days for an accurate idea of baby's milk intake per feed and per day.
- Use average milk intake per day. For nursing babies older than 1 month this is about 25 oz. (750 mL) and average milk intake per feed is about 3 to 4 ounces (89 to 118 mL).

The ABM protocol suggests that when babies use a "small volume frequent feed" style of nursing that parents measure baby's blood sugar every 3 hours and give insulin doses as needed to correct high blood sugar. Another way to check milk intake at a feed over time is to ask to do before- and after-feed weights at regular health checkups.

DOWN SYNDROME is a genetic birth defect caused by the presence of an extra chromosome that causes developmental delays and other characteristics, such as low muscle tone (hypotonia). Babies with Down syndrome have a greater incidence of respiratory tract infections and heart and bowel problems.

Rates of nursing among babies with Down syndrome vary from country to country, with babies in some countries nursing at the same rate as other babies. Not so in other countries. Health outcomes are better with exclusive human-milk feeding.

When a baby is born with Down syndrome, the skin-to-skin contact enhances neurodevelopment. The physical contact and hormones released during nursing also promote emotional attachment while the family adjusts to the birth of a special-needs baby. The nursing parent's responsiveness to the baby's cues are the same skills families need to help the baby best realize her potential as she grows.

Not all newborns with Down syndrome have difficulty nursing. But low muscle tone and health problems can contribute to early nursing challenges. A baby with low muscle tone may have trouble cupping her tongue during nursing. If baby's tongue stays flat, milk slides to the sides of the mouth rather than being swallowed. Suggest families allow extra time for feedings during the early weeks.

Admission to the special-care nursery also affects nursing outcomes. If the nursing couple is separated after birth when baby is in special care, discuss effective milk-expression strategies (p. 214).

If a baby with Down syndrome can feed by mouth, health outcomes are better when she is fed expressed milk. If the baby is tube-fed, she can begin to nurse even before transitioning off the tube.

When the baby begins latching, suggest thinking of early nursing as practice sessions and focus on enjoying their time together. Expect that it may take time for baby to catch on.

If the baby is sleepy most of the time, suggest keeping her on the parent's body as much as possible to trigger innate feeding behaviors. Help the baby latch when she goes into light sleep (squirming, eyes moving under eyelids, any body movements). Keep the baby skin-to-skin as much as possible, so parents can feel from the baby's movements and changes in breathing when she is ready to feed.

Low muscle tone can leave a baby's airway unprotected during swallowing, which causes the gasping and coughing common among babies with Down syndrome. If this happens, nursing may go more smoothly when the baby feeds in positions with her head higher than the nipple (p. 6). A low-tone, protruding tongue may make latching more challenging.

If despite the nursing parent's efforts, the baby does not nurse effectively or often enough, supplements may be needed, as gaining weight means gaining strength, too. A baby who gains weight slowly despite good milk intake needs to be checked for a health problem, such as a heart defect.

GALACTOSEMIA AND PKU are metabolic disorders that affect babies' ability to break down certain components of human milk. Exclusive nursing is impossible for many babies born with these disorders, but partial nursing is possible for many. Because these milk components are not broken down, they accumulate in the baby's body, which can cause serious health problems and eventually become life-threatening.

False positives are common with tests used to screen newborns for galactosemia and PKU, especially during the summer when blood samples are not always kept cool, which affects the results. If a baby's test results are positive, first ask the baby's healthcare provider to evaluate the baby for symptoms of the disorder and arrange for a second blood test as soon as possible. Sometimes several retests are needed. By being proactive with the healthcare provider and the testing facility, a family may get the second test results faster. One way might be to ask the baby's healthcare provider to call the testing facility and request special handling of the test. Overnight delivery is an option, or if the family is within driving distance of the facility, they may be able to arrange for someone trustworthy to drive the baby's blood sample there.

After evaluating the baby's health, the healthcare provider can advise the family on whether to begin feeding the baby a lactose-free or phenylalanine-free formula until the second test results are received.

If nursing is interrupted, suggest expressing milk to stay comfortable and safeguard the milk production until the final results are available.

GALACTOSEMIA is a rare, inherited metabolic disorder in which the liver does not produce the enzyme that metabolizes galactose (a byproduct of the milk sugar lactose), causing it to accumulate in the baby's system.

Classic Galactosemia   Too much galactose usually becomes apparent on about the third day of life as jaundice, an enlarged liver, vomiting, and lethargy. If treatment is not begun soon, it can progress to failure-to-thrive, liver and kidney damage, convulsions, and mental retardation. Human milk is high in lactose, so with classic galactosemia, nursing is contraindicated and the baby must be fed a lactose-free formula. If classic galactosemia is diagnosed, provide strategies for reducing milk production gradually.

Duarte Galactosemia is one of more than 100 mutations of this disorder in which the baby may produce varying levels of the liver enzyme needed to break down galactose. The baby who is a carrier of Duarte galactosemia may produce 75% of the needed enzyme, while babies with Duarte galactosemia may produce between 25% and 50%. A blood test can determine the baby's enzyme level. Some of these babies can partially or exclusively nurse. The range of treatment options is broad, from complete removal of human milk from the baby's diet to partial nursing to full nursing.

PKU (phenylketonuria) is a rare metabolic disorder in which the baby lacks the liver enzyme needed to break down the essential amino acid phenylalanine, an ingredient of both human milk and most infant formulas. If untreated, this amino acid accumulates in the blood, causing brain damage. Treatment consists of a lifelong diet of low-phenylalanine foods. But even when the special diet is maintained, those with PKU may still have cognitive impairment.

Continued partial nursing is an option because the baby with PKU needs some phenylalanine for normal growth. Nursing the baby with PKU has advantages. Nursing babies with PKU have better health outcomes than those exclusively formula-fed. Human milk is lower in phenylalanine than regular formula, so parents need less expensive phenylalanine-free formula. Human milk also improves cognitive development, which is vital to quality of life for these babies.

Through their entire lifespan, people with PKU must be carefully monitored to avoid unsafe phenylalanine blood levels. After diagnosis, nursing is usually interrupted for a few days to bring the baby's blood levels down to normal. During this time, the nursing parent can express milk to safeguard their milk production. After this, nursing can be combined with special formula in several ways.

- Alternate all-nursing with all-formula feeds, letting baby take as much of each as desired.
- At each feed, first give a predetermined volume of special formula (65% of the baby's 24-hour milk intake divided by number of feeds) and then nurse unrestrictedly.
- At each feed, give the baby first a predetermined volume of expressed milk, followed by as much special formula as the baby wants.
- Feed the baby a bottle of special formula every 3 hours and nurse as desired during the intervals between.
- Estimate the baby's total daily milk intake by age and calculate the volume of formula needed to maintain safe phenylalanine blood levels. Give the baby this volume of formula every 24 hours (however it is most convenient). Schedule biweekly blood tests to monitor baby's blood levels and make adjustments as needed.

NEUROLOGICAL IMPAIRMENT can occur with obvious and serious health issues, such as a brain bleed, abnormal brain structure, a birth defect or syndrome. A neurological impairment can compromise a baby's ability to feed effectively, learn, and stay alert.

If nursing does not come easily to the baby, think of it as a normal behavior to be encouraged, like walking and talking. Unless the baby has a degenerative neurological disorder, with patience and persistence, as baby grows and matures, she will become stronger and more coordinated, which makes nursing easier. Time spent learning to nurse helps improve a baby's neuro-muscular coordination. If the baby's neurological problem is so severe that it is impossible for her to nurse, expressed milk contains components missing in formula that may enhance her development.

Suggest nursing families seek out healthcare providers supportive of nursing and early intervention programs to prevent or minimize developmental delay.

Even when a neurological impairment affects a baby's ability to coordinate sucking, swallowing, and breathing, with practice and patience, many of these babies can learn to nurse, and some can learn to feed effectively. Babies bottle-fed have higher stress responses and lower oxygen levels than during nursing. The baby's ability to bottle-feed should not be used to determine when the baby can nurse.

In severe cases, if the baby needs to be tube-fed, expressed milk is the first choice. Even in babies who are tube-fed for months, feeding competence can improve with maturity and time spent nursing. Nursing can often begin even before tube-feeding ends.

HIGH AND LOW MUSCLE TONE Babies with a neurological impairment often have high or low muscle tone, which can contribute to feeding problems. Some babies have high muscle tone in their body and low muscle tone in their mouth, and vice versa. The next two sections describe strategies that can help babies achieve a "middle tone" during feeds that enhances both their feeling of well-being and their feeding effectiveness.

High Muscle Tone may cause baby to over-respond to sensory stimulation. Babies with high tone may arch their bodies, over-extend their heads, over-respond to stimulation, and bite or clench during nursing. They are often fussy during feeds.

Most high-tone babies nurse more effectively if feeds start before they are too hungry. The high-tone baby may have an unusually sensitive mouth, which can cause gagging during feeds. Use only those strategies that work well and discontinue any that don't or that the baby doesn't like:

- Before feeds, hold baby in the colic hold (Figure 8.3) or gently swing baby from head to foot in a blanket gathered up at the corners (blanket swing) until she relaxes and flexes.

- During feeds, avoid movement, such as rocking or swaying, and try a stable semi-reclined starter position (p. 6), with baby lying tummy down on the parent's body, or try nursing in a snug sling, swaddled, lying on a firm pillow, or side-lying on a firm surface.

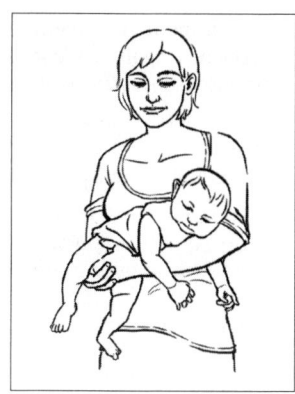

Figure 8.3 The colic hold
©2021 Nancy Mohrbacher Solutions, Inc.

- Use deep, firm touch rather than light touch.
- Keep lights and sound low.

If the baby gags easily during nursing, try a more "baby-driven" approach to positioning and latch so baby can take a more active role (p. 6).

Skin-to-skin contact helps calm and comfort some high-tone babies. If the baby is so ineffective at feeds that she is gaining too little weight, supplement as needed.

Low Muscle Tone may cause baby to under-respond to sensory stimulation, including feeding triggers, which can lead to ineffective nursing. Both high- and low-tone babies may have trouble coordinating sucking, swallowing, and breathing, and they may take very little milk, even after nursing for a long time. When a neurologically impaired baby with low oral muscle tone nurses, she may suck weakly and dribble milk out of the sides of her mouth. When not nursing, her mouth may stay open and her tongue protrude. Reflux disease is also common among these babies due to the low-tone sphincter muscle that is supposed to keep food in the stomach.

When trying the following strategies with a low-tone baby, use only those that work well and discontinue any that don't work or the baby doesn't like:

- Before feeds, increase muscle tone by sitting baby on the nursing parent's knee and bouncing gently or leaning her forward and backward in a non-rhythmic way. If milk was dribbling out of baby's mouth during feeds, try firmly patting her lips before nursing.

- Experiment with feeding positions, trying first the more upright versions of the starter positions (image on p. 7), which provide the full-body support low-tone babies need.

- Use a "baby-driven" approach to latching, by triggering baby's inborn feeding behaviors to stimulate a wide-open mouth and gravity to help maintain a stable position (p. 6).

- Experiment with the baby's head position. In neurologically normal babies, nursing with the head tilted slightly back makes swallowing and breathing easier. But some babies with a neurological impairment or anatomical abnormality find swallowing easier with their chin tucked slightly toward their chest. Use whichever head position works better for the baby.

- If upright or side-lying positions are used and the baby can't stay latched or uses unusually wide jaw movements, try the Dancer Hand position (p. 109) to support baby's jaw.

- If the baby's tongue movements are weak, apply gentle pressure with a fingertip under the baby's chin. Do this by gently pressing upward, with a fingertip on the soft tissue behind the baby's jawbone, with a steady, gentle traction toward the mammary gland.

More Nursing Strategies for Babies with High/Low Tone may be needed if a baby with a neurological impairment nurses ineffectively due to one or more of the following: unusual piston-like tongue movements, wide jaw excursions, low or non-existent vacuum, uncoordinated sucking due to breathing or swallowing problems, and/or other deviations from the norm. Even with adequate milk production, during nursing, the baby may take only 10% to 60% of the milk the parent can express.

Until the baby is exclusively nursing and gaining adequate weight, try a silicone nipple shield during feeds to see if that improves the baby's effectiveness. In some cases, the firmer nipple shield can push past the tensed tongue of the high-tone baby and the protruding tongue of the low-tone baby , providing the right stimulation for more effective sucking. For the low-tone baby, the firmer feel of the shield may trigger a stronger sensory response. If the baby's milk intake increases when the shield is used, the need to supplement may be reduced or eliminated. It also provides positive reinforcement for direct nursing. See p. 329 for shield application and fit.

With the shield in place, if the baby cannot get milk, try filling the tip of the shield with expressed milk (either by expressing milk into it or inserting milk with a curved-tip syringe). This gives baby milk during the first sucks, which may lead to more active sucking.

Until the baby can take full feeds with the shield, express milk to maintain milk production. If the shield does not improve baby's milk intake, discontinue using it.

Babies nurse best when milk flow is fast enough to keep them interested and active, but not so fast that it overwhelms them. The baby's specific issues will determine which milk flow is right for her. For example, a baby with breathing or swallowing problems (dysphagia) may be easily overwhelmed and do best with a very slow milk flow, whereas a baby with low tone who needs more sensory stimulation to stay active during feeds may feed better with a faster flow. Except for the times a baby needs a little squirt of milk to "jumpstart" sucking, ideally the baby should control the milk flow, either through her own efforts or the feeder should coordinate the milk delivered to the baby as she sucks. Unless a baby's efforts affect the milk flow, the feeding method will not promote more effective nursing.

For a baby who feeds better with a faster milk flow, try breast compression (p. 309) or a nursing supplementer, which uses a thin tube at the nipple to deliver the supplement during nursing. The baby's natural response to a swallow is to suck. Some babies learn a more effective sucking pattern when the steady milk flow from the tube stimulates more active and consistent sucking and swallowing. When a baby sucks more vigorously, she also takes more milk directly, stimulating more milk production.

Commercial nursing supplementers require suction, which means the baby must actively suck the milk through its thin tubing from the container. Makeshift nursing supplementers that do not require suction can be created using a periodontal syringe or a syringe attached by a port to thin tubing. These "suction not required" devices allow the feeder to push the milk to the baby while she is sucking. Depending on the baby's issue, one or the other may be a more effective tool. For more details, see p. 311.

A nursing supplementer may not improve a baby's nursing effectiveness if the baby learns to take the milk "like a straw" from the supplementer tube without sucking vigorously. In this case, it may help to make the end of the tube flush with the nipple, rather than extending it past the nipple, which is usually recommended. But if this doesn't help, the nursing supplementer may not be a useful tool. In some cases, the baby may do better if the nursing supplementer is used with a nipple shield to provide both a faster milk flow and a firmer feel. In some cases, a different strategy, such as finger-feeding may be more effective.

When creating a lactation plan, families should plan to spend no more than about 40 minutes on all things feeding-related, including nursing, expressing milk, and feeding a supplement. If they spend much more time than that, it becomes impossible to fit in the number of feeds per day baby needs.

If a baby is ineffective during nursing, most parents appreciate some guidance in structuring their day to maximize their milk production, while keeping the rest of their life manageable. How much time a baby spends nursing will depend on how effectively she takes milk. If she consumes little or no milk while nursing, nurse for "practice" whenever the baby seems interested and alert, rather than using a fixed schedule. Then the nursing parent can focus most of the "feeding time" on expressing milk and feeding the baby in other ways.

On the other hand, if the baby takes most milk while directly nursing, make time spent nursing the priority. In this case, spend less time on milk expression and more time on maximizing the baby's effectiveness during nursing. In these cases, use of a nipple shield and/or a nursing supplementer may increase milk taken during direct nursing, which reduces the need to supplement after feeds.

As the baby's nursing improves, it's time to gradually reduce supplements. If a nursing supplementer is used, the flow can be slowed by lowering the level of the container, the tube can be kinked to stop flow for part of the nursing session, or the device can be used at gradually fewer feeds during the day. Usually, the first nursing in the morning (or whenever the nursing parent is fullest) is the first feed to stop supplementing.

If other feeding methods are used, less supplement can be given at each feed or supplements can be gradually given fewer and fewer times each day.

HOSPITALIZATION OF THE NURSING BABY

INFORMATION GATHERING involves asking the following:

- The baby's age
- How much she was nursing before the hospitalization (partial/exclusive?)
- The reason the baby was hospitalized
- Estimated length of baby's hospital stay
- How far the nursing parent lives from the hospital and the transportation options
- Any other responsibilities (employment/other children and their ages)

WHILE BABY IS HOSPITALIZED, ask what the baby's healthcare provider said about nursing and how much time each day the nursing parent can spend with the baby. Is the baby being fed by mouth? If not, discuss milk expression to safeguard milk production and stay comfortable. If the baby can take anything by mouth, mother's milk is the best first choice.

If the baby's healthcare provider recommends against nursing, suggest discussing their wishes. If a mutually acceptable solution can't be found, suggest a second opinion.

Help brainstorm ways to spend as much time as possible at the hospital (take sick or vacation time from work, arrange childcare for other children). If the hospital is far from home, ask if the baby can be transferred to a closer hospital after her condition is stabilized.

Is rooming-in an option? Nursing is easiest when parent and child can be together day and night and can nurse without restrictions, but circumstances (other children at home, job responsibilities) may interfere. Some hospitals encourage parents to stay with their children, but even if the hospital doesn't usually allow 24-hour rooming-in, they may if the family requests it. If the baby's healthcare provider is supportive, the family can ask for an order for unlimited access. Suggest getting all special orders in writing and have them on hand while at the hospital.

If the baby is not yet nursing or they cannot be together, ask about the family's feeding goals and help them plan ahead. When oral feeds begin, is the goal to provide exclusive human milk for the baby, even when they can't be with her? If so, discuss the practical details. Talk about a typical day and the times and places milk expression may be possible.

If the plan is for baby to be fed formula at missed feeds, be sure the family knows:

1. Depending on the level of milk production, some milk expression may be needed to stay comfortable and prevent mastitis.
2. If the baby was exclusively nursing and the goal is to resume this after the baby is discharged, to maintain milk production, plan to express milk as many times per day as the baby was nursing or if exclusively nursing, at least 6 or 7 times per day.

A temporary drop in milk production or a delay in milk ejection during stressful times is not unusual. But frequently nursing and/or expressing milk usually causes milk production to rebound.

The following suggestions may make baby's hospital stay easier.

Environment
- If the baby is in a semi-private room, request the bed farthest from the door for more privacy and less traffic.
- Look into the possibility of a private room.

The parent's comfort
- If a large part of each day is spent at the hospital, bring drinks and snacks or ask about receiving hospital meals.
- Bring extra pillows or cushions from home for added comfort.
- Wear comfortable shoes and clothes that make nursing easy.

Medical equipment and procedures
- If the baby is on an IV, ask for longer tubing for more freedom of movement while nursing.
- If the baby needs an oxygen tent, can the parent nurse inside it?
- If painful procedures must be done, can the baby nurse during the procedure? Alternatively, could topical anesthetics be used to numb the site and multiple procedures be done at once, rather than spreading them out over the course of the day?

Nursing is a potent pain-reliever, which helps speed baby's recovery. Better pain management improves health outcomes. When a baby undergoes a painful medical procedure, nursing is the most effective non-drug pain reducer. For a complete overview of pain-reducing options for preterm and term newborns and older babies, download ABM Clinical Protocol #23 at: **bfmed.org/protocols**.

A baby's usual nursing rhythms may change during illness or injury. Some babies want to nurse more often when very sick or injured. When illness makes a baby lethargic, they may have less interest in nursing. If a baby loses interest, express milk to stay comfortable and maintain milk production for when the baby is feeling better. A lethargic baby can be fed mother's milk by tube (gavage feeding).

COPING WITH SURGERY is stressful. The most stressful time for a nursing child may be the period before the surgery when all food and drink stops so that her stomach is empty during the procedure. This is known as "preoperative fasting" or being "NPO," which is meant to decrease the risk the child's stomach contents will enter her lungs (aspiration) during or after surgery.

The length of time recommended for preoperative fasting decreased over the decades, from "no food or drink after midnight" to much shorter periods, which vary by food, depending on how quickly that food leaves the stomach. In the ABM Clinical Protocol #25, these preoperative fasting times are listed for different foods:

- Light meal: 6 hours
- Non-human milks: 6 hours
- Infant formula: 6 hours
- Human milk: 4 hours,
- Clear liquids: 2 hours

Suggest the family talk to the baby's surgeon and anesthesiologist before the day of the surgery to reach an agreement on the fasting time. During those difficult hours before surgery, one possible option is to ask about pumping first and then nursing the baby for comfort up to 2 hours before the surgery.

After surgery, it may be possible to nurse in the recovery room. Ask the baby's healthcare provider about this option. Whenever the baby is ready to be fed by mouth, nursing should resume.

Discuss possible milk-expression strategies based on the baby's need for milk and how long nursing will be restricted.

DIGITAL RESOURCES

bfmed.org/protocols—Download the Academy of Breastfeeding Medicine Clinical Protocols:

- #11 Neonatal ankyloglossia
- #16 Breastfeeding the hypotonic infant
- #17 Guidelines for breastfeeding infants with cleft lip or palate
- #23 Non-pharmacologic management of procedure-related pain in the breastfeeding infant
- #24 Allergic proctocolitis in the exclusively breastfed infant
- #25 Preprocedural fasting for the breastfeeding infant
- #27 Breastfeeding an infant or young child with insulin-dependent diabetes

CHAPTER 9   HEALTH ISSUES: NURSING PARENT

NURSING WITH HEALTH ISSUES

Despite common myths, lactation is not physically draining for nursing parents. Nursing relieves stress, enhances sleep, metabolism, and the immune system, and in many cases, provides a greater sense of control and normalcy during a difficult time.

When nursing parents are ill, those supporting them may look for ways to reduce their stress and workload and suggest weaning. But if a parent wants to continue nursing through an illness, this may aid in their recovery. Follow the parent's lead.

Ways to make nursing easier during an illness include bringing the young baby into bed while resting and nursing in starter or side-lying positions. If the nursing child is older and more active, parents may be able to keep them contained by closing the door and having toys available during rest periods. If the parent has a disability, see p. 162.

In nearly all cases, continuing to nurse is better for baby. If nursing parents are contagious, using good personal hygiene, including regular handwashing, can decrease the baby's chances of catching the illness. Parents can also try to avoid breathing on the baby by limiting face-to-face contact. In cases of a highly contagious or serious illness, wearing a face mask when holding the baby can help prevent transmission. Fever can reduce body fluids, which increases the chances of becoming constipated and dehydrated. When parents are feverish, encourage them to drink plenty of fluids.

BACTERIAL ILLNESSES

FOOD POISONING occurs after consuming a food or drink contaminated with specific bacteria or toxins, such as botulism, listeriosis, salmonella, and *E. coli*. Symptoms include vomiting, abdominal cramps, and diarrhea. Recovery usually occurs within a few days.

Lactation issues: If nursing parents are vomiting and have diarrhea, suggest drinking plenty of fluids to avoid dehydration. Depending on the bacterium involved, if the food poisoning is severe enough to require antibiotics, precautions to prevent airborne or skin-contact transmission between parent and baby, such as handwashing and wearing a face mask while nursing, may be needed.

Medication issues.   If food poisoning is so severe that antibiotics are prescribed, check their compatibility with lactation.

GROUP B STREPTOCOCCUS (GBS) is a major cause of serious infection in newborns and their parents. Up to 40% of pregnant U.S. parents are colonized with GBS. Without treatment, 1% to 2% of their newborns become ill. Nearly 90% of newborns ill with GBS develop symptoms within the first 6 days after birth, which may become pneumonia, meningitis, and sepsis.

Lactation issues: It is rare for GBS to be found in human milk and when it is, it's unrelated to the nursing parent's GBS status. Transmission of GBS via milk is only of concern in very preterm or compromised babies. The GBS organism can be passed between parent and baby, especially when the baby becomes colonized. In this case, both need treatment at the same time. If the milk cultures positive for GBS and the baby is ill or preterm, the milk can be pasteurized (heat it to 62.5° [145° F] for 30 minutes) or discarded until the milk cultures are clear.

Medication issues: In the U.S., GBS is treated during labor with IV antibiotics that are also used to treat babies, which makes them compatible with lactation.

LYME DISEASE is transmitted by the bite of an infected tick. Most human cases occur in late spring and summer, when people spend more time outdoors. Symptoms start with a painless circular rash at the tick-bite site, which expands in size, reaching up to 12 inches (30 cm) in diameter. Symptoms may include fever, headache, chills, muscle and joint pain, and swollen lymph glands.

Lactation issues: None, as the Lyme spirochete can be transmitted to an unborn baby in utero but there are no reports of Lyme disease being spread through human milk.

Medication issues: None. The antibiotics used to treat Lyme disease are compatible with lactation.

METHICILLIN-RESISTANT STAPHYLOCOCCUS AUREUS (MRSA) refers to a virulent strain of the bacterium staph aureus that does not respond to the usual treatments. Once found rarely and only in hospitals, it is now common in communities in some areas. MRSA is spread mostly by direct contact and can be harbored in the nose and throat. It begins as a skin infection that may look like a spider bite, boil, or abscess. It is usually swollen, red, and painful and can progress to a fever, shortness of breath, cough, and chills.

Lactation issues: None. If a parent has MRSA, the baby was already exposed before symptoms appear, so there is no reason to stop nursing. If the parent has an open sore that the baby could touch during nursing, completely cover it with a clean, dry bandage. If it can't be fully covered during nursing, nurse the baby on the unaffected side, and express milk from the affected side. If the baby is ill or preterm, the milk can be cultured, and if MRSA is found, it can be killed by pasteurizing the milk (heat it to 62.5° C [145° F] for 30 minutes) before feeding. If heat treatment is not an option, expressed milk for compromised babies may be discarded until it is clear, within 48 hours of starting treatment.

Medication issues: None. The same antibiotics used to treat babies with MRSA are also used to treat parents, making them compatible with lactation.

TUBERCULOSIS (TB) is caused by a bacterium that is transmitted via droplets in the air from coughing. TB usually attacks the lungs but can also spread to other parts of the body. Symptoms include weight loss, fever, cough, night sweats, and chills.

Lactation issues: Parents contagious with active pulmonary TB are separated from their babies, no matter how they are fed, at least until parent and baby are started on drug therapy. Initiation of prophylactic treatment of the baby is effective in preventing TB infection, so continued separation is unnecessary after therapy is started in both parent and child. After birth, if treatment of the nursing couple is delayed or healthcare providers recommend separation, parents can use a pump to establish milk production (p. 214). If an active case of TB develops during pregnancy and the parent receives appropriate drug therapy, separation after birth is unlikely and nursing is encouraged.

Medication issues: TB requires long-term drug therapy. Many anti-tubercular drugs—such as isoniazid, rifampin, and ethambutol—are compatible with lactation.

VIRAL INFECTIONS

COLDS AND MILD INFECTIONS Before parents notice the symptoms of these illnesses, they are already contagious. Their body begins producing antibodies specific to that illness that pass into the milk to protect the nursing baby. Continued nursing is the baby's best protection from the illness, but if he does catch it, the antibodies he receives usually make his illness less severe.

Lactation issues: None

Medication issues: There are some reports of reduced milk production in those who take decongestants or antihistamines for relief of congestion.

COVID-19 AND SEASONAL INFLUENZA Nursing parents with an active case of COVID-19 or the seasonal flu can continue nursing but should take precautions to avoid transmitting these viruses to their baby. Getting the flu is a problem for babies younger than 6 months because there is a risk of severe complications. Precautions include avoiding touching their eyes and mouth and contact with sick people, as well as frequent handwashing before touching the baby, using clean blankets and burp cloths at each feed, and wearing a face mask while nursing. Cleaning and disinfecting the living area often is also recommended. If the nursing couple is separated, when recommended hygiene practices are followed, feed any expressed milk to the baby.

For parents giving birth with an active case of the flu or COVID-19, the nursing couple may be separated until 24 hours after the parent's fever is gone. In this situation, express milk and a healthy caregiver can feed it to the newborn.

Lactation issues: None.

Medication issues: None. According to the U.S. CDC, the antiviral medications used to treat the flu are compatible with lactation.

HEPATITIS A is an acute illness in which the liver becomes tender and swollen and bilirubin accumulates in the bloodstream causing jaundice (yellowish skin). Fever and nausea are also common. Hepatitis A can be transmitted by contact with infected blood or feces. In most people, it resolves completely without long-term damage. Contracting hepatitis A confers lifelong immunity to it.

Lactation issues: Nursing can continue in parents who contract hepatitis A. If the baby is a newborn when the parent contracts it, suggest arranging for the baby to receive the hepatitis A vaccine, immune globulin, or both.

Medication issues: None. Symptoms may be treated with fever-reducers or pain medications.

HEPATITIS B symptoms are similar to hepatitis A, but in up to 10% of cases, hepatitis B becomes a chronic illness. It is spread when body fluids (saliva, mucus, blood, etc.) containing the virus come into contact with broken skin, as well as by contaminated food and sexual contact.

Lactation issues: During birth, the newborn is exposed to hepatitis B through contact with body fluids. Nursing is not affected if the baby receives the first dose of the hepatitis B vaccine and the hepatitis B immune globulin within 12 hours after birth. If nursing parents contract hepatitis B after birth, the same course of action is advised. The baby (and other family members) should be vaccinated and nursing continue.

Medication issues: Treatment with some antiviral medications, such as telbivudine, are compatible with lactation.

But other antiviral medications (entecavir, tenofovir, and lamivudine.) are either potentially hazardous (L4) or contraindicated (L5).

HEPATITIS C may start as a mild infection, or there may be no symptoms, but it becomes a chronic liver infection in up to 85% of those who contract it. Hepatitis C is transmitted through sexual contact and infected blood. It occurs most often after blood transfusions or an accidental needle stick in healthcare settings, in drug users sharing needles, those with many sexual partners, and babies infected before or during birth. Only about 6% of babies born to hepatitis C-positive parents acquire the virus during pregnancy or birth. It is not transmitted by nursing.

Lactation issues: Nursing is not contraindicated during hepatitis C. But because it is transmitted via blood, controversy exists about whether infected nursing parents with bleeding nipples should interrupt nursing until their nipples heal. There are no documented cases of a baby contracting hepatitis C this way. The rare exception is the nursing parent who becomes infected with hepatitis C after birth and has acute symptoms while nursing but before their levels of antibodies are high enough to provide protection to the baby. In this situation, suggest parents talk to their healthcare provider about their options in light of their unique situation.

Medication issues: The antiviral regimens used to cure hepatitis C are usually taken for at least 8 weeks and are targeted to specific genotypes of the virus. Many of these drugs are relatively new. Some, such as ledipasvir, sofosbuvir, and simeprevir, are rated as L3 drugs, meaning they are considered compatible with nursing even with little research available. Others are not yet rated in reliable resources.

HEPATITIS D, E, and G are much less common types of hepatitis. Hepatitis D may cause acute or chronic infection only in those who are already infected with hepatitis B and is most common in South America, west Africa, Russia, Pacific islands, central Asia, and the Mediterranean region. Hepatitis E is transmitted primarily via contaminated food and water, is usually short-term and self-limiting, but has a high mortality rate when contracted during pregnancy. Hepatitis G is associated with blood transfusions.

Lactation issues: Because hepatitis D occurs only with hepatitis B infections, protecting baby from contracting hepatitis B by giving him the hepatitis-B vaccine and immune globulin also provides protection from hepatitis D, making the risk from nursing negligible. There is no evidence of transmission of hepatitis E or G through human milk.

Medication issues: Not applicable.

HERPES VIRUS: CHICKENPOX is a highly contagious illness common in childhood that is caused by the same herpes varicella-zoster virus that later in life causes shingles. Chickenpox can cause lifelong health problems if the infection occurs in an unborn baby, in a very preterm baby, or during the first 10 days after birth. After this vulnerable period, its symptoms are usually more severe in adults than in children. It is spread by contact with the sores or by inhaling droplets in the air. Infected people are contagious for about 7 days, beginning about 2 days before the lesions appear. It is no longer contagious when there are no new eruptions for 72 hours and all lesions are crusted.

If parents exposed to chickenpox during pregnancy are uncertain if they had it as a child (which confers lifelong immunity), a blood test can determine their immune status. If they are exposed and not immune, suggest they get the varicella vaccine. If they contract chickenpox between 5 days before birth and 10 days after birth and the baby is born without the disease, special precautions are needed. Up to 50% of newborns in this situation catch chickenpox, and if infected during their first 10 days, the mortality rate is up to 30%. After birth, to reduce the risk to the newborn, he needs to get the high-titer varicella immune globulin (VZIG) and the nursing couple should be kept together but isolated from other patients. If siblings at home are infected, parents can keep them away from the baby to minimize transmission risk. If nursing parents are immune, the baby received antibodies to chickenpox in utero, and the risk of the newborn catching it is greatly reduced.

Lactation issues: None.

Medication issues: None. Symptoms may be treated with fever-reducers or pain medications.

HERPES VIRUS: COLD SORES AND GENITAL HERPES are caused by herpes simplex virus 1 (cold sores) and 2 (genital herpes), which are spread by contact with the sores. These sores are small, painful, fluid-filled, red-rimmed blisters that dry after a few days and form a scab. Genital herpes sores can be spread to the mammary gland by touching the sores and then touching the gland. Herpes infections are very dangerous, even fatal, to a newborn up to 3 weeks old, although with quick hospitalization and quality care, a few newborns survived and went on to nurse after discharge.

Lactation issues: During pregnancy, suggest parents with recurrent herpes sores talk to a healthcare provider about precautions to take. If a sore on the nipple or mammary gland is suspected of being herpes, have it cultured. If herpes sores appear on the nipple or gland after birth, nursing can continue if the sores can be completely covered to prevent the baby from touching them. If the sores are on the nipple, areola, or anywhere else the baby might touch while nursing, express milk from that side until the sores heal, while continuing to nurse on the unaffected side. During hand expression or pumping, if the parent's hand or breast-pump parts touch the sores, the milk should be discarded. If the parent's hand (if hand-expressing) or pump parts do not touch the sores, the baby may be fed the milk. Although an older baby is not likely to develop life-threatening complications from herpes, if herpes sores appear after the newborn period, suggest parents take steps to avoid spreading it to a child, as the sores can be very painful and may make eating and drinking difficult.

Medication issues: Antiviral drugs compatible with nursing, such as acyclovir (L2), famciclovir (L2), and valacyclovir (L1), can be used to treat these herpes viruses in parents and children.

HERPES VIRUS: CYTOMEGALOVIRUS (CMV) is the most widespread herpes virus that infects humans. By 40 years of age, up to 80% of U.S. adults are infected with CMV for life. Few who become infected experience symptoms, which may include fatigue, fever, and swollen lymph glands. If the initial CMV infection occurs before pregnancy, the CMV virus is in parents' urine, tears, saliva, and milk, and during pregnancy, the baby is exposed in utero to both the virus and its antibodies. In healthy term babies, the parent's milk acts like a vaccine, with more than two-thirds of term babies born to CMV-positive parents testing positive, despite having no symptoms. But if the initial CMV infection occurs during pregnancy, about half of babies are born infected (congenital CMV), with 10% with symptoms, such as hearing loss, developmental delays, and other problems.

Lactation issues: Concerns about CMV and lactation only pertain to the compromised or very preterm baby. If at birth both parent and baby are CMV-negative or CMV-positive, there is no concern about nursing or feeding expressed milk. But when a baby born before 32 weeks and with a birth weight less than 1500 g (3 lbs. 5 oz.), is CMV-negative and his nursing parent is CMV-positive, there is a small risk the baby could become seriously ill from exposure to the CMV virus in the milk. Being born CMV-negative means the baby did not receive antibodies to the virus in utero. Plus, an immature or compromised immune system makes a baby more vulnerable to infections of all kinds. Expressed milk can be pasteurized to eliminate the risk of CMV transmission (p. 263) or frozen to reduce the virus.

Medication issues: None.

HERPES VIRUS: SHINGLES is caused by the same varicella zoster virus responsible for chickenpox. It occurs most often in an adult who had a mild case of chickenpox as a child and didn't become completely immune to the virus, which lays dormant until it is reactivated later in life. Several days before the shingles rash erupts, the infected person may notice burning pain and sensitive skin. The rash starts as small blisters on a red base that continue to form for 3 to 5 days. They often appear in a band- or belt-like pattern on an area of skin and can be very painful. The blisters will pop, ooze, crust over, and heal. A person with shingles can transmit chickenpox to someone who never had it or was never vaccinated against it. It is contagious when the rash appears and until it is crusted over. The shingles episode may last 3 to 4 weeks in total.

Lactation issues: If parents contract shingles while nursing, suggest the baby receive the varicella zoster immune globulin as soon as possible, as it is most effective when given soon after exposure. To prevent spreading it to others, parents can cover their rash, avoid touching or scratching it, wash their hands often, and avoid contact with vulnerable people, including preterm babies.

Medication issues: Antiviral drugs may be given. See "Cold Sores and Genital Herpes" about specific antiviral drugs and their compatibility with lactation.

HIV (human immunodeficiency virus) can lead to Acquired Immune Deficiency Syndrome (AIDS), which destroys parts of the immune system, leaving those affected unable to fight off illness. HIV is transmitted by the exchange of body fluids from parent to child during pregnancy and birth, from sexual contact, sharing needles, and blood transfusions. HIV can also be transmitted by nursing. Major advances in treating HIV improved survival rates and made nursing much safer.

Lactation issues: Before modern treatments were available, 18 months of nursing led to an HIV mother-to-child transmission (MTCT) rate of 14%. But the combined use of antiretroviral therapy (ART) significantly reduced MTCT from 18 months of nursing to 1% or less. Due to wide availability of ART, HIV is no longer a death sentence. Current recommendations on nursing with HIV in developing countries (where risk of death from infection is high) are for HIV-positive birthing parents to receive ART and exclusively nurse for 6 months and continue nursing for 1 to 2 years. In developed countries (where risk of death from infection is low), health organizations recommend HIV-positive birthing parents exclusively formula feed. Mixed feeding increases risk of MTCT of HIV. If HIV-positive parents in developed countries who are on effective ART with undetectable viral loads nurse their babies, it is recommended they consult a pediatric HIV specialist on best practices for minimizing risk. Minimizing risk means in part taking ART drugs as directed, nursing exclusively, and following best lactation practices to prevent nipple trauma and mastitis.

Medication issues: None. ART drugs are compatible with lactation and many are also given directly to nursing babies and children to prevent HIV infection.

HTLV-1 (human T-cell leukemia virus type 1) is spread through contact with body fluids from blood transfusions, through sexual contact, from parent to child during pregnancy and birth, and through nursing. It is rare in the U.S. and Europe, with most cases in the Caribbean, Africa, South America, and southwestern Japan. When HTLV-1 infections occur during infancy, 1% to 5% of those infected develop in adulthood adult leukemia, a malignant and usually fatal disease.

Lactation issues: As with HIV, in developed countries, when birthing parents are diagnosed with HTLV-1, some recommend against nursing. But in developing countries where death from infection is high, nursing is a better option. Because the risk of adult-onset leukemia from HTLV-1 infection is relatively small (1% to 5% of those infected), each carrier parent should discuss the risks with the baby's healthcare provider in light of their specific situation. Another option is to avoid any risk of transmission by freezing expressed milk to -20 degrees C (-4° F) and then thawing it, which greatly reduces the HTLV-1 virus in the milk.

Medication issues: None. Symptoms appear long after lactation.

MEASLES is spread by contact with infectious droplets or in the air. During the first 3 to 4 days, symptoms include fever, watery eyes, congestion, and cough. At about the fourth day, the rash appears. Measles is no longer contagious about 72 hours later, when the rash and cold symptoms are gone. If a baby is infected in utero (congenital measles), this can be serious and even fatal. If parents exposed to measles during pregnancy are unsure of their immune status, suggest asking for a blood test. If the baby contracts measles more than 2 weeks after birth, the illness will likely be mild. If siblings at home are infected and the parent is immune, the parents can keep them away from the baby to avoid contact. If the nursing parent catches measles after the newborn period, the baby can be given the measles immune globulin. If the parent is immune to measles, the baby will receive antibodies in utero, and the risk of the newborn catching measles from his siblings is greatly reduced.

Lactation issues: If at birth the exposed parent and baby have no symptoms, give both the measles immune globulin, and they can begin nursing. Although rare, if parents give birth with acute measles and the baby is born uninfected, they may be separated. If so, until the parent is no longer contagious, the baby can be fed expressed milk, which contains protective antibodies that help prevent this illness or lessen its severity. Even with separation, about half of newborns will become infected with disease.

Medication issues: None. Symptoms may be treated.

RUBELLA, also known as German measles, is a mild infectious disease. The biggest risk of rubella is catching it during pregnancy (congenital rubella), when it can damage the unborn baby. At any other time, it is likely to be short-lived and without complications. Symptoms include a generalized rash, swollen lymph glands, and a slight fever. Up to 50% of cases are asymptomatic.

Lactation issues: None. The nursing baby of a parent with active rubella was already exposed to it before the symptoms appeared. Nursing provides the baby with antibodies, so if he does become ill, he will likely have a milder case. If nursing parents previously had rubella or received the rubella vaccine, their milk may provide the baby with a partial immunity to rubella.

Medication issues: None. Symptoms may be treated.

WEST NILE VIRUS, which can become a serious illness, is most often transmitted by an infected mosquito, making it most common during summer and fall. It can also be spread by blood transfusions, transplants, and from parent to child during pregnancy. Symptoms include fever, headache, and neck stiffness. If severe, it can lead to disorientation, coma, tremors, and paralysis.

Lactation issues: West Nile virus was found in the milk of infected parents, but no nursing babies became ill.

Medication issues: None. Symptoms may be treated.

ZIKA is transmitted by the bite of an infected mosquito and if contracted during pregnancy, is known to cause birth defects, such as microcephaly. A zika infection is often asymptomatic, but when symptoms occur, such as fever and rash, they are mild.

Lactation issues: Much like other viruses, the Zika virus can be found in the milk of infected parents and in the blood of their nursing babies. However, this exposure does not result in infection. The World Health Organization recommends nursing for parents infected with the Zika virus and for those who live in areas where the virus is endemic. Holder pasteurization of expressed milk (heating milk to 62.5° C [145° F] for 30 minutes) deactivates the Zika virus, as does refrigerating the expressed milk at 4° C (39° F) for 2 to 3 days, during which the antiviral properties of human milk deactivate the virus.

Medication issues: None. Symptoms may be treated.

CANCER

All forms of cancer start with out-of-control growth of abnormal cells. Instead of eventually dying, like normal cells, cancer cells continue to grow and form new, abnormal cells. Cancer cells may invade other tissues, which normal cells cannot do. If found and treated early, many cancers can be completely cured. As the cancerous cells spread from the original tumor through the body, the chances for a cure decrease.

DIAGNOSTIC TESTS AND CANCER SURGERY For details on diagnostic tests and biopsy for breast cancer, see p. 38. Before having surgery, discuss nursing with the surgeon and ask that medications be chosen that are most compatible with lactation.

RADIOACTIVE TESTS AND TREATMENTS If radioactive materials are used to diagnose or treat cancer, ask what specific materials will be used. Some radioactive materials accumulate in human milk, and temporary or permanent weaning is necessary. After some tests or treatments, nursing (or even holding the baby) may expose him to radioactivity. The specific substance, its form, and the dose will determine whether nursing can continue, if weaning is necessary, whether the weaning will be permanent or temporary, and if temporary, its duration and when the baby can resume nursing.

For a listing of radioactive substances and recommended length of weaning after use in diagnosis or treatment, see Clinical Protocol #31 from the Academy of Breastfeeding Medicine (ABM) at **bfmed.org/protocols**.

Radioactive Iodine ^{131}I Some substances can be used for diagnostic tests without interrupting nursing, but when radioactive iodine ^{131}I is used for a thyroid scan or tumor imaging, weaning is necessary due to potentially harmful effects on both parent and baby. According to the ABM Clinical Protocol #31, when this substance is used, at the very least, several months of weaning is required. After procedures with this substance, even holding or sleeping close to the baby is risky, because it exposes him to radiation. Nursing parents need to completely wean at least several weeks before the treatment because about 40% of the radiation dose will be deposited in active mammary tissue, putting parents at higher risk for later breast cancer. Weaning several weeks in advance gives parents' mammary tissue time to involute, so it is no longer active during the treatment. After this treatment, it may take months before the radioactivity in the milk drops to safe levels.

Questions to Ask If Radioactive Materials Are Recommended
If parents do not want to wean, suggest sharing this with the provider, ask if other options are available, and ask the following questions:

- Is the radioactive procedure for diagnosis or treatment?
- What will happen if the procedure is not done or if it is postponed?
- Is there an alternative that does not involve weaning?
- If the baby is younger than 12 months, can the procedure be delayed until they can express enough milk for the baby during the temporary weaning?
- Was a radioactive material chosen that will clear the milk in the shortest time possible?
- Is there a local testing facility available to determine when the milk is clear of radioactivity?
- Will the radioactive material be concentrated in one organ (i.e., the thyroid), and if so, will parents need to keep their baby away from that part of their body for a time?

If parents are not satisfied with the healthcare provider's answers, suggest seeking a second opinion.

MILK EXPRESSION AFTER RADIOACTIVE PROCEDURES
After radioactive testing and temporary weaning, parents can maintain milk production by pumping (p. 215). Unlike medications, milk expression eliminates the radioactivity from the body more quickly.

CHEMOTHERAPY used to treat cancer was once considered incompatible with lactation. But chemotherapy has evolved, and more information is available on using these drugs during lactation, allowing for a more nuanced approach. For example, continued nursing may be possible for some nursing parents receiving low-dose chemotherapy. If the chemotherapy is given for short periods with longer periods in between, some may wean temporarily and go back to nursing after the drugs are eliminated from the body. This may be an option with drugs with shorter half-lives but not with more toxic drugs with longer half-lives.

RADIATION THERAPY Like diagnostic x-rays, cancer radiation therapy does ***not*** make human milk radioactive, and nursing can continue. During treatment for breast cancer, the unradiated mammary gland will not be affected. But radiation damages mammary tissue, which may destroy tissue and reduce milk production during treatment and with subsequent pregnancies and lactations.

DECISIONS ABOUT NURSING Healthcare providers often advise breast cancer patients to wean, even when no contraindication exists. If nursing parents diagnosed with cancer do not want to wean or feel that weaning would not make life easier, suggest discussing this with their provider.

Common lactation worries of parents who survived breast cancer are:

- Nursing will cause a recurrence (no evidence supports this).
- Because lactation makes mammary tissue denser, a recurrence might be more difficult to detect.
- If surgery decreased sensation of the areola and nipple, this may inhibit milk ejection.
- Low milk production from previous radiation may reduce baby's ability to latch and suck well.

These parents may need extra lactation help and support while establishing nursing.

Cancer diagnosis during pregnancy may or may not affect lactation outcomes. When chemotherapy is not required, nursing outcomes are not affected. But when chemotherapy is used during pregnancy, this may negatively affect lactation outcomes.

CARDIAC ISSUES/HYPERTENSION

The impact of lactation on cardiovascular health, both short- and long-term, is positive. Nursing also reduces risk of stroke and improves health outcomes in parents with active cardiovascular disease.

Lactation issues: None

Medication issues: Some low-dose diuretics used to treat hypertension by increasing the volume of urine and keeping fluid levels low, are compatible with lactation. But high-dose diuretics may decrease milk production. Other cardiac drugs, such as beta-blockers, are compatible with lactation.

DEPRESSION, ANXIETY, AND MENTAL HEALTH

POSTPARTUM DEPRESSION More than half of new parents have occasional bouts of crying, irritability, and fatigue referred to as the ***baby blues***. Postpartum depression refers to more consistent and severe symptoms. During the first year of new parenthood, the incidence is 12% to 25% overall and 35% to 60% among high-risk parents, including those who experience racial and economic discrimination.

Depressive symptoms include feelings of sadness, an absence of pleasure from activities once enjoyed, sleep problems unrelated to baby care, inability to focus, feelings of hopelessness, changes in appetite, anxiety, and greater anger or hostility, including thoughts of death. Before considering treatment for depression, parents should see a healthcare provider to rule out physical causes, such as thyroid problems and anemia. Symptoms considered **red flags that parents need immediate medical attention** include suicidal or bizarre statements, substance abuse, days without sleep, fast weight loss, lack of normal grooming, and inability to get out of bed.

CAUSES AND RISK FACTORS FOR POSTPARTUM DEPRESSIVE SYMPTOMS Inflammation is the risk factor that underlies the others. When other risk factors are present—sleep disturbance, stress (a fussy baby, a household move away from family and friends), physical pain, psychological trauma, or a history of trauma or abuse—these cause the immune system to release **proinflammatory cytokines**, cells that trigger physical inflammation and depressive symptoms. This can go both ways: parents with inflammation from other risk factors are at increased risk for depression, and depressed parents release more of these proinflammatory cells, causing more inflammation.

LACTATION AND POSTPARTUM DEPRESSION When going well, nursing is protective of mental health. Nursing lowers stress and increases sleep, which decreases the risk of depressive symptoms. Nursing decreases inflammation and increases feelings of well-being. While nursing parents have a lower risk of postpartum depressive symptoms, nursing is not a guarantee against depression. And if nursing problems develop, this can add to inflammation and depressive symptoms.

If nursing parents become depressed, they are at increased risk of nursing less often and weaning earlier. Higher anxiety levels at 3 months reduces the odds of exclusive nursing at 6 months. Depressed parents may interpret their baby's fussiness when hungry as a rejection of them or their milk rather than being due to a physical cause. Depressed parents may also be less sensitive to their babies' cues. They may see nursing as the cause of their problems. If so, explain that caring for a newborn can be stressful, and the challenges of a fussy baby, fatigue, and feeling overwhelmed are not confined to nursing parents.

WHY TREATING DEPRESSIVE SYMPTOMS MATTERS Depression and anxiety negatively affect parents' health, well-being, and their relationships. Parents' depressive symptoms also affect their baby physically, emotionally, and socially and can impair the way they interact with their baby. But never imply that their depression "damaged" their baby. Emphasize instead that when parents seek treatment, it benefits both them and their baby.

NON-PHARMACOLOGICAL TREATMENTS FOR POSTPARTUM DEPRESSION Depression should be treated rather than ignored, but many parents hesitate to seek treatment for fear they might have to choose between treatment and nursing. That's not usually the case. Most antidepressant medications are compatible with nursing. For parents reluctant to use medications, many non-drug strategies can effectively treat depression. Non-pharmacologic treatments include:

- **Long-chain omega-3 fatty acids** can be taken alone or with antidepressants. DHA and EPA, both anti-inflammatories, are safe during pregnancy and lactation. To treat depressive symptoms, take daily 1000 mg of EPA and 200-400 mg of DHA.
- **Exercise** also reduces inflammation and improves mood after childbirth. Exercise is as effective at resolving major depression as antidepressants. For moderate depression, suggest 20 to 30 minutes of exercise 2 to 3 times per week. For major depression, suggest 45 to 60 minutes of exercise 3 to 5 times per week.
- **Bright light therapy** alleviates up to 75% of depressive symptoms when professionally created light boxes are used. The time of day light therapy is used makes a difference, with light therapy early in the day more effective than light therapy later in the day.
- **Psychotherapy** also has an anti-inflammatory effect. Cognitive behavioral therapy is as effective as medications in treating depression, with a lower incidence of relapse.
- **St. John's Wort**, used to treat depression since the Middle Ages, is as effective as prescribed antidepressants, with fewer side effects. The recommended dose is 300 mg 3 times per day, standardized to 0.3% hypericin and/or 2% to 4% hyperforin.

ANTIDEPRESSANTS AND LACTATION Most antidepressant medications are compatible with lactation, but even after parents are told this, many still have concerns about addiction, side effects, and possible harm to their nursing baby. Suggest discussing concerns with their healthcare provider. When deciding which antidepressant to use, consider these factors.

- Have they used an antidepressant before that worked well for them?
- Do they find particular side effects especially concerning?
- Are they taking any other medications that might interact with the drug?

POSTPARTUM PSYCHOSIS is relatively rare (up to 0.2%, of birthing parents). It usually strikes during the first month after birth but can occur any time within the first year. When it does, parents and babies need immediate help because they are at risk of serious harm. Parents with postpartum psychosis have a distorted perception of reality, hallucinations, delusions, and/or suicidal or homicidal thoughts. Immediate treatment is needed.

HOSPITALIZATION is usually required when postpartum psychosis is diagnosed. In some countries, hospitals have units where parents being treated can care for their babies. Keeping the nursing couple together allows nursing to continue and can boost s parents' often-fragile self-esteem, while recognizing the baby's need for them as a nurturer. Suggest looking into this possibility.

Medication issues: Many of the antipsychotic medications used to treat postpartum psychosis are compatible with lactation.

IF WEANING IS NECESSARY due to parents' drug therapy being incompatible with lactation or when nursing ends for any reason, weaning carefully is an important part of any treatment plan for postpartum psychosis. The physical, hormonal, and emotional changes during weaning can affect parents' mental and emotional state. In rare cases, weaning may trigger a mental-health crisis. When weaning is necessary, discuss ways to wean gradually. If the baby must stop nursing abruptly, discuss milk-expression strategies that allow a gradual and comfortable reduction of milk production.

PAST SEXUAL ABUSE OR CHILDHOOD TRAUMA About 25% of women and 15% of men have a history of sexual abuse or assault that occurred within their families or by peers. These experiences can affect their birth, nursing, and early parenting. The more types of abuse and trauma children experience, the greater their long-term effects.

NURSING WITH A HISTORY OF SEXUAL ABUSE Some assume that abuse survivors will not want to nurse, but in some studies, significantly more abuse survivors intend to nurse and initiate nursing compared with others. But incidence of nursing problems, such as pain and mastitis, may be higher among abuse survivors and rates of exclusive nursing lower. Those with past trauma may find skin-to-skin contact challenging. Some hate the visceral sensation of their baby's mouth on their nipple. Some have post-traumatic flashbacks during birth and nursing. A common challenge is the increased risk of depressive symptoms, which puts nursing at risk. After the fact, some say they never learned to like nursing, but they learned to tolerate it, which they considered an important goal. For others, nursing was a positive and healing experience. There is a large range of possible reactions to nursing. In parents who struggle with nursing for seemingly unexplained reasons, a history of abuse may be one possible root cause.

BE FLEXIBLE ABOUT NURSING OPTIONS when nursing triggers negative reactions related to past trauma. If this happens, discuss possible triggers. If parents are unsure, suggest keeping a diary for a few days to try to pinpoint the problem and modify nursing to increase their comfort with it. This might include reducing the amount of skin-to-skin contact during feeds. If the problem occurs only at night, partial nursing just during the day may be workable. To avoid the intimate contact of nursing, some parents express their milk and bottle-feed it at some feeds. Be flexible, keeping in mind that some nursing is nearly always better than none.

TREATMENT OPTIONS TO REDUCE TRAUMA SYMPTOMS include:

- **Education and peer counseling** to help parents understand their reactions to trauma so they can avoid their triggers and reduce their stress responses.
- **Trauma-focused psychotherapy** to better cope with past trauma include cognitive-behavioral therapy and eye-movement desensitization and reprocessing (EMDR).
- **Medications**, including some SSRIs, SNRIs, SARIs, and atypical antipsychotics, many of which are compatible with lactation.

ENDOCRINE, METABOLIC, AND AUTOIMMUNE DISORDERS

A chronic illness or disorder may be present at birth (congenital) or it may develop over time. Most ill parents are well-educated about their health issues, so if needed, ask questions about the illness or any limitations that might affect nursing. For more details about an illness, visit the websites of national and international organizations supporting those with chronic illnesses.

CYSTIC FIBROSIS is a genetic disease that causes secretion of a thick, gluey mucus that clogs the bronchial tubes, interfering with breathing and blocking digestive enzymes from leaving the pancreas, causing incomplete digestion. Parents may have a mild or severe form. Some cases are so mild they can be detected only through laboratory tests. Some are serious enough to be life-threatening. During pregnancy, 25% of those with cystic fibrosis deliver preterm.

Lactation issues: Parents with cystic fibrosis produce milk with normal composition. Babies cannot "catch" this genetic disease by nursing. Babies born with cystic fibrosis who do not nurse have poorer health outcomes and earlier and more severe symptoms. (For nursing the baby with cystic fibrosis, see p. 120.) Many parents with cystic fibrosis have difficulty maintaining a healthy weight due to their issues with incomplete digestion of food. Parents may take digestive enzymes to break down the food more completely and vitamin and mineral supplements. As long as these parents can maintain a healthy weight, nursing can continue.

Medication issues: Some parents with cystic fibrosis decide not to nurse due to medication concerns, but most drugs prescribed for cystic fibrosis are compatible with lactation. As a result, these parents may need extra lactation help and support to meet their feeding goals.

DIABETES MELLITUS TYPE 1 (insulin-dependent diabetes mellitus or IDDM) accounts for 5% to 10% of diabetics and occurs when the insulin-producing beta cells in the pancreas are destroyed, leaving the body unable to produce insulin, a hormone needed to convert sugar, starches, and other foods into fuel for the body. Without insulin, blood sugar can rise to dangerous levels and cause health complications. Parents with Type 1 diabetes need to check their blood-sugar levels regularly and receive daily insulin replacement therapy via injections or subcutaneous pump, so their blood sugar doesn't become dangerously high.

Lactation issues: Babies cannot "catch" Type 1 diabetes by nursing. After birth, newborns whose birthing parent has Type 1 diabetes are at greater risk for low blood sugar (hypoglycemia), which can be prevented or minimized by early skin-to-skin contact and frequent nursing. In parents with this condition, milk increase after birth is delayed on average by about 1 day. To reduce the need to expose a newborn to cow-milk based formula, which can sensitize baby to allergies, if the baby needs a supplement, suggest families consider hand-expressing and storing colostrum during the last month of pregnancy (see **firstdroplets.com**). Other alternatives include providing pasteurized donor human milk or using elemental or amino-acid-based infant formula, such as Nutramigen AA or Neocate.

When parents' blood sugar is in good control, long-term milk production is not affected. However, diabetic parents are at greater risk of bacterial and fungal infections, including mastitis and candida (thrush), so suggest they learn how to prevent these infections and their symptoms, so if needed, they can seek treatment immediately.

Medication issues: The insulin replacement needed daily by parents with Type 1 diabetes does not affect the nursing baby. Insulin molecules are too large to pass into the milk, but even if they did, they would be broken down in the baby's gut. Lactation increases insulin sensitivity, which decreases the amount of insulin the nursing parent needs by 27% to 50%. During weaning, suggest parents wean as gradually as possible to more easily maintain blood-sugar control.

TYPE 2 DIABETES (non-insulin dependent diabetes mellitus or NIDDM) either reduces production of insulin or the body's insulin receptors do not respond normally to insulin (insulin resistance). When sugar builds up in the blood instead of being used as fuel by cells, this can affect the eyes, skin, feet, heart, and other systems. Type 2 diabetes is one part of a constellation of health problems known as metabolic syndrome (which includes obesity, high cholesterol, and high blood pressure) that increases the risk of cardiovascular disease.

Lactation issues: Exclusively nursing babies have a reduced risk of Type 2 diabetes later in life. For the parent, lactation improves glucose metabolism, increasing insulin sensitivity, which reduces the severity of Type 2 diabetes. The insulin resistance that accompanies Type 2 diabetes may delay milk increase after birth. Immediately post-delivery, newborns whose birthing parent has Type 2 diabetes are at greater risk for low blood sugar (hypoglycemia), which can be prevented or minimized by early skin-to-skin contact and frequent nursing. Suggest expectant parents learn and follow optimal early nursing practices (Chapter 2).

Medication issues: None. The most commonly used antidiabetic drugs, such as insulin, metformin, and some second-generation sulfonylureas are compatible with lactation.

GESTATIONAL DIABETES is a glucose intolerance that occurs in up to 9% of pregnancies. About half of those who develop gestational diabetes will later develop Type 2 diabetes. Any lactation after birth prevents or delays the development of Type 2 diabetes in nursing parents, and this effect increases with longer duration and greater exclusivity of nursing. Later in life, duration of lactation is also associated with a lower prevalence of metabolic syndrome, of which Type 2 diabetes is a part. Not only does lactation increase parents' insulin sensitivity while nursing, it appears to positively program their metabolism for years afterwards. Lactation seems to prime the metabolic system, making the body more energy efficient. Children whose birthing parents have gestational diabetes are also more likely to develop Type 2 diabetes, but at least 8 months of nursing is associated with healthier A1C levels (a measure of blood sugar) in childhood.

Lactation issues: Even with the positive effects of lactation on health, parents with gestational diabetes are less likely than others to start nursing after birth, be nursing at hospital discharge, and exclusively nurse. They are more likely to nurse for a shorter duration. These same results are found worldwide. Targeted lactation help and support may be needed by these families.

As with the other diabetics, early milk increase after birth may be delayed in parents with gestational diabetes. Treatment with insulin during pregnancy is associated with this delay, as well as obesity and suboptimal nursing in the hospital. Suggest following the optimal early nursing practices described in Chapter 2.

Medication issues: None. The most commonly used antidiabetic drugs, such as insulin, metformin, and some second-generation sulfonylureas are compatible with lactation.

GALACTOSEMIA AND PKU (phenylketonuria) are genetic metabolic disorders that make it impossible to completely metabolize specific components of human milk. Babies with galactosemia cannot metabolize galactose, a milk sugar, and its accumulation in their system causes severe health problems. Babies with PKU cannot easily metabolize the essential amino acid phenylalanine, also causing severe health issues unless diet is modified. No matter their age, these individuals must remain vigilant about diet to avoid dangerously high blood levels of these substances. When people with galactosemia or PKU reach childbearing age, they can become pregnant and nurse.

Lactation issues: None. During lactation, the milk composition of these parents is normal.

Medication issues: None. These conditions are managed by diet, not medications.

GESTATIONAL OVARIAN THECA LUTEIN CYSTS are benign cysts that develop on the ovaries during pregnancy that produce testosterone at levels 10 to 150 times higher than normal. When testosterone levels are very high, body or facial hair may develop and the voice may deepen. If testosterone levels are elevated to more moderate levels, there may be no obvious symptoms, and parents and their healthcare provider may be unaware they have this condition. After birth, these cysts disappear without treatment, and within several weeks, the affected parent's testosterone levels return to normal.

Lactation issues: High testosterone levels after birth can inhibit milk production. If a blood test reveals high testosterone levels (a "high normal" level is 67-70 ng/dL), an ultrasound can confirm the presence of the cysts. When testosterone levels fall below 300 ng/dL, milk increase occurs. (In case reports, this occurred between 10 to 31 days after birth.) In the meantime, nursing with a nursing supplementer or pumping at least 8 times per day helps eventually achieve normal milk increase when testosterone levels drop far enough.

Medication issues: None. No drug treatment is available.

MULTIPLE SCLEROSIS (MS) is a chronic, often disabling disease that attacks the central nervous system. Symptoms may be mild or severe. The development, severity, and symptoms of MS vary from person to person. Although the cause of MS is not yet known, it is thought to be a type of autoimmune disorder. It involves damage to the fatty substance (***myelin***) that surrounds the central nervous system. It may also damage the nerve fibers and form scar tissue (***sclerosis***). When any part of the myelin sheath or nerve fiber is damaged, nerve impulses traveling to and from the brain and spinal cord are distorted or interrupted, producing its symptoms, such as numbness, fatigue, trouble walking, vision problems, pain, vertigo, and even paralysis.

In mild cases, the affected person may completely recover after the symptoms pass and have long periods of remission. In severe cases, the symptoms may become progressively worse and not subside, or there may be repeated relapses that leave those affected permanently and increasingly disabled. It is common for MS to occur during the childbearing years.

Lactation issues: MS cannot be transmitted by nursing. In fact, nursing decreases baby's risk of developing pediatric MS. Nursing longer than 6 months decreases risk more than nursing less.

Lactation issues: During pregnancy, many of those with MS enjoy a remission from its symptoms. But the first 3 months after birth often bring a major increase in symptoms. The more exclusively parents nurse after delivery, the longer the period of remission from MS symptoms.

Medication issues: Many of the first-line drugs used to slow the progression of MS (disease-modifying treatments or DMTs) are considered compatible with lactation. Some exceptions include mitoxantrone (Novantrone), which is contraindicated during lactation. But in most cases, parents with MS can take their medications and nurse.

POLYCYSTIC OVARY SYNDROME (PCOS) is not a disease but a syndrome (a constellation of symptoms) that is still poorly understood. It affects up to 15% of women and is one of the leading causes of infertility. Common symptoms of PCOS include:

- High levels of estrogen and androgens (testosterone and other male hormones), which can cause severe acne, skin discoloration, and excess hair growth

- High insulin levels that contribute to the obesity affecting about half of those with PCOS
- Multiple ovarian cysts
- Menstrual abnormalities, which usually begin in adolescence and contribute to infertility

Many with PCOS also develop insulin resistance and Type 2 diabetes during their childbearing years. Insulin resistance (insulin receptors not responding normally to insulin in the body) appears to be a pivotal issue, as when insulin resistance is treated, it resolves many other PCOS symptoms. Some with PCOS experience low thyroid levels (hypothyroidism), which may contribute to infertility.

Lactation issues: Because its hormonal disruptions vary in type and degree, the effect of PCOS on milk production is inconsistent. Some with PCOS produce overabundant milk, others have low milk production, while still others produce milk in the normal range. Studies found some with PCOS had hypoplastic breasts made mostly of fat with few milk-making glands while others had breast tissue abnormalities. Insulin is known to affect mammary growth and development during pregnancy and to play an important role in increasing milk production after birth. When a parent's body does not respond normally to insulin, this has the potential to affect milk production. It is possible that higher levels of testosterone and other androgens during pregnancy may affect mammary development. When a parent with PCOS is also obese, has high blood pressure, and is insulin resistant, this increases the chances of having milk-production problems. But not all of those with PCOS have issues with mammary function and milk production. As with other lactation red flags, when a parent has PCOS, the nursing couple should be monitored after birth without undermining their confidence in nursing.

Medication issues: A common treatment for PCOS, the hypoglycemic medication metformin, decreases the hormonal disruptions in some of those affected, even those without insulin resistance. Regarding lactation, metformin is rated an L1 (safest) drug, and little transfers into human milk. For some with PCOS, treatment with metformin through pregnancy and lactation help normalize milk production. Doses start at about 500 mg per day and increase up to 1,000 to 2,500 mg per day.

RHEUMATOID ARTHRITIS AND LUPUS (the most common type is systemic lupus erythematosus) are autoimmune disorders caused by the immune system attacking body tissues with unusual antibodies known as "autoantibodies." Autoimmune disorders are more common in women than men and often occur in periods of flares and remissions. During the flares, symptoms include joint swelling, pain, fatigue, and fever. In those with lupus, neurological problems can occur and organ function may be affected. In severe cases, organ failure may occur.

Lactation issues: The baby cannot "catch" rheumatoid arthritis or lupus by nursing. In fact, nursing babies are less likely to contract these disorders than babies not nursed. Nursing also offers parents some protection from developing these autoimmune disorders later in life, with longer nursing providing greater protection than shorter nursing. Many parents with rheumatoid arthritis experience a remission from their symptoms beginning in the second trimester of pregnancy and ending with their return about 3 to 4 months after delivery. When a chronic illness goes into remission during pregnancy and symptoms return during nursing, parents may think nursing is the cause. This is not the case. In fact, for many parents, the hormonal changes of nursing actually help prolong their remission. In parents with lupus, symptoms during pregnancy are more unpredictable, and pregnancy may be a difficult time.

Parents with lupus are less likely than others to initiate nursing, and they wean earlier. A common reason for weaning is concern about starting a new medication, even when told it is compatible with nursing. Parents report finding it difficult to access reliable information about medications and lactation.

Joint pain, nipple pain from Raynaud's phenomenon, and fatigue are common among nursing parents with these conditions. For strategies to make nursing easier with these physical challenges, see p. 162.

RA medication issues: Many pain drugs used to treat rheumatoid arthritis are compatible with lactation, such as ibuprofen, acetaminophen, and meperidine. The disease-modifying antirheumatic drugs (DMARDs) include steroids, antimalarial drugs, and others, many of which are compatible with lactation. But some cytotoxic drugs in this category, such as methotrexate, are questionable during lactation. Although only small amounts of these drugs pass into the milk, they are retained in the tissues.

Lupus medication issues: The drugs used depend on its severity and the organ involvement. Non-steroidal anti-inflammatories like ibuprofen may be used for inflammation and/or pain. DMARDs may also be prescribed, many of which are compatible with lactation.

THYROID DISEASE may be triggered by the hormonal changes of pregnancy. Located in the neck, the butterfly-shaped thyroid gland releases hormones (T_3 and T_4) that regulate much of the body's activities: metabolism, heat generation, brain and heart function, and more. When the thyroid gland becomes overactive (**hyperthyroidism**), it releases too much hormone. When it becomes underactive (**hypothyroidism**), it releases too little hormone. Both too much and too little thyroid hormone may affect parents' mood and energy level, as well as their health and milk production. Encourage parents with a history of thyroid problems to have their thyroid levels tested every few weeks during pregnancy and after birth so their medication can be adjusted as their levels change.

POSTPARTUM THYROIDITIS is a temporary change in parents' thyroid levels after birth, which occurs in 5% to 10% of pregnancies. This autoimmune condition can occur even in parents without a history of thyroid problems. It is most common among those with autoimmune disorders and a history of thyroid disorders. It usually starts with a period of overactive thyroid (hyperthyroidism), sometime between 1 and 4 months after birth. Symptoms may include fast heartbeat, insomnia, anxiety, weight loss, and irritability. This overactive phase may last a few weeks to a few months, and then in some (but not all) parents it is followed by a period of underactive thyroid (hypothyroidism), usually between 4 to 8 months after birth. Symptoms in this phase may include weight gain, fatigue, dry skin, constipation, depression, and decrease in milk production. Postpartum thyroiditis may be diagnosed from its symptoms alone or blood tests may detect thyroid levels that are too high or too low. Depending on its severity, treatments described in the following two sections for hypo- and hyperthyroidism may be used to bring thyroid levels back into the normal range until the thyroid function normalizes over time. In 80% of parents with this condition, its symptoms resolve within 12 to 18 months after they began. If thyroid replacement therapy is used, it is tapered off gradually as the parent's thyroid begins functioning normally.

HYPOTHYROIDISM, or underactive thyroid, may be caused by autoimmune disorders such as Hashimoto's thyroiditis, medical treatments such as surgery or radiation of the thyroid gland, medications, illness, or damage to the pituitary gland, the "master gland" that tells the thyroid how much hormone to release. With clinical hypothyroidism, lower-than-normal levels of thyroid hormones cause symptoms that indicate the body is slowing down. Parents with low thyroid may feel cold, lack energy, be forgetful, and depressed. Constipation and low milk production are other possible symptoms. Because some symptoms may be vague and start slowly, it is not unusual for hypothyroidism to be missed or misdiagnosed. This condition is usually diagnosed from a combination of symptoms, medical history, physical exam, and blood tests. If the blood TSH (**thyroid stimulating hormone**) levels are high and the T_3 (**triiodothyronine**) and T_4 (**thyroxine**) levels are low, this indicates underactive thyroid. Before any new parent is treated for depressive symptoms, first rule out hypothyroidism. Taking St. John's wort (an herbal depression treatment) can mask hypothyroidism.

Lactation issues: The connection between low thyroid function and low milk production is well known. Low thyroid may also affect the release of oxytocin. In some parents with low milk production, a "low-normal" thyroid test result may not lead to treatment. But sometimes more extensive testing may lead to a diagnosis of subclinical hypothyroidism (abnormal lab results with no symptoms) and treatment. For information to share with a healthcare provider from the American Thyroid Association that provides treatment recommendations, see the 2017 guidelines at **bit.ly/BA2-Thyroid**. Recommendations 74 and 75 in these guidelines address treatment for hypothyroidism to address lactation-related issues. If a galactogogue is used to boost low milk production, avoid those that decrease thyroid function, such as fenugreek and moringa.

Medication issues: Hypothyroidism is usually treated with synthetic thyroid replacement hormones, such as levothyroxine (Synthroid), which bring parents' levels up to normal by providing the hormones their body should produce naturally. This drug is rated an L1 (safest). With treatment, many parents with hypothyroidism not only feel better, their milk production increases, sometimes dramatically.

HYPERTHYROIDISM, or overactive thyroid, is caused in 70% of cases by Graves' disease, an autoimmune disorder in which autoantibodies stimulate overproduction of the thyroid gland. It can also be caused by thyroid nodes or lumps or a temporary condition called thyroiditis, which may be triggered by a virus. When parents produce higher-than-normal thyroid levels, symptoms indicate the body is running faster: racing heartbeat, anxiety, insomnia, irritability, more perspiration, and weight loss. Their eyes may bulge and their thyroid gland may swell into a visible lump (goiter) on their neck. Diagnosis is usually made first with a physical exam, which reveals a swollen thyroid gland, and confirmed by a blood test. When parents' TSH (thyroid-stimulating hormone) levels are low and T_3 and T_4 levels are high, this indicates an overactive thyroid.

Lactation issues: In cases of severe, untreated hyperthyroidism, parents may experience early, rapid milk increase after delivery but be unable to remove milk by either nursing or milk expression. If so, seek treatment for hyperthyroidism, and consider oxytocin nasal spray after birth to trigger milk ejection to aid in milk removal.

Radioactive diagnostic tests: Once hyperthyroidism is confirmed, to determine its cause, the healthcare provider may order a thyroid scan to check for lumps. The radioactive iodine uptake test requires an interruption of nursing until it clears the parent's system, usually at least 12 hours. If a radioactive scan is recommended, suggest parents ask if a material can be used that has the shortest half-life, which requires the shortest interruption of nursing. The Academy of Breastfeeding Medicine (ABM) Clinical Protocol #31 (at **bfmed.org/protocols**) includes this information and is suitable for sharing with healthcare providers. Hyperthyroidism can be a serious health problem that stresses the heart muscles and nervous system, so if a parent's condition is serious, quick treatment may be critical.

Medication issues: Antithyroid medications, such as propylthiouracil (PTU) and methimazole (Tapazole), and the beta-blocker propranolol (Inderal) are all compatible with lactation. In many cases of Graves' disease, medication alone for 12 to 18 months is enough to cause a remission of symptoms.

Radioactive iodine treatment: Unfortunately, the above medications are not always effective for all types of hyperthyroidism and in all people. Other treatment options include surgical removal of all or part of the thyroid gland, which is compatible with continued nursing, or radioactive iodine treatment, which is not. For details, see p. 145. Radioactive iodine is also used to treat thyroid cancer.

HEADACHES AND LACTATION

Some types of headaches, such as migraines, are affected by hormonal fluctuations. Migraines tend to occur less often during pregnancy, lactation, and after menopause than during other times. However, some types of headaches, such as tension headaches, are not affected by hormonal fluctuations, so nursing will likely have no effect on them.

In rare cases, rather than preventing headaches, the hormonal changes of lactation trigger them. In two case reports, migraines became worse during lactation. In one case, migraines occurred only during weaning when the glands became overly full. The author noted that lactational headaches occurred either during the first milk ejection (early in a nursing session) or when the mammary glands feel full. For an overview on types of headaches occurring during pregnancy and lactation and treatment options, including non-drug therapies, see **bit.ly/BA2-Headaches**.

HOSPITALIZATION AND SURGERY

HOSPITALIZATION of the nursing parent can be incredibly stressful and complicated to navigate. Before discussing possible options, first ask for the following basic information.

- The reason for the hospitalization and how long it is estimated to last
- The ages of any nursing child and any other children
- Their long- and short-term nursing goals
- Plans for the nursing child. Will the child stay with them in the hospital (with an adult helper)? If not, can he visit, and if so, for how much of the day? (Some hospitals will make exceptions to policies if asked.) Will he be cared for elsewhere?
- Available help from family and friends while in the hospital and after
- What the healthcare provider said about nursing
- Availability of lactation consultants and breast pumps at the hospital. If parents need help expressing milk, is the nursing staff knowledgeable and willing?

For information about the lactation services and equipment available at the hospital, suggest contacting the lactation consultant or patient liaison. Parents—or their advocate—can explain to hospital staff that nursing or expressing milk is a vital part of the parent's medical care, as it will help avoid complications, such as pain and mastitis. If parents are told their child cannot stay with them, suggest asking if arranging for a room in another area, such as the post-birth unit, would make a difference. If the healthcare providers are concerned about a young baby being exposed to organisms in the hospital, explain that a private room will decrease risk.

Feeding goals. If the family's goal is to continue nursing and parents will be separated from their baby for all or part of the hospitalization, discuss milk-expression strategies for maintaining milk production (see p. 215). If parents want to wean or slow milk production temporarily until they are feeling healthier, discuss how to use milk expression to reduce milk production gradually and avoid painful mammary fullness and mastitis (p. 29). If the baby is exclusively nursing, discuss strategies for helping the baby accept another feeding method (p. 93). If parents are concerned their baby may not return to nursing later, reassure them that even if the baby is reluctant to nurse at first, with patience and persistence, he will likely be persuaded to nurse again (p. 72).

Medication issues: Suggest parents ask for the names and spellings of all medications to check their compatibility with lactation.

SURGERY will be less stressful if parents have realistic ideas about what to expect during and afterwards. After surgery, the parents' condition and level of pain will determine their ability and desire to nurse and care for their child. If parents can plan ahead, are motivated, and have help, it may be possible to directly nurse soon after surgery. While some healthcare facilities put lactation programs in place for nursing parents undergoing surgery, this is the exception rather than the rule.

Suggest parents ask their healthcare provider how they will feel after surgery. Depending on the procedure and the parent's condition, some will be alert and in little pain, while others will be completely incapacitated and in need of intensive medical care. Knowing what to expect will help them decide how they want to handle nursing or milk expression after surgery. Some may want to nurse as soon as possible, while others may want or need to wait. If there will be a wait, suggest making arrangements to have an effective breast pump available, and if needed, help expressing.

Anesthesia and lactation: After surgery, in most cases when the nursing parent is alert and awake enough to hold the baby, it is safe to resume nursing. An interruption of nursing for 6 to 12 hours after the anesthesia was administered is recommended only for parents whose babies are at risk for apnea, low blood pressure, or low muscle tone, such as some preterm or ill babies. If healthcare providers have concerns about the effects of anesthesia on the nursing baby, suggest sharing ABM Clinical Protocol #15 at **bfmed.org/protocols**.

PHYSICAL IMPAIRMENT OR CHALLENGE

Physical limitations may be present at birth, such as a missing limb. They may occur after an accident, a spinal cord injury, or stroke. Temporary or permanent loss of function, including swelling, weakness, numbness, and fatigue can occur with autoimmune disorders, such as lupus, multiple sclerosis, and rheumatoid arthritis.

BASIC STRATEGIES FOR PARENTS WITH DISABILITIES include:

- Create a "nursing nest" at home where everything is within easy reach and the parent can nurse comfortably.
- Use as needed slings, pillows, strollers, and other tools to simplify baby care and nursing.

Parents who have difficulty supporting the baby's weight in arms or have chronic fatigue can try nursing in the side-lying (p. 12) or starter positions (p. 6) described in Chapter 1. Some lean over an elevated surface (like a crib or the drawer of a tall dresser). If a comfortable nursing position cannot be found, pumping exclusively is another option parents with disabilities can consider.

CARPAL TUNNEL SYNDROME occurs when repetitive hand movements cause swelling in the wrist, which compresses nerves leading to the hand. Symptoms include hand numbness, tingling, and pain that extends from wrist to shoulder. When carpal tunnel syndrome develops during pregnancy, it usually resolves without treatment after birth, sometimes taking a month or two to resolve completely. A small number of parents develop carpal tunnel syndrome during the first month of nursing, with symptoms that only completely resolve after weaning.

Lactation issues: If nursing is painful when supporting baby's weight in arms, suggest as much as possible using the side-lying (p. 12) or starter positions (p. 6) described in Chapter 1. Suggest using pillows or cushions as needed in upright positions or nurse baby in a sling or baby carrier.

Medication issues: An effective treatment for carpal tunnel syndrome is wearing a splint at night, keeping the hand elevated, and taking diuretic medications, which are compatible with lactation.

EPILEPSY AND OTHER SEIZURE DISORDERS Each year, about 20,000 parents with epilepsy give birth in the U.S. Medication is usually so effective at preventing seizures that they are rare, but during pregnancy, many experience more frequent seizures as their body changes and their usual dosage of medication becomes less effective. A baby cannot "catch" epilepsy by nursing. In fact, babies who are not nursed are at greater risk for developing epilepsy as they grow.

To create a nursing environment that is safe during seizures (important no matter how baby is fed), suggest choosing a feeding area with padding to protect the baby, such as a bed or a chair with padded arms. If the chair's arms are not padded, suggest folding two towels, wrapping and securing them around the chair's arms. This creates a cushion for baby's head during a seizure. Padding and extra pillows may also help parents avoid bruising. Other strategies include:

- In upright feeding positions, keep their feet elevated (i.e., use a footstool) so that if a seizure occurs, the baby rolls back into their lap, not onto the floor.
- If nursing in bed, use guardrails and pillows for padding. A mattress or futon on the floor away from walls would be safer.
- Have a safe surface available on each level of the home, such as a pram, stroller, or portable crib, where parents can lay the baby if they feel a seizure coming.

- Change the baby's diaper/nappy on the floor, or if using a changing table, strap the baby securely, and bathe the baby only when another adult is present.
- When babies and toddlers are crawling and walking, use gates at staircases and doorways to prevent accidents.
- When away from home, attach a tag or sticker to the pram or stroller with information about epilepsy, the baby's name, and contact information for a friend or relative.

Medication issues. Parents' major concern is the compatibility of their medications with lactation. The amount of anti-seizure medication the baby receives while nursing is much less than what he received while in utero. Although each nursing couple must be evaluated individually, most of these medications have been thoroughly studied and used in nursing parents for years. Yet despite this, many of these parents decide not to nurse because of their medication concerns. One way to address this is to provide education about drugs and lactation to epileptic specialists so they can support nursing among these parents rather than giving contradictory messages. Some anti-epileptic medications, such as phenobarbital, have infrequently been associated with sedation in newborns.

SPINAL CORD INJURY OR STROKE may cause physical limitations, depending on its severity and with a spinal-cord injury, its location and extent. The lower the spinal cord injury, the less function is lost, and the higher and more complete the injury, the more function is lost.

Lactation issues: If a spinal cord injury causes complete loss of mammary sensation, milk ejection may be inhibited because the nerve pathways between nipple and brain that trigger milk ejection are no longer functional. Some parents with this issue have successfully nursed. In one case, the act of nursing triggered milk ejection. Others used visualization and relaxation exercises to trigger it. Without full use of the hands and arms, a parent will need help getting baby into a nursing position.

A stroke can cause partial paralysis and affect parents' vision and judgment. The physical effects of the stroke depend upon its severity and which side of the brain is affected. Due to a stroke's effects on judgment, parents may need help knowing when to nurse the baby. They may need extra pillows for support, and if paralysis is involved, help holding their baby. When nursing, it may help to suggest parents lie on their affected side so they can use the unaffected arm and hand to help the baby latch. As with any disability, creativity and an open mind can help find the best strategies.

VISUAL IMPAIRMENT includes different degrees of vision loss. If parents are completely blind, a sling or baby carrier can help them learn to read the baby's hunger cues through movements and changes in breathing. Nursing is likely to be easier to manage than formula-feeding, which involves (both at home and in unfamiliar places) measuring, preparing, pouring, and cleaning.

When suggesting educational materials, ask how they usually access information. Some have partial vision and can read large print materials or use magnifying lenses. Others use audio materials, Braille, or computer screen reading programs with a voice synthesizer. Many handouts on positioning and latch rely on photos and drawings to convey information, which blind parents may not be able to access. Use words and ask permission before touching parent or baby.

DIGITAL RESOURCES

bfmed.org/protocols—Free, downloadable, fully referenced clinical protocols from the Academy of Breastfeeding Medicine, ideal for sharing with healthcare providers:

- #15: Analgesia and anesthesia for the breastfeeding mother
- #18: Use of antidepressants in nursing mothers
- #30: Breast masses, breast complaints, and diagnostic breast imaging
- #31: Radiology and nuclear medicine studies in lactating women

CHAPTER 10 HYPOGLYCEMIA AND JAUNDICE

NEWBORN HYPOGLYCEMIA

Hypoglycemia refers to low blood glucose levels. Glucose, a simple sugar, provides most of a newborn's brain fuel. In utero, the baby stores glucose in the form of glycogen in her liver and muscles. After birth, hormones are released that help her use her glycogen stores for brain fuel while she adapts to life on the outside. About 70% of a baby's brain glucose needs are met this way, with the other 30% coming from alternative fuels. A newborn's blood sugar levels normally drop after birth and then rise again as she adapts to life outside the womb.

NORMAL BLOOD SUGAR FLUCTUATIONS AFTER BIRTH
In a healthy term newborn, normal blood sugar levels are at their lowest at about 1 to 2 hours after birth. They begin to rise, independent of feeding, within 2 to 4 hours and continue rising until about 96 hours after birth. There are no short- or long-term benefits to testing and treating newborns for this normal dip in blood-sugar levels.

By 12 hours after birth, a newborn's glycogen stores are gone, and milk feedings and fat stores provide a baby with the glucose her brain needs. In addition, newborns can access other fuel sources, such as lactate (aka lactic acid) and ketone bodies. Healthy term exclusively nursing babies are not considered at risk for hypoglycemia, in part because they have greater access to these alternative fuels. Routine blood-sugar testing is not recommended, even when a healthy term newborn without symptoms goes 8 hours without nursing.

The first nursing session has little effect on blood-sugar levels, so if the first nursing is delayed, the baby will not benefit from being fed a supplement. In fact, formula supplements can suppress a baby's ability to use ketone bodies as an alternative brain fuel. But in newborns with low blood glucose levels, lactate appears to have a larger role as an alternative brain fuel.

SYMPTOMS OF HYPOGLYCEMIA include tremors, irritability, jitteriness, a high-pitched cry, irregular breathing, low body temperature, and refusal to feed, as well as low muscle tone, lethargy, and seizures. Jitteriness can be difficult to distinguish from normal newborn behavior, and some researchers recommend against doing blood tests if this is the only symptom.

The normal and temporary dip in blood sugar after birth that occurs in most mammal species is distinctly different from the more serious type of hypoglycemia that can develop in at-risk newborns. Prolonged and severe if untreated, it can cause brain damage and lead to vision problems, neuromotor retardation, epilepsy, cerebral palsy, and in rare cases, death.

DEFINING HYPOGLYCEMIA AND MEASURING BLOOD SUGAR There is no generally agreed-upon definition for hypoglycemia, and many common testing methods are inaccurate. Its definition varies among healthcare providers and in different parts of the world. One common guideline is less than 40 mg/dL or 2.2 mmol/L (whole blood glucose level lower than 35 mg/dL or 1.9 mmoL). But when this guideline is used, more than 20% of healthy term newborns with normal blood-sugar levels are misidentified as hypoglycemic. Even so, in many hospitals even higher levels, such as 50 mg/dL (2.8 mmol/L), are now being used.

No matter what specific blood-sugar level is used, there are problems with defining hypoglycemia as one single measurement for all newborns. One blood glucose level does not reflect the many factors that determine the effect of that level on an individual baby, such as her gestational age, her health, her age in hours—which determines where she falls on the normal blood-sugar curve after birth—and her symptoms or lack of symptoms. Some researchers suggest instead thresholds be used that take these influencing factors into account (Table 10.1).

Confusion about the differences among the methods of measuring blood sugar contributes to overtreatment of hypoglycemia. For example, when whole blood is tested, the results are 10% to 18% higher than when plasma is tested. Also, all of the methods of measuring blood sugar levels at the bedside have limited accuracy. The American Academy of Pediatrics and World Health Organization recommend against using these as the sole screening method for hypoglycemia.

SCREENING AT-RISK NEWBORNS (risk factors listed in the last two rows of the first column in Table 10.1) The Academy of Breastfeeding Medicine recommends that the first blood-sugar screening begin after the first nursing session after birth but before the second, no later than 2 hours after birth. When possible, monitor blood-sugar before feeds until at least two consecutive measurements are within the healthy range.

EFFECTS OF POST-BIRTH PRACTICES ON BLOOD SUGAR Early skin-to-skin contact and frequent nursing reduce a newborn's risk of hypoglycemia. Skin-to-skin contact prevents cold stress, a risk factor, and is more effective than mechanical warmers at maintaining newborn body temperature even among preterm babies. To reduce the risk of both hypoglycemia and jaundice during the first days, after nursing, express a little colostrum into a spoon and feed it to the baby (**firstdroplets.com**). Colostrum enhances a newborn's ability to use alternative brain fuels and improves gut function, allowing nutrients to be absorbed more quickly.

Table 10.1. When to Treat Hypoglycemia

Baby's status	Baby's age in hours	Glucose levels indicating need for treatment
No symptoms Born 35-40 weeks Healthy Taking milk feedings No risk factors	≤24 hours	<30-35 mg/dL (1.7-1.9 mmol/L)
	>24 hours	<40-50 mg/dL (2.2 -2.8 mmol/L)
Symptoms of hypoglycemia	Any age	<45 mg/dL (2.5 mmol/L)
Illness or birth-related issues Low birth weight Preterm Respiratory distress, failure Sepsis (blood infection)	≤24 hours	<45-50 mg/dL (2.5-2.8 mmol/L)
	>24 hours	<40-50 mg/dL (2.2-2.8 mmol/L)
At risk Diabetic birthing parent Low birth weight Cold stress Metabolic, endocrine or blood disorder	Any age	<36 mg/dL (2.0 mmol/L)
Low blood-glucose levels <20-25 mg/dL	Any age	Start treatment and monitor

TREATING HYPOGLYCEMIA Oral dextrose gel with continued nursing is now the recommended first treatment. This involves inserting into baby's cheek a 40% dextrose gel. This treatment was found to be effective in randomized controlled trials done worldwide. It also reduces hospital costs without impairing later nursing sessions. Another treatment is IV glucose therapy, which is recommended in babies who are still hypoglycemic after treatment with dextrose gel or who have very low blood glucose levels. Nursing can continue during IV glucose therapy if baby is willing and able to nurse.

NEWBORN JAUNDICE

JAUNDICE BASICS More than 80% of newborns become visibly jaundiced during the first week of life. In utero, babies have extra red blood cells to transport the oxygen received via the placenta. After a baby is born and breathing air, these extra red blood cells are no longer needed, and they are broken down and eliminated. Bilirubin, a yellow pigment, is a byproduct of the breakdown of these extra red blood cells.

Jaundice occurs as bilirubin accumulates in baby's blood and enters the skin, muscles, and mucous membranes, giving her a yellow tinge. Jaundice is more common among newborns than in older children and adults for several reasons.

- Newborns make more bilirubin as extra red blood cells are broken down.
- Newborns process bilirubin more slowly because their liver is immature.
- Newborns absorb bilirubin more easily through their gut.

Among nursing babies, bilirubin levels can remain elevated for as long as 12 to 15 weeks. Mild to moderate bilirubin levels may have health benefits. But high levels can be dangerous.

EFFECT OF EARLY NURSING ON BILIRUBIN LEVELS Most cases of mild to moderate newborn jaundice, known as normal or *physiological jaundice*, are temporary and do not require treatment. This type of jaundice usually resolves on its own. With this type, bilirubin levels in healthy term babies usually peak between the third and fifth days of life at less than 12 mg/dL, (204 µmol/L) and rarely go higher than 15 mg/dL (255 µmol/L).

Bilirubin levels are more likely to become concerning when a baby isn't feeding well and often. It was once thought that more stooling was vital to lowering high bilirubin levels. Rather than lack of stooling, though, inadequate feeding was found to causes high bilirubin levels. Nursing early and often after birth stimulates an earlier increase in milk production, which in healthy term babies keeps bilirubin levels in the safe and moderate range.

PATHOLOGICAL JAUNDICE If a baby becomes visibly jaundiced during the first 24 to 48 hours or if the jaundice quickly becomes severe, this is likely a sign of an underlying health problem that may require treatment. Known as *pathological jaundice*, another indicator is bilirubin levels rising faster than 5 mg/dL (85 µmol/L) per day and higher than 17 mg/dL (290 µmol/L) in a full-term baby.

Possible underlying causes for pathological jaundice include diseases or conditions that cause increased red blood cell breakdown, interfere with bilirubin processing in the liver, or increase reabsorption of bilirubin by the gut. Examples include infection, blood disease, rubella, Rh or ABO incompatibility, inborn errors of metabolism, congenital thyroid deficiency, serious bruising or cephalohematoma, and intestinal obstruction or defect.

With only rare exceptions, such as some types of galactosemia, nursing can and should continue. Tests that can pinpoint treatable causes include those that identify blood and Rh type, direct antibody (Coombs) test, complete blood count, and red blood cell smear, as well as both a total bilirubin and a direct-reacting fraction.

PROLONGED JAUNDICE after the first 2 weeks was once thought to be a separate and distinct type of jaundice (called *late-onset* or *breast-milk jaundice*) that affected only a small percentage of nursing babies. But this is now recognized as an extension of normal newborn jaundice in which bilirubin can remain in the moderate range for many weeks, especially among babies who had higher bilirubin levels earlier.

By 2 to 3 weeks of age, the vast majority of newborns fed non-human milks have adult bilirubin levels of less than 1.3 to 1.5 mg/dL (22 to 26 µmol/L). But at 2 to 3 weeks of age, this is very different among nursing babies:

- One-third of nursing babies are visibly jaundiced with bilirubin levels above 5 mg/dL (85 µmol/L).

- One-third of nursing babies still have elevated bilirubin levels of between 1.5 and 5 mg/dL (26 to 85 µmol/L), even though their jaundice is not visible

In healthy term babies, as long as bilirubin levels stay below about 20 mg/dL (342 µmol/L) and are not rising rapidly, this prolonged jaundice will eventually clear without treatment within about 12 to 15 weeks. Sometimes a temporary weaning is recommended, but as long as bilirubin levels stay moderate, this is neither beneficial nor necessary. If a baby's healthcare provider recommends temporary weaning, share the Academy of Breastfeeding Medicine Clinical Protocol #22 on jaundice at: **bfmed.org/protocols**.

With few exceptions, once a baby's bilirubin levels have reached their peak and begun to decline, they are unlikely to rise again. A slight rebound in bilirubin levels is common after phototherapy is stopped or when the baby begins nursing again after a temporary interruption. Any rebound should be slight but closely followed.

DANGERS OF HIGH BILIRUBIN LEVELS Monitoring bilirubin levels in newborns is vital, because although rare, high bilirubin levels can cause severe health problems. While mild-to-moderate bilirubin levels may be beneficial, at the rare times when it exceeds 25 mg/dL (425 µmol/L), it may cross the blood-brain barrier, causing a condition known as **bilirubin encephalopathy**. Its early symptoms include lethargy and disinterest in feeding and can eventually progress to a high-pitched cry and neurological symptoms, such as seizures, head- and spine-arching, and fever. If not treated promptly, the baby may develop **kernicterus**, a yellow staining of the brain that causes permanent neurological damage and potentially lifelong problems such as cerebral palsy, hearing loss, developmental delays, paralysis, mental retardation, and even death.

Not all newborns with bilirubin levels higher than 25 mg/dL (425 µmol/L) develop bilirubin encephalopathy, but treatment should be started before it becomes a risk. In developed countries, very high bilirubin levels are rare among healthy term babies, as well as preterm and ill babies.

The outcomes from newborn jaundice are vastly different in the developing world, where good medical care is often scarce and phototherapy is less available. In developing countries, bilirubin encephalopathy, exchange transfusions to treat severe jaundice, and death are common.

Several factors, including baby's health and race, affect the course of newborn jaundice, with babies of Asian origin having higher bilirubin levels than non-Asian babies.

MONITORING BILIRUBIN LEVELS Not long ago, bilirubin levels could only be reliably monitored through painful blood tests that often needed to be done repeatedly. But now there are other, less-invasive ways to monitor baby's bilirubin levels.

CHANGES IN BABY'S SKIN COLOR Jaundice is not usually visible to the eye until bilirubin levels reach at least 4 mg/dL (68 µmol/L). As bilirubin levels rise, the yellow color spreads from the head to the chest (about 10 mg/dL [170 µmol/L]) to the abdomen and finally (usually at more than 15 mg/dL [255 µmol/L]) to the palms and the soles of the feet. The color of the baby's body are a rough indicator of jaundice. But bilirubin levels cannot be reliably gauged visually from baby's skin color alone, as room lighting and racial differences affect perception of skin tone.

NON-INVASIVE TOOLS TO MONITOR BILIRUBIN LEVELS are now available that are more reliable than visually checking baby's skin color and can reduce the need for painful blood tests.

- **Transcutaneous bilirubinometry** (TcB). An instrument is gently pressed against the baby's skin and reflects light through the skin to the underlying tissues and back into the instrument to calculate the intensity of the skin's yellow color. They are more reliable than the eye alone and are often used first so blood is drawn only from babies in need of medical follow-up. Often used as a first screening for healthy term babies, TcB is not as accurate as blood tests and is even less accurate among some races.

- **Bilicam smartphone app** uses the phone's camera to gauge skin tone. Studies found it reliable enough to use in low-risk newborns instead of TcB by healthcare providers and parents.

- **Bili-ruler** is a simple tool validated for measuring bilirubin levels in low-resource, high-risk areas to prevent delays in identifying babies with high bilirubin levels. Along the ruler are six circles of gradually intensifying colors with a number above each. The user gently presses the ruler into the bridge of baby's nose to blanch the skin and compares the baby's color with the six color choices. For more, see **bit.ly/BA2-BiliRuler**.

In many countries, all healthcare institutions routinely screen newborns for jaundice before hospital discharge. This screening often involves a combination of visually checking babies' skin color, determining any risk factors, and/or using one or more of the methods above for checking bilirubin levels. Close follow-up with a healthcare provider after discharge is strongly recommended.

JAUNDICE TREATMENTS include a range of options.

OPTIMIZING NURSING Nursing itself does not increase a baby's risk for severe jaundice, but inadequate milk intake does. Baby's weight loss after birth and stool color can help gauge early milk intake. Using baby's 24-hour weight as a baseline (rather than birth weight), the nursing newborn should lose no more than about 10% of this weight. Weight loss of more than 10% by Day 4 in exclusively nursing newborns or continued weight loss after Day 4 increases baby's risk for exaggerated jaundice and indicates the need for skilled lactation help. Dark meconium stools after Day 4 is another red flag to check baby's weight and take a closer look at nursing dynamics.

To increase milk intake, first make sure baby is latching deeply. Second, nurse at least 10 to 12 times each day during baby's wakeful periods. Express colostrum after nursing and feed it by spoon (**firstdroplets.com**). Between feeds and before latching, make sure baby is in full frontal contact with the nursing parent's body so that her innate feeding behaviors are activated (p. 6). Laying a swaddled baby in a separate bed for much of the day can lead to more sleep, suppress feeding behaviors, and decrease total number of daily feeds. If the baby latches but does not nurse actively, suggest trying breast compression (p. 309).

If high bilirubin levels make the baby lethargic, lay baby tummy-to-tummy on the semi-reclined parent's body to trigger feeding behaviors, with her head near the nipple. When baby is in light sleep (any movement) and begins rooting, without waking her, guide her to the nipple and help her latch. Babies in light sleep can nurse actively.

If the baby is unresponsive and not nursing actively, start milk expression to stimulate healthy milk production. Discuss feeding methods. Expressed milk can be fed using a nursing supplementer, spoon, cup, eyedropper, feeding syringe, or bottle.

FEEDING FORMULA When bilirubin levels rise high enough to be of concern in a healthy term baby, it is usually due to low milk intake, which is likely from one or more of the following reasons:

- **Too little time spent nursing effectively**, either too few feeds or too little time actively nursing
- **Nursing ineffectively due to oral variations**, such as tongue-tie, unusual palate, or others (p. 101)
- **Low milk production**, possibly related to lack of stimulation or other factors

Whatever the reason for insufficient milk intake, the baby still needs to be fed. When considering a supplement, the first choice is expressed milk. If the baby is willing to take larger volumes than the nursing parent can express, the second choice, if available, is donor human milk. The third choice is elemental (casein–hydrolysate or extensively hydrolyzed) formula, such as Alimentum and Nutramigen, because they are less likely to sensitize newborns to allergy and they reduce bilirubin levels faster than other formulas by preventing bilirubin in the baby's intestine from being reabsorbed. If formula is given, take steps to increase milk production by expressing milk and nursing frequently until the baby's needs are met from nursing alone. Another way to promote a quicker transition to exclusive nursing is to use a nursing supplementer to stimulate milk production while formula is fed.

Formula may be recommended as a supplement or as a temporary replacement for nursing. Because phototherapy (next section) can be costly and lengthen the hospital stay, some healthcare providers recommend giving jaundiced newborns formula when low milk intake is the cause, even before the baby's bilirubin reaches the level at which phototherapy is recommended. Depending on the baby's bilirubin levels, a 12-hour trial or a 24-hour interruption of nursing with or without phototherapy may be recommended, which may be extended to 48 hours if the baby's bilirubin levels do not decrease significantly. If these strategies are suggested, share Clinical Protocol #22 from the Academy of Breastfeeding Medicine at **bfmed.org/protocols**.

A temporary weaning puts nursing at risk. Express milk to stay comfortable and to establish or maintain milk production. Make sure families know that formula is not recommended because their milk is "bad" for their baby.

PHOTOTHERAPY uses special white, blue, or green fluorescent or spotlights to quickly lower bilirubin levels. The baby is laid nearly naked with her eyes covered under bili-lights. Their light is absorbed by the bilirubin under baby's skin, changing it to a water-soluble form that allows the baby to eliminate it without needing to first process it in her liver. Phototherapy has fewer side effects than exchange transfusions, can be used for all types of jaundice, and is sometimes combined with other treatments.

Criteria for Starting Phototherapy The bilirubin level at which phototherapy should be started depends on the baby's age, her risk factors, and her location. As with hypoglycemia, one bilirubin level does not reflect the many factors that determine its effect on an individual baby. Factors that affect when phototherapy begins include the baby's gestational age, how soon after birth her jaundice appeared, how fast her bilirubin levels are rising, the compatibility of her blood type with the birthing parent, any bruising, a sibling with a history of jaundice, her race, and the country's jaundice guidelines.

The U.K. phototherapy interactive guidelines for jaundiced babies younger than 28 days and born at least 38 weeks are online at: **bit.ly/BA2-UKJaundice**.

The American Academy of Pediatrics' (AAP) practice guidelines for starting phototherapy on hospitalized newborns born at least 35 weeks gestation (Table 10.2) first divides newborns by risk into three groups:

- Lower risk (≥38 weeks at birth and healthy)
- Medium risk (≥38 weeks at birth with risk factors or 35 to 35 6/7 weeks at birth and healthy)
- Higher risk (35 to 35 6/7 weeks at birth with risk factors)

The AAP defines major risk factors as:

- Bilirubin levels in the high-risk zone (if 3 days or older >16 mg/dL)
- Jaundice visible during the first 24 hours
- Blood group incompatibility or other blood disease
- An older sibling received phototherapy

- Significant bruising or cephalohematoma
- Exclusive breastfeeding with feeding problems and/or weight loss ≥12%
- East Asian race

Along with the baby's bilirubin level, a rise of more than 0.5 mg/dL (8.5 µmol/L) per hour increases risk.

Like the U.S., the Canadian Paediatric Society divided newborns into groups based on risk factors. The Canadian guidelines are available online at: **bit.ly/BA2-CPS**.

Table 10.2   U.S. Guidelines for Phototherapy in Babies Born ≥35 Weeks Gestation

Baby's Age in Hours	Lower Risk	Intermediate Risk	Higher Risk
24 Hours	12 mg/dL (204 µmol/L)	10 mg/dL (170 µmol/L)	8 mg/dL (136 µmol/L)
48 Hours	15 mg/dL (255 µmol/L)	13 mg/dL (221 µmol/L)	11 mg/dL (187 µmol/L)
72 hours	17 mg/dL (289 µmol/L)	15 mg/dL (255 µmol/L)	13 mg/dL (221 µmol/L)
96 hours	20 mg/dL (340 µmol/L)	17 mg/dL (289 µmol/L)	14 mg/dL (238 µmol/L)
5 days or older	21 mg/dL (357 µmol/L)	18 mg/dL (306 µmol/L)	15 mg/dL (255 µmol/L)

Safe bilirubin levels are lower in babies born earlier than 35 weeks. A preterm baby is at greater risk of brain injury at lower bilirubin levels because her immature liver is less effective at processing bilirubin and her blood-brain barrier is less effective at blocking it. Adding illness (infection, oxygen deprivation, and blood imbalances) to prematurity increases the risk of injury at lower bilirubin levels. Safe bilirubin levels for the preemie are determined individually based on the baby's gestational age, weight, and health.

Alternatives to Separating the Nursing Couple   If separation is suggested, discuss alternatives. For example, if the baby is in the hospital nursery:

- Can the nursing parent sit near the baby and nurse when she shows feeding cues?

- Can the bili-lights be set up in the nursing parent's room to make it easier to nurse under the lights or to take the baby out from under the lights to nurse?
- Can a phototherapy unit (a fiberoptic blanket) be rented for hospital or home use?

In babies who are otherwise healthy, intermittent phototherapy (12 hours on and 12 hours off) is as effective as continuous phototherapy in reducing bilirubin levels. Nursing often during phototherapy can help meet the baby's need for extra fluids while under the lights. Massage may also help, as babies who are massaged during phototherapy have significantly lower bilirubin levels than others.

Formula Use During Phototherapy is recommended in some cases, either as a supplement or as a replacement for nursing. See p. 175 for more details. The Academy of Breastfeeding Medicine noted that temporarily replacing nursing with formula during phototherapy is recommended only in extenuating circumstances.

EXCHANGE TRANSFUSIONS are recommended only when a baby's bilirubin levels are dangerously high (Table 10.3 for U.S. guidelines and **bit.ly/BA2-UKJaundice** for U.K. guidelines) or baby has neurological symptoms. An exchange transfusion is the fastest way to bring down bilirubin levels. During an exchange transfusion, small amounts of the baby's blood are continuously replaced with donor blood. Because safe bilirubin levels are lower in sick or very preterm babies, exchange transfusions may be recommended at lower levels in these at-risk babies.

Table 10.3 U.S. Guidelines for Exchange Transfusions in Babies Born ≥35 Weeks Gestation

Baby's Age in Hours	Lower Risk	Intermediate Risk	Higher Risk
24 Hours	19 mg/dL (323 µmol/L)	17 mg/dL (289 µmol/L)	15 mg/dL (255 µmol/L)
48 Hours	22 mg/dL (374 µmol/L)	19 mg/dL (323 µmol/L)	17 mg/dL (289 µmol/L)
72 hours	24 mg/dL (408 µmol/L)	21 mg/dL (357 µmol/L)	18 mg/dL (306 µmol/L)
96 hours or older	25 mg/dL (425 µmol/L)	22 mg/dL (374 µmol/L)	19 mg/dL (323 µmol/L)

Exchange transfusions are used less often today than in years past due to the use of RhoGAM to prevent severe jaundice from Rh incompatibility. There are more health risks associated with exchange transfusions than phototherapy, so phototherapy is routinely used first to prevent the need for this procedure.

Nursing can continue before and after exchange transfusions, as withholding feeds can increase bilirubin levels.

OTHER JAUNDICE TREATMENTS   Some medications can bring down bilirubin level, but some, such as tin-mesoporphyrin, have not yet been approved for this purpose. Other drugs used to treat jaundice include the anti-seizure medication phenobarbital, but this drug has significant drawbacks.

WHAT TO AVOID DURING JAUNDICE   Some drugs or other treatments should be avoided because they may increase the risk of injury from jaundice when used by the baby or the nursing parent. Examples include aspirin, other salicylates, ibuprofen, and certain sulfa drugs because they prevent bilirubin from binding to the protein in the baby's blood. Other substances to avoid while baby is jaundiced include the antibiotic sulfisoxazole (Gantrisin), benzyl alcohol, and its byproduct, benzoic acid, a preservative in some IV fluids. If they are needed, a substitute should be considered.

Glucose or plain water supplements—once commonly recommended— should be avoided, because they do not prevent jaundice and may increase bilirubin levels.

Putting the baby in indirect sunlight is not recommended to treat jaundice in developed countries, but filtered sunlight treatments may be an effective strategy in developing nations. See **bit.ly/BA2-NEJM**.

DIGITAL RESOURCES

www.bfmed.org/protocols/   Download the current versions of the following Academy of Breastfeeding Medicine Clinical Protocols, which are available in multiple languages:

- #1 Hypoglycemia
- #22 Jaundice

CHAPTER 11 MAKING MILK

ANATOMY OF THE MAMMARY GLAND

Mammary development begins in the womb, but the mammary gland doesn't become fully functional until lactation begins. The gland consists of:

- Glandular tissue, which makes milk and transports it to the nipple
- Connective (muscle) tissue, which provides mechanical support
- Adipose (fatty) tissue, which supports the growth of milk ducts during puberty and provides protection from outside injury
- Nerves, which provide the sensitivity to touch and temperature needed for milk ejection
- Blood, which provides nourishment and the ingredients needed to make milk
- Lymph, which transports waste products away from the gland

The size of the mammary gland is determined mainly by the amount of fatty tissue, which is unrelated to milk production. On average, there is about twice as much glandular tissue as fatty tissue, and they are intermixed within the gland. The glandular or milk-making tissue is composed of:

- Alveoli: milk-making factories that draw nutrients from the blood. Resembling clusters of grapes, the surrounding muscles squeeze during milk ejection to push the milk into the ducts.
- Ducts and ductules: small tubes that carry the milk from the alveoli to the nipple. The ducts near the nipple are the same diameter as elsewhere.
- Lobes and lobules: a lobule consists of one branch of alveoli and milk ducts that deliver milk to a lobe, which leads to a single nipple pore. On average, there are 9 lobes per gland.
- The nipple has between 4 and 18 nipple pores connected to the lobes. There may be many more nipple pores that are not connected to functional ducts. The nipple and areola contain smooth muscle erectile tissue that contracts with stimulation, firming and protruding it. Its flexibility allows it to stretch and conform to the inside of the baby's mouth.

- The areola is the darker pigmented area from which the nipple protrudes and where the Montgomery glands are located.
- Montgomery glands are a combination of sebaceous and mammary glands located on the areola that enlarge and become more prominent during pregnancy. Their number varies from 1 to 15 and their secretions protect the skin from sucking friction, reduce bacterial counts by altering the pH of the skin, and help the baby find the nipple after birth via their fluid's odor.

Nursing does *not* cause the mammary glands to sag. Changes in gland occur whether or not baby nurses as a result of the hormones of pregnancy.

MILK EJECTION

Milk ejection is triggered by the release of the hormone oxytocin and is responsible for most of the milk removal during nursing and milk expression. Oxytocin causes the band-like muscles around the milk-producing alveoli to squeeze and the milk ducts to shorten and dilate, pushing the milk out of the nipple pores. Because its trigger is hormonal, milk ejection occurs in both glands within about 10 seconds of each other and lasts for an average of 2 minutes.

During early nursing, milk ejection may take a few minutes to occur. But with time and conditioning, milk ejection becomes faster and more automatic, sometimes even occurring outside of nursing.

The average number of milk ejections per nursing session is 3 to 4, with a range of 1 to 17. Nearly 9 out of 10 nursing parents notice the first milk ejection, but not subsequent ones. Those who feel milk ejection may perceive it as a tingling, pressure, a pins-and-needles sensation, a feeling of "drawing" or "rushing down," increased thirst, milk leakage from the other side, even pain, while others feel nothing. Soon after birth, milk ejection may also be felt as uterine cramping or as tension across the shoulder blades. Parents feel milk ejection at varying levels of intensity.

On average, it takes about a minute of nursing for milk ejection to occur. The most reliable signs of milk ejection during nursing are longer, slower jaw movements or audible swallowing. When expressing milk, visibly faster milk flow is a reliable sign of milk ejection.

Sensations and emotions unrelated to nursing can trigger milk ejection, such as hearing another baby cry or having loving thoughts about the baby. Conversely, feeling upset, frustrated, stressed, or angry can delay milk ejection. Other stimuli that can inhibit milk ejection include the feeling of ice against skin, excessive alcohol intake, and some medications. The normal stresses of parenthood, fatigue, and lack of sleep do not affect milk ejection or milk volumes.

STRATEGIES TO SPEED DELAYED MILK EJECTION include relaxation techniques, warm compresses, and mammary massage. If strong negative emotions are a factor, try waiting a few minutes for a calmer time. In a crisis, if the milk ejection is consistently delayed, keep nursing and/or expressing milk. With time and stimulation, milk ejection and production will quickly rebound.

D-MER, short for ***dysphoric milk ejection reflex***, is an abrupt emotional drop just before milk ejection that continues for no more than a few minutes. These feelings can be mild, moderate, or severe and include wistfulness, hopelessness, dread, anxiety, and anger. For some, the intensity of these feelings increases as more milk accumulates in the glands. D-MER is a physical response (as yet unexplained), not a symptom of psychological issues.

When these upsetting feelings arise, share with parents the following strategies:

- Visit the website **d-mer.org** and read the personal stories. It can be helpful just knowing this condition has a name and that others have experienced it.
- Try the approaches other families reported on the website that worked for them.
- Know that D-MER seems to be physical rather than psychological.
- Post experiences on the website to increase the general knowledge about this condition.

MILK PRODUCTION

Each mammary gland produces milk independently from the other, and milk volume can vary greatly between left and right sides. Nearly 75% of nursing parents report significant milk-production differences between the two sides. Even if there is a large difference in size, the glands will usually return to prepregnancy size after weaning.

BASIC INGREDIENTS NEEDED FOR MILK PRODUCTION include the following, and if any are missing, milk production may be compromised.

   Sufficient glandular tissue

   + Enough intact nerve pathways and milk ducts

   + Adequate normal hormones and receptors

   + Adequate lactation-critical nutrients

+ Frequent and effective milk removal/transfer and mammary stimulation

+ No lactation inhibitors

= Ample milk production

AMOUNT OF GLANDULAR TISSUE   This is not a common issue, but some parents lack enough milk-producing glands to achieve full milk production.

Mammary hypoplasia or insufficient glandular tissue (or IGT, p. 41) refers to a lack of the glandular tissue needed to achieve full milk production. A few areas of glandular tissue may be felt in a mostly soft gland. The glands may appear widely spaced (more than 1.5 inches or 4 cm apart), with large differences in size (asymmetry); tubular, irregular, or cone-shaped glands rather than rounded, and bulbous-looking areolae. No tissue changes or growth may occur during pregnancy.

Never assume from mammary shape or lack of changes during pregnancy that a parent will not produce enough milk. Consider parents with these physical traits at risk for insufficient milk production, and monitor baby's weight closely during the early weeks after birth.

Hyperplastic (or hypertrophic) mammary glands are the opposite issue: too much glandular tissue or glandular overdevelopment, which may occur in one side or both. Not all types of hyperplasia cause problems. See p. 42 for one that does: gestational gigantomastia.

CONDITION OF NERVES AND MILK DUCTS   Breast or chest surgery or injury (p. 43) can damage nerves and milk ducts, possibly affecting milk production and milk ejection. In rare cases, prolonged, severe engorgement can damage a gland enough to affect milk production. With nerve damage, the parent may lose some or all sensation in the nipple and areola. If the parent can feel both touch and temperature on the nipple and areola, problems with milk ejection are unlikely. When nerve pathways are damaged, milk ejection may only be possible with the help of techniques like mental imagery, acupressure, the use of a synthetic oxytocin nasal spray, or by applying pressure to the gland.

HORMONAL LEVELS AND RECEPTOR FUNCTION   Except for the early days after birth, hormones are not usually a major factor in milk production. But if a parent's hormonal levels deviate enough from the normal range, this can lead to too much or too little milk. The parent's body response to a hormone is partly determined by the number of receptors for that hormone and how many of them are **upregulated** (activated and responsive) and whether the hormone and its receptors, like a lock and key, work together well.

During pregnancy, high blood levels of estrogen, placental lactogen, prolactin, and progesterone stimulate the growth of the milk-making tissue. Insulin and thyroid hormone also play a role. This growth of glandular tissue and the production of colostrum, beginning mid-pregnancy, is called **secretory differentiation** or **lactogenesis I**. Progesterone inhibits milk production until delivery.

After birth, the delivery of the placenta triggers the hormonal chain of events that causes milk production to rapidly increase, called **secretory activation**, **lactogenesis II**, or the milk "coming in" or "coming to volume." Secretion of placental lactogen ends with the delivery of the placenta. Estrogen and progesterone blood levels also fall quickly and stay low for the first months of nursing, while prolactin levels start high and then decrease over the weeks but remain higher overall (Table 11.1). Other hormones that affect lactation are cortisol, thyroid-stimulating hormone, and insulin.

During the first 2 weeks after birth, the prolactin response to mammary stimulation is at its peak. With every milk removal (nursing or milk expression), the nursing parent's blood prolactin levels rise sharply. Due to this intense hormonal response, during the early weeks, it takes the least amount of mammary stimulation to boost milk production and upregulate prolactin receptors. The number of prolactin receptors upregulated during this time may influence the peak long-term milk production for that baby. During the early months, blood prolactin levels are at their highest about 10 to 15 minutes after the end of a nursing or pump session and return to baseline levels within 3 hours.

After the first 2 weeks, less prolactin is released during mammary stimulation, requiring more time and effort to boost milk production. As the weeks and months pass, even with ample milk production, baseline prolactin blood levels and prolactin surges after nursing gradually decrease. Even with this decreased response, the prolactin levels of nursing parents are higher than non-nursing parents, but the difference is not nearly as great (Table 11.1).

Hormonal disruption during puberty from health or metabolic issues may lead to abnormal mammary development and low milk production after birth. Health conditions that affect hormonal levels and potentially milk production include obesity, diabetes, insulin resistance, and thyroid issues.

Table 11.1. Prolactin Levels Expected During Full or Nearly Full Lactation

Stage	Baseline (ng/mL)	After Nursing (ng/mL)
During childbearing years (not lactating or pregnant)	2-20	n/a
Third trimester of pregnancy	150-250	n/a
Pregnant at term	200-500	n/a
First 10 days after birth	200	400
1 month	100-140	260-310
2 months	100-140	195-240
4 months	60-80	120-155
6 months	50-65	80-100
7-12 months	30-40	45-80

Adapted from Marasco & West,. (2020). *Making More Milk*, New York: McGraw-Hill.

Emotions and the baby's touch have a hormonal effect on milk production. Early skin-to-skin contact after birth can enhance early milk production, as can early hand expression after nursing.

LACTATION-CRITICAL NUTRIENTS A perfect diet is not necessary for making adequate, good-quality milk (p. 237), but lactation requires a minimum of 1,500 to 1,800 calories per day. Anecdotally some parents report an increase in milk production when they eat more, so if milk production is low, consider making the following dietary adjustments: more protein, calcium, omega-3 fatty acids, and fiber. If the nursing parent is deficient in these nutrients, consider supplements: vitamin B_{12} (especially in vegan parents), iron (if anemic), zinc, and iodine.

A history of an eating disorder, weight-loss surgery, or nutrient malabsorption conditions like Crohn's disease, or other health issues should be considered red flags of possible nutrient deficiencies.

HOW WELL AND OFTEN MILK IS REMOVED is the primary driver of milk production after delivery. Milk production is usually best regulated when the baby drives the process by feeding on cue. Unless there are problems, efforts to manipulate the baby's feeding pattern are more likely to lead to milk-production challenges.

Degree of Mammary Fullness is one of the two main dynamics affecting the rate of milk production. Simply put: drained glands make milk faster and full glands make milk slower. As the mammary gland fills with milk, this slows its rate of milk production due to:

- FIL. As the volume of milk in the gland increases, so does the amount of the substance known as "feedback inhibitor of lactation" (FIL), possibly serotonin, which slows milk production.
- Internal pressure from the milk also slows milk production by reducing blood flow to the gland and compressing the milk-making cells, temporarily slowing production.

A nursing parent with overabundant milk production can slow it by restricting baby to one side for longer stretches of time (p. 203). The opposite is also true. Draining the glands more often and more fully, cause milk to be produced faster.

On average, nursing babies take 67% of the milk in the glands, leaving 33%. If a growing baby wants more milk, he nurses more often and drains the glands more fully, taking a larger percentage of the available milk, which speeds the rate of milk production. When baby nurses on each side more than once, by draining each side more fully, this causes milk production to speed even more.

Frequent and effective milk removal triggers three physical processes that speed milk production.

- **Short-term:** It minimizes FIL and pressure in the gland, speeding milk-making.
- **Medium-term:** Faster milk production speeds the metabolic activity of key enzymes used in milk-making to make milk even faster.
- **Long-term:** Over time, it stimulates the growth of more milk-making tissue, which increases the speed of milk production.

Storage Capacity is the second main milk-production dynamic, which is defined as the maximum volume of milk available to the baby when the mammary gland is at its fullest time of the day. It is unrelated to mammary size (which is mostly determined by amount of fatty tissue) and differs among parents and from one baby to the next. The range of storage capacity measured so far is 74 to 606 g (2.6 to 20.5 oz.).

Storage capacity determines how long it takes for mammary glands to become full enough of milk for the rate of milk production to slow. Parents with both large and small storage capacities can make ample milk for their babies, but their feeding patterns may vary greatly. The parent with a large storage capacity can hold more milk, so the baby may be satisfied with one side at most feeds, feed fewer times per day overall, and sleep longer at night. The parent with a small storage capacity holds less milk, so to consume the same daily milk intake, the baby may take both sides at each feed, nurse more times per day, and feed more often at night.

Simple observations can provide clues to a parent's storage capacity, such as volume of milk expressed at a session. Exclusively pumping parents with a large storage capacity who do not pump at night may express 300 mL (10 oz.) or more at their first morning pump session. The exclusively pumping parent with a small storage capacity, on the other hand, may awaken before morning with mammary discomfort, yet be unable to express more than 89 to 150 mL (3 to 5 oz.).

LACTATION INHIBITORS include lactation-suppressing "dry-up" medications, such as bromocriptine and cabergoline. Even with all other milk-making dynamics working well, exposure to these drugs can undermine milk production. Other medications (estrogen, progesterone, testosterone), vitamins (B_6 in large doses), and herbs (sage, parsley, peppermint) may slow milk production in some users but not others. In cases of low milk production when no other contributing factors are identified, ask about their use.

No studies yet directly linked low milk production to the use of alcohol, tobacco, or cannabis. But alcohol consumption reduces milk intake and delays milk ejection. Nicotine reduces prolactin and oxytocin levels. Use of tobacco and cannabis are linked to shorter nursing duration (see p. 243-246).

COMMON MISCONCEPTIONS ABOUT MILK PRODUCTION include:

- Drinking more fluids increases milk production (not found)
- A less-than-perfect diet will decrease milk production (not unless it is severely restricted)

Common "false alarms" that parents misinterpret as signs of low milk production include:

- Baby wants to feed frequently (normal in young babies)
- Can't express much milk (milk expression is a learned skill)
- Glands feel softer and less full (happens naturally several weeks after birth)
- No milk leakage (some parents never leak)
- Don't feel the milk ejection (some never do)
- Expressed milk looks thin (this is normal)

- Baby will take a bottle after nursing (not a sign of milk issues)

Even if a family's concerns seem unwarranted, acknowledge them and discuss reliable ways to gauge adequate milk production.

MILK PRODUCTION NORMS In mid-pregnancy birthing parents begin producing colostrum, which is limited in volume by high blood levels of progesterone. No link has been found between colostrum leakage and milk production later.

MAKING MILK IN THE FIRST YEAR AND BEYOND After delivery of the placenta, within 30 to 40 hours after birth, milk production begins to increase dramatically. The average volume of colostrum consumed per nursing session on the first day of life is 5 to 7 mL. Mean daily milk intake among nursing newborns during the first 4 days of life are:

- Day 1: 56 mL
- Day 2: 185 mL
- Day 3: 393 mL
- Day 4: 580 mL

Birthing parents who nursed a previous baby are about 1 day ahead of first-time nursing parents, who produced about 3 to 4 ounces (89-142 mL) less milk on Day 3. Nursing parents' perception of milk increase after birth (feelings of fullness and heaviness) is usually reliable. Feelings of fullness usually last several weeks after delivery.

How early, often, and effectively milk is removed after birth is the main driver of milk production.

- ***Early.*** After premature birth, those who began expressing milk within 1 hour of delivery expressed significantly more milk at the first expression and over the entire first 6 weeks.
- ***Often.*** During the first 2 weeks, the more times each day milk is effectively removed via nursing or expressing, the faster milk is produced. Suggest at least 8 milk removals per day.
- ***Effective.*** Early and frequent milk removals will not stimulate faster milk-making unless the milk is removed effectively. During nursing, ineffective feeding may occur if baby has a shallow latch. With exclusive pumping, hands-on techniques to remove milk more fully boosted milk yields by nearly 50% compared with using the pump alone.

During the first 2 to 3 weeks, the milk changes gradually from colostrum to transitional milk to mature milk. Colostrum, transitional milk, and mature milk are not distinct types of milk. They reflect a continuum of changes as the mammary gland makes more milk and more water is drawn into the alveoli, diluting the components of the milk.

At birth, a steep drop in blood progesterone levels with stable blood prolactin levels causes the spaces between the milk-making cells (lactocytes) to close, so the milk and its components can no longer leak out of the alveoli. Because more of the milk stays in the alveoli, more fat, lactose, citrate, and potassium remain there and their concentration increases. The immunoprotective proteins, sodium, and chloride decrease in concentration.

Colostrum may be clear, golden, white, and other colors. As many as 24% of nursing parents have blood in their colostrum ("rusty-pipe syndrome," p. 39). It may appear very thick or it may be thinner.

Over the first 2 to 3 weeks, as the milk undergoes these changes, the milk becomes whiter and thinner-looking. Babies 2 to 3 weeks old usually take about 2 to 3 ounces (59 to 89 mL) during nursing sessions, taking daily about 20 to 25 ounces (591 to 750 mL) of milk. To increase milk production to meet their growing needs, babies often have periods of longer, more frequent feeds, which are sometimes termed "growth spurts" or "frequency days."

During weeks 4 and 5, most babies continue to take more milk per feed as their stomachs grow in size. An average nursing is about 3 to 4 ounces (89 to 118 mL), with daily milk intake increasing to an average of about 25 to 30 oz. (750 to 887 mL) per day. Nursing babies' milk intake increases rapidly during the first 3 weeks of life, increasing slightly during Weeks 4 and 5, and staying relatively stable from Weeks 5 to 6 until a decline occurs when baby begins consuming other foods.

Normal milk volumes cover a wide range. What's important is not the exact volume of milk baby consumes per day, but baby's weight gain and growth. In thriving nursing babies, daily milk intake may vary threefold, from 15.5 to 43 oz. (440 to 1220 g).

Milk composition varies among nursing parents. Milk fat content may vary as much as tenfold, averaging just under 18 kcal/oz. The type of milk fat also varies, depending on the parent's diet (p. 237). Nursing parents who eat fish regularly have higher levels of omega-3 fatty acids in their milk than those who don't eat fish. Milk metabolites and its microbiome vary by country of residence. Early research suggests that milk composition also may vary by sex of the baby.

Milk composition changes over time. One example is the ratio of whey proteins to casein proteins. During the first month, when the baby's digestive system is most immature, the ratio of whey (which is easier and faster to digest) to casein in human milk is about 90:10. By about 6 weeks, it is 80:20. At 6 months, it is 60:40. In later lactation, it is 50:50. There are also day and night variations in milk melatonin levels, with melatonin (linked to ease of falling asleep) levels in milk higher at night than during the day.

During the second year and beyond, the milk older babies receive during nursing is significantly higher in fat than the milk received by younger nursing babies. Over time, there is an increase in the concentrations of total protein, lactoferrin, lysozyme, IgA, sodium, and oligosaccharides (a milk sugar that feeds the "good bacteria" in a baby's gut). But from 11 to 17 months there is a decrease in zinc and calcium. After 18 months, milk fat and protein content increase and carbohydrate content decreases. Between 24 and 48 months, the level of fat, protein, and carbohydrates remain stable, with the calories in the milk primarily coming from fat, as opposed to carbohydrates during early infancy.

Milk volumes vary after 1 year, depending on how often the baby nurses. In an Australian study, at 15 months, daily milk production was between 95 and 315 mL (3 to 10 oz.) per day. In Zaire at 30 months (where nursing older babies is the norm), milk production averaged 300 mL (10 oz.) per day.

With exclusive nursing, mammary tissue is densest at its peak between 1 and 6 months. As the baby starts other foods, density decreases significantly between 6 and 9 months. By 15 months, the glands return to their prepregnancy size, even when they are producing significant volumes of milk.

With weaning, milk production stops and the glandular tissue involutes. As milk production ends, the milk increases in sodium, chloride, fat, and protein and decreases in lactose and potassium. During involution, first the milk-making cells (lactocytes) die, and the fat cells in the glands differentiate to fill the spaces they occupied. Finally, the blood vessels recede. After involution, parents can often express drops of milk weeks, months, even years after their baby stopped nursing.

MAKING MILK FOR TWINS, TRIPLETS, AND MORE By nursing on cue, most nursing parents can produce enough milk for two, three, even four babies. Parents who give birth to multiple babies have the advantage of more placenta, which releases more mammary-stimulating hormones to grow more glandular tissue during pregnancy.

Each family needs to work out their own way of managing nursing multiples, because there is no one right way. As a time-saver, some prefer to always nurse two babies at once, while others nurse them separately at least some of the time. One baby may nurse more often than the other(s).

If one baby does not nurse as effectively as his sibling(s), nursing both babies together allows the more effective baby to better stimulate milk ejection, and the faster flow of milk may help the less effective baby get more milk more quickly.

Which baby gets which side when? Some parents nurse with no particular plan, offering whichever side feels fuller to whichever baby seems hungriest. Others keep each baby on the same side for an entire day, alternating sides every day. Some parents of twins assign each baby a particular side at every feed that never varies. If one baby nurses less effectively, alternating sides ensures both sides are well stimulated to maintain milk production.

Tracking nursing is a good idea at least the first few weeks. This can be done digitally or in writing. Track number of daily nursing sessions for each baby along with diaper output. If the babies gain weight well, no record-keeping is needed. If a baby is not gaining weight well, try recording frequency and length of feeds and diaper output for a few days. Life with multiples is hectic, and if a baby is placid or sleepy, he may not be nursing often or long enough to meet his needs.

Handling night nursing may be easier if the parent finds well-supported feeding positions that allow resting during nursing (see Chapter 1). Multiples may sleep in one crib or bed because they sleep better when they are touching. If a crib is used, for easy access at night, consider keeping it in the parent's room and fastening it to the side of the parent's bed, adjusting the mattress levels to the same height, and removing the side rail closest to the adult bed.

If due to health issues one or more babies aren't nursing or aren't nursing effectively, discuss milk expression (see Chapter 12).

Nursing multiples does not have to be all or nothing; partial nursing is almost always a better option than no nursing.

LGBTQ NURSING   The same basic milk-making principles apply to LGBTQ families as to cisgender families.

SAME-SEX FEMALE PARTNERS   If same-sex female partners plan to co-nurse, breastfeeding may happen in different ways

- Both women give birth within a short time of each other and breastfeed both babies.
- One partner gives birth and the other relactates or induces lactation.

- Neither woman gives birth, and the couple adopts a baby or the baby is born via surrogacy, with both women inducing lactation.

TRANSGENDER WOMEN were assigned as male at birth but identify as female and transitioned to female. Their transition may involve undergoing hormone therapy to suppress male traits and enhance female traits. In one reported case (at **bit.ly/BA2-BFTransWoman**), a transgender woman exclusively nursed for 6 weeks. She received female hormone therapy for 6 years and developed breast tissue before her partner (who did not want to breastfeed) became pregnant. See the article for the details on how hormones were used to prepare for nursing. During the pregnancy, she pumped a few times each day. After 3 months of pumping, she produced 8 oz (240 mL) per day. After the baby was born, she breastfed exclusively for 6 weeks.

A transgender woman may produce more milk if she has previously undergone female hormone therapy. Another option is following the induced lactation protocols on p. 275. If milk production is not the top priority, she may consider **dry nursing**, for parents who produce no milk but want to experience nursing.

TRANSGENDER MEN were assigned as female at birth but identify as male and transitioned to male. As with transgender women, the transition from female to male may involve hormone treatments and surgery. "Top surgery" (p. 49) involves the removal of mammary tissue. Not all transgender men have this surgery. Some bind their mammary tissue to appear more masculine, which needs to be done carefully to avoid plugged ducts and mastitis.

In some families, transgender men get pregnant, give birth, and some nurse (or **chestfeed**) their babies. Experiencing the biologically female experiences of pregnancy, mammary growth, birth, and nursing may be stressful for some, leading to a type of distress or anxiety known as **gender dysphoria.** Because transgender men fall on different points of the gender spectrum, how pregnancy and nursing fit into their gender identity will vary from person to person.

The use of male hormones, such as testosterone, which enhances male traits such as facial hair, may also suppress mammary growth and milk production. In some cases, transgender men prefer to nurse in private and if milk production is less than full, use a nursing supplementer or supplement in other ways. For details, see **bit.ly/BA2-Transmasculine**.

LOW MILK PRODUCTION is not always the cause of a nursing baby's slow weight gain. Some health problems cause babies to gain weight slowly even with ample milk intake (p. 120).

DETERMINING MILK PRODUCTION   Aside from the baby's weight gain (which if in the expected range is a sure sign he's getting enough milk), two other strategies can be used to evaluate milk production.

- Test-weighing is a reliable gauge of milk intake when a scale accurate to 2 g is used. Because feeding volumes vary by time of day, one test-weight does not reveal baby's 24-hour milk intake. It can, however, rule out ineffective nursing at that feed and low milk production. Only if it's done at every feed over 24 hours, will it show if baby's nursing is consistently effective.

- Milk expression can rule out low milk production as a cause of slow weight gain if the nursing parent can express ample milk at several sessions. (The first session alone is not enough, because milk may accumulate in the mammary gland.) But milk expression cannot confirm low milk production, because some parents do not express milk effectively, especially at first.

Commercial devices that claim to measure milk intake are now available, but their accuracy has not yet been validated. And they may be even less reliable when milk production is low.

INHIBITED MILK INCREASE AFTER BIRTH   Milk production is considered delayed when the nursing parent notices no mammary changes or fullness by about 72 hours after delivery. A delay may be due to hormonal or mammary issues and/or ineffective milk removal, such as:

Parent factors

- First time nursing
- Obesity, overweight, excessive weight gain
- Mammary/nipple issues (hypoplasia, anatomy issues, previous surgery/injury)
- Health conditions (diabetes, PCOS, pregnancy hypertension, prolactin resistance, pituitary issues, gestational ovarian theca lutein cysts, history of infertility)
- Medications that suppress or inhibit lactation

Baby Factors

- Conditions that reduce nursing effectiveness (birth injury, variations in oral or airway anatomy, health or neurological issues)

Birth-related factors

- Long, traumatic, or stressful birth
- Preterm delivery
- Placental issues, including retained placenta
- Blood loss of ≥1000 mL (>2 pints)

Post-delivery factors

- A late start to nursing or infrequent milk removal
- Separation (little or no skin-to-skin or body contact)

LOW MILK PRODUCTION IN THE EARLY WEEKS In addition to the previous factors at birth, other factors contribute to low milk production during the early weeks.

Less-Than-Optimal Nursing Dynamics

- Shallow latch
- Too little active nursing time (scheduled, limited, or infrequent sessions)
- Less-than-optimal milk removals, delaying milk increase
- Supplementing baby with other liquids or foods

Baby Factors

- Temperament (placid/sleepy, difficult to settle for feeds)
- Health issues (cardiac defect, cystic fibrosis, other genetic or metabolic disorders)

Parent Factors

- Health or medication issues (serious illness, drugs/herbs that suppress or are incompatible with lactation, conditions that affect the parent's hormonal levels)

STRATEGIES FOR MAKING MORE MILK With low milk production, the first priority is to feed the baby. The second is to safeguard the milk production. Supplementing baby with extra milk boosts nursing effectiveness. When a baby is underfed, this can lead to poor feeding.

With an ineffectively nursing baby, milk expression may be necessary to safeguard milk production. The number of effective expressions per day needed will depend on the baby's age, the volume of supplement needed, and how far the parent is from full milk production. Finding the cause(s) of low milk production will help determine the most effective strategies for making more milk.

The most common cause of low milk production is too little time spent actively nursing. But if low milk production is caused by ineffective nursing or physical issues in the parent, increasing the time spent nursing may not necessarily solve the problem. In nursing parents with hormonal issues, such as thyroid imbalance, polycystic ovary syndrome (PCOS), and other physical conditions, medical treatment may be the best milk-enhancing strategy. (See Table 11.2 for medical tests to determine possible hormonal causes.) Rather than testing for all possible hormonal causes, suggest the parent's provider order tests based on reasonable suspicions. If milk production is compromised by surgery or insufficient glandular tissue, using the basic strategies described in the next section may not be enough to stimulate full milk production, but they may increase baby's daily intake of human milk.

If the baby's feeding effectiveness is compromised by tongue-tie, airway abnormality, neurological impairment, prematurity, or other health conditions, treating or addressing the baby's health issue directly while using milk expression to boost production may be the best option.

Offer to help the family formulate a daily plan that will maximize the time spent boosting milk production while giving them the time needed to nurture their relationship with their baby, care for other children, and handle any other responsibilities.

Using Basic Dynamics to Boost Milk Production When considering strategies to boost milk production, start by asking parents:

- How many times each day does baby nurse and do you express milk?

- At each session, about how long on each side does baby nurse or is milk expressed? Does baby nurse effectively? Has this changed recently? Are you single or double pumping?

- What is the longest stretch between milk removals? Stretches longer than about 6 to 8 hours may cause production to slow over time.

- If expressing milk, what method or pump do you use? Ask for the brand name and model of any pump(s) used and if pump fit was checked.

- What else might be affecting milk production? Meds? Previous breast or chest surgery?

Table 11.2 Tests for Hormonal Causes of Low Milk Production

	Reason to Test	**Tests to Consider**	**Levels**
Prolactin	Insufficient milk with normal mammary tissue, no other risk factors History of excess blood loss, pituitary tumor, head injury	Test levels before and 10-15 min. after nursing to check for prolactin surge	See Table 10.1
Testosterone	Excess hair on face or body, thinning head hair, and acne are signs of excess male hormones that tests may not find	Bioavailable testosterone	If elevated, an ultrasound can confirm presence of gestational ovarian theca lutein cysts
Thyroid	Personal or family history of thyroid issues Extreme fatigue (hypothyroidism) Weight gain (hypothyroidism) Weight loss and jittery (hyperthyroidism)	TSH T4 T3 levels may reveal a T3 to T4 conversion issue: TPO antibody test may reveal a problem before it becomes obvious	Ideal: 0.5-2.5 Okay: 0.3-3.5
Retained placenta	No milk increase in 1st week Vaginal birth in which tension was applied to umbilical cord during delivery of placenta	hCG (beta human chorionic gonadotropin)	High levels may indicate retained placenta
Insulin resistance	Family history of diabetes Borderline glucose tolerance test or gestational diabetes High-birth-weight baby	Hemoglobin A1C 2-hr glucose tolerance test	

Adapted from Marasco & West,. (2020). *Making More Milk*, New York: McGraw-Hill.

Help parents formulate a daily plan that's not overwhelming. Encourage them to revisit the plan if some aspect is an issue. Focus on aspects of the plan that are working and jettison those that aren't.

To make milk faster, it's vital to drain the glands more often and more fully.

- Help baby latch deeper to transfer milk more effectively.
- At each feed, offer each side more than once.
- While nursing, use breast compression or alternate massage.
- Nurse more times each day, for example, help the baby latch while in a light sleep.
- Avoid soothers and restrict all sucking to nursing.
- Use milk expression to drain the gland more fully and/or more often.

If the baby is not nursing effectively or will not nurse more often, express milk after nursing or between feeds (whichever parents prefer), using massage and compression. The following intensive pumping strategies may help boost milk production faster.

- Power pumping: put the pump in an area the parent passes often and is comfortable sitting or standing. Over several days, every time the pump is passed (as often as every 45 to 60 minutes), pump for 5 to 10 minutes, pumping into the same bottle with the same pumping pieces without cleaning them for 4 to 6 hours (how long milk is safe at room temperature). Combine and cool the milk and wash the pump parts. Use only with healthy term babies.
- Cluster pumping: spend an hour pumping 10 minutes on and 10 minutes off.
- Pump like crazy: pump every hour for 5 to 10 minutes from 8 am to 9 pm or another convenient period.

Keep the longest stretch between milk removal no more than 6 to 8 hours. Stretches that are too long (usually at night) can slow milk production.

Other strategies that can be used with these basics include breast massage, acupuncture and acupressure, chiropractic, mental imagery, music, and audio relaxation techniques.

Galactogogues are any substance—drug, herb, food, drink—that speeds milk production.

Some were passed down by word of mouth. A few have been scientifically studied. Galactogogues alone are likely to have little effect on milk production. They are most likely to boost production by a small to moderate amount when used in combination with frequent and effective milk removal.

Galactogogues are not all equally effective in all cases of low milk production. When considering a plant-based preparation, consult with a trained specialist and ask the user's healthcare provider to review its safety in light of their health history.

In most cases, if a galactogogue is going to work, it takes at least 2-5 days to see results. If a week goes by with no change, it likely won't work. If it is used to boost a temporary dip in milk production from less-frequent nursing, it may be taken short term and gradually reduced over a couple of weeks. In more difficult cases, a galactogogue may be needed long term.

The drugs domperidone and metoclopramide are used "off-label" as galactogogues, because one of their side effects is increased blood prolactin levels. These drugs boosted production only about 1 oz. per day in parents exclusively pumping for babies in the NICU.

Domperidone (Motilium™) is used to treat nausea and reflux disease. It prevents the release of dopamine which increases blood prolactin levels. Unlike metoclopramide, domperidone does not cross the blood-brain barrier, so central nervous system side effects are less likely. Very little passes into the milk, so domperidone is compatible with nursing. Due to serious reactions in chemotherapy patients who received high doses of domperidone by IV, the U.S. FDA advises it not be prescribed for nursing parents. Women are at higher risk than men of its more serious side effects, and the risk of side effects is higher if the user is obese or has a history of cardiac arrythmias.

The Academy of Breastfeeding Medicine (ABM) recommends any parent considering it be screened for a history of cardiac arrhythmia, and if there's concern, do an EKG. It is not recommended if the nursing parent is using any drugs that increase its effect, such as fluconazole and erythromycin.

If domperidone is used, take the smallest effective dose for the shortest time possible. Recommended dose is 30 to 60 mg per day. Typically, it takes 2 to 4 weeks for it to achieve its peak effect.

Metoclopramide (Reglan™ or Maxeran™) is usually taken 10 to 15 mg 3 times per day (30 to 45 mg per day total). It was not found effective when taken during the first 96 hours post-birth, when the parent's blood prolactin levels should be naturally high.

Metoclopramide crosses the blood-brain barrier and may cause depression, so it is not recommended for those with a history of depression. Its other side effects (restlessness, irritability, headache, fatigue) increase when taken longer than a month, which is not recommended. Although compatible with lactation, it puts parents at risk for **tardive dyskinesia**, a neurological problem involving involuntary movements that may become permanent in a small percentage of those who take it.

Weaning gradually from domperidone and metoclopramide is suggested to avoid a steep drop in milk production. To minimize this drop, taper off these drugs gradually by 10 mg per week.

Metformin (Glucophage™) is another drug that may improve milk production in some lactating parents by sensitizing insulin receptors in those with insulin resistance.

Plant-based galactogogues have been used to increase milk production throughout human history. But they need to be used with caution, as some contain the same active ingredients used in prescription medications, which may affect the nursing baby and interact with other herbs or drugs. They should be taken only under the guidance of someone with expertise in their use, such as a certified herbalist, practitioner of traditional Chinese medicine, or a naturopath. In the U.S. no regulatory agency monitors herbal preparations, and their quality can vary widely. Some were found to contain dangerous levels of the heavy metals mercury and lead.

Herbal preparations are available in powders, tablets, capsules, tinctures, and teas. A parent may respond better to one form than another and to lower or higher doses. With teas, the amount of active ingredient increases with longer steeping.

Fenugreek (*Trigonella foenum-graecum*) is used in seed form and is the most common herbal galactogogue in the West. Doses high enough to boost milk production are usually three capsules three to four times per day or about 6,000 mg per day. It can be taken alone or with other herbal galactogogues or conventional medications. It usually takes 24 to 72 hours to notice a boost in milk production. Fenugreek is generally recognized as safe (GRAS) by the U.S. FDA but research on its efficacy in increasing milk production is mixed. In animal research, fenugreek in high doses lowered blood level of thyroid hormone T3 in rats. For this reason, it is not a good choice for those with low thyroid or at risk of hypothyroidism. As with any other substance, an allergic reaction to fenugreek is possible. Fenugreek may boost milk production in part because it reduces the effects of insulin resistance, so caution is recommended among diabetic nursing parents.

Malunggay (*Moringa oleifera*), is commonly used to boost milk production in the Philippines. Malunggay leaves from the drumstick tree are added to soups or stews. It may be taken as a capsule or in powder form, with 0.5 to 1 teaspoon (5 to 7 g) added to smoothies. Unlike other plant-based galactogogues, many studies (including meta-analyses) are available on its safety (no adverse effects) and efficacy.

Other herbal galactogogues include blessed thistle, goat's rue, alfalfa, fennel, nettle, and shatavari. Not all herbal galactogogues are safe during pregnancy. For more on plant-based galactogogues, their dosages and quality sources, see the book *Making More Milk: The Breastfeeding Guide to Increasing Your Milk Production* by Lisa Marasco and Diana West and their website **lowmilksupply.org**.

In some cultures, specific foods and drinks are recommended to enhance milk production.

- Eastern India: pumpkin, sunflower, and sesame seeds, rice pudding with milk and sugar
- China: foods thought to regulate body warmth and fluids, chicken and seaweed soups, cooked papaya, millet, rice, anise, fennel, dill, cumin, caraway, and ginger
- North America: grains, such as oatmeal, have a reputation for speeding milk production
- Mexico: grain-based drinks containing oats or cornmeal simmered in milk.
- Europe: coffee-substitutes made from roasted grains, especially barley

For more details, see **mother-food.com**.

Some claim that consuming the placenta after birth can improve mood and milk production, but these claims have not been verified. The U.S. CDC recommends against this practice after it received a case report of a baby who acquired a late-onset *Group B Streptococcus agalactiae* (GBS) infection that was eventually traced to the mother's ingestion of placental capsules.

STRATEGIES FOR SUPPLEMENTING THAT ENHANCES MILK-MAKING The volume of supplement needed depends on the baby's age, weight gain, and condition. If the baby is in good condition and an effective nurser, the goal is to strike a delicate balance between giving the least amount of supplement needed while actively nursing as much as possible to stimulate faster milk production. If the baby was underfed, provide as much milk as he wants to boost his energy for effective nursing. For details on supplement choices and volume of milk needed by age, see Table 20.1 on p. 305.

Discuss possible feeding methods and the advantages of using a nursing supplementer to increase mammary stimulation.

Also known as a feeding-tube device, this method provides needed supplement while baby nurses, keeping the baby actively feeding longer to stimulate faster milk production. Its use also eliminates the need to feed the baby again after nursing. Discuss the options and support parents in their choice. The feeding method chosen may depend in part on the level of milk production: close to full production, making some milk, or making little or no milk, as well as the baby's nursing effectiveness. For the pros and cons of each feeding method, see p. 311.

If the baby is supplemented by bottle, encourage the family to use techniques that reinforce nursing. Suggest using a slow-flow teat, and make bottle-feeding more like nursing by holding the baby more upright and the bottle horizontal to keep milk flow manageable.

When full nursing is not an option, discuss partially nursing with supplements. Depending on how much milk-making tissue is present and the nursing dynamics, the parent may find—like the parent inducing lactation—that with frequent nursing, milk production may continue to increase over time. Frequent nursing causes more glandular tissue to grow, so they may eventually be able to eliminate the supplement after solid foods are started or exclusively nurse later babies.

OVERABUNDANT MILK PRODUCTION, also known as oversupply or hyperlactation, is defined as producing so much milk that the lactating parent experiences discomfort and the need to express milk beyond what the normally growing baby takes during nursing. If the parent and baby are happy and comfortable, their situation does not meet this definition and is not a problem. Although some parents are just naturally larger milk producers than others, in the West, over-pumping and attempts to manipulate baby's nursing patterns may contribute to too much milk.

GALACTORRHEA is a condition in which milk production occurs outside the context of pregnancy, birth, and lactation and is usually caused by a health problem or medication. A person with this condition should see a healthcare provider for evaluation. Although some refer to this condition as "overproduction," because nursing is not involved, this is an entirely different category from the overabundant milk production described in this section. Galactorrhea may be a sign of elevated prolactin levels caused by a benign pituitary tumor (adenoma), an overactive thyroid (thyroxicosis), or other health problem. It may occur in people with normal prolactin levels and is a side effect of breast augmentation surgery in less than 1% of cases. Galactorrhea can also be a side effect of some medications, such as tricyclic antidepressants, theophylline, and some contraceptives.

COPING WITH TOO MUCH MILK can be difficult for the baby, especially during the first milk ejection, when milk flow can be very fast.

Baby Struggles with Fast Milk Flow In an attempt to cope with or slow fast flow, baby may pull back, clamp down, or use biting or chewing mouth movements, come on and off during nursing sessions, and/or keep the nipple loosely in his mouth. Some babies fuss during milk ejection, coughing, sputtering, or arching away. Many swallow lots of air when gulping milk, spit up regularly, and pass lots of gas.

To make fast milk flow more manageable for the baby, try:

- Nursing in starter or side-lying positions to give baby more control over milk flow.

- The "milk shake" by spending half a minute before nursing massaging each side like warming modeling clay or kneading dough, only gentler. Massage and compression dislodge some fat sticking to the walls of the alveoli, nearly doubling the milk-fat content, so baby feels full longer.

- Nursing more often, before feeling too full.

- Nursing when the baby is drowsy or sleepy for calmer feeds.

- Frequent burping and breaks so the baby can pace himself.

Rather than offering the baby a full gland, try expressing the first milk ejection to decrease flow and make nursing more manageable. The drawback to this strategy is that on average about 45% of the available milk is expressed with the first milk ejection, so if done regularly, it can boost milk production more. If pumping is necessary for comfort, try pumping slightly less milk over time until it is no longer needed. If pumping 3 oz. (89 mL), stop after 2.5 oz. (75 mL). After a day or two, cut back more.

Baby Struggles with Large Volume, Low-Fat Milk Intake The excess gas many of these babies have is not due to swallowed air (air cannot pass from the stomach into the intestines) but rather by a large volume of low-fat milk passing quickly through baby's intestines. Other symptoms include an unwillingness to nurse while falling asleep and fussy behaviors. If fussiness occurs during feeds, it is most likely due to difficulty coping with fast milk flow. If it occurs after feeds, it may be from taking too much low-fat milk. Other symptoms include not feeding even when obviously hungry, not taking the second side, and an unwillingness to nurse at all (p. 71). Some of these symptoms may also occur in the baby with reflux disease and hypersensitivity, intolerance, or allergy.

Other symptoms of high-milk-volume, low-fat feeds may include:

- Very fast weight gain, with some babies exceeding by double, triple, or more the average weight gain of 2 pounds (900 g) per month during the first 3 months
- Fussiness between feeds
- Explosive green, frothy, or watery stools
- Continuous feeding cues even after taking ample milk

Some of these babies always seem ravenous and unsatisfied despite large weight gains, which convinces many families that their problem is not too much milk but too little. There may be so much milk in a full, overproducing gland that the baby cannot reach the fattier hindmilk. Fat triggers the release in a baby's gut of a peptide called cholecystokinin (CCK), which aids in digestion and in regulation of intake, leaving baby feeling satisfied and relaxed after a full meal. Nursing babies release more CCK than formula-fed babies, but a nursing baby taking mostly high-volume, low-fat milk presumably releases less CCK, leaving baby feeling unsatisfied, despite consuming large volumes.

Why do these babies' stools sometimes appear green, frothy, watery, or contain mucus or blood? The sugar in this high-volume, low-fat milk is mostly lactose (milk sugar), and if the baby receives enough, it may overwhelm his gut, causing watery, frothy, or green stools. Green stools may also be a normal variation or a symptom of the baby's sensitivity to a food or medication received directly or indirectly through mother's milk (p. 238). To determine if the combination of colicky symptoms and mucus or blood in the stools is due to allergy or overabundant milk production alone, consider baby's weight gain, and if way above normal, try slowing milk production (next section) to see if it resolves these symptoms.

Nursing Parent Struggles with Too Much Milk Overabundant milk production can contribute to some or all of the following symptoms in the nursing parent.

- Profuse milk leakage during and between feeds
- Painful nipples from an overwhelmed baby clamping down, chewing, or clenching his jaw to slow milk flow, which may cause pinched, injured, or infected nipples
- Painful mammary glands from "knife-like" milk ejections (especially the first) or fullness and tenderness leading to discomfort, even shortly after nursing.
- Recurring mastitis from regularly occurring and prolonged periods of mammary fullness

STRATEGIES FOR MAKING LESS MILK can eliminate the symptoms of overabundant milk production, but before slowing milk production, be absolutely sure it is the cause of the symptoms, as some of these symptoms may have other causes. A baby with an airway abnormality, tongue-tie, or neurological impairment, for example, might find it difficult to cope with even an average milk flow. Recurring mastitis and painful nursing can occur when a baby latches shallowly or nurses ineffectively for other reasons. Slowing milk production when overproduction is not the cause will not address the real issue and can lead to slow weight gain and low milk production.

Use Baby's Weight Gain and Milk Intake as a Gauge In most cases of overabundant milk production, a baby will gain weight at double, triple, or more of the expected early weight gain of 2 pounds (900 g) per month. Although a small percentage of babies shut down or feed poorly with fast milk flow, if a baby gains weight in the normal range or below, overabundant milk production may not be the cause of the symptoms. No matter what the underlying cause (reflux disease, cystic fibrosis), if a baby is not gaining more weight than average, slowing milk production is unlikely to help.

It may be difficult to convince nursing parents to slow milk production because they may interpret the baby's behaviors as signs of hunger and low—not high—milk production. Pre- and post-feed test weights may help show parents how much milk their baby is consuming to provide objective information that links the baby's unhappiness with too much milk.

Using the "Full Glands Make Milk Slower" Dynamic to Make Less Milk Two different dynamics cause full glands to make milk slower: 1) internal pressure from milk filling the gland, which reduces blood flow and compresses milk-making cells, and 2) higher levels of the substance known as feedback inhibitor of lactation, or FIL, which some think is serotonin in the milk. As the glands become fuller, the combination of increasing FIL and increasing internal pressure cause milk production to become slower and slower. These dynamics can be used to slow milk production without limiting the baby's nursing time with the following strategies.

One side per feed or for 3-hour periods. This involves offering the same side whenever baby wants to nurse within a 3-hour time window, alternating sides every 3 hours. During this 3-hour period, if the unused side feels full, the parent removes (by nursing or expressing) the minimum milk needed to stay comfortable. If that's not enough to decrease symptoms, the following measures may be needed.

Full drainage and block feeding (FDBF) method starts at the beginning of the first treatment day by using an effective breast pump to drain both sides as fully as possible, then latch the baby immediately. Any time during the next 3 hours the baby wants to nurse, offer the same side. After 3 hours, offer the other side at all feeds for the next 3 hours. Depending on the severity of the overproduction, the time blocks can be increased to 4, 6, 8, or even 12 hours. For some, no further use of the pump is needed; for others, draining the glands fully one or two more times helps.

Modified block feeding is a variation of block feeding developed by Christina Smillie, MD, IBCLC to help parents learn to use as their guide their own and their baby's comfort. As above, this approach alternately drains each gland well, and then leaves it full to slow milk production. The parent uses a pump once each day to drain the glands as fully as possible to minimize the risk of mastitis and give the baby access to the high-fat milk for longer intervals between feeds. The parent offers the same side for periods of time, but rather than doing this by the clock, each day is divided into unequal blocks of time based on the family's lifestyle (Table 11.3). Each morning, the parent alternates the side used to avoid uneven stimulation and slow milk production faster. "Morning" starts when the parents are up for the day until lunch, "afternoon" is lunch to dinner, "evening" is dinner to bedtime, and "night" from bedtime until the next morning. These times can vary from day to day. The side listed in each block of time (L=left, R=right) is favored, with the side in parentheses used whenever it feels right. During parents' usual sleeping hours, the parent does what feels right. This strategy is limited to 5 days only to avoid families continuing it for weeks or months. The goal is for parents to learn to nurse by "feel" by responding to their baby and avoid external nursing rules, one cause of overproduction.

Table 11.3. The More Intuitive "Modified Block Feeding" to Slow Milk Production

	Day 1	Day 2	Day 3	Day 4	Day 5:Done
Morning	L (R)	R (L)	L (R)	R (L)	L (R)
Afternoon	R (L)	L (R)	R (L)	L (R)	R (L)
Evening	L (R)	R (L)	L (R)	R (L)	L (R)
Night	Any	Any	Any	Any	Any

(C. Smillie, personal communication, August, 2019)

Using Herbs or Drugs to Slow Milk Production If the previous methods do not resolve the symptoms of overabundant milk production, parents can consult with their healthcare provider about using drugs or herbs ("anti-galactogogues") to slow milk production.

Herbs to slow milk production. As with galactogogues, it's important when using herbal preparations during lactation to consult with someone knowledgeable in their use, such as an herbalist, a practitioner of traditional Chinese medicine, or a naturopath.

- *Sage* (*Sativa officinalis*) should be used with special caution, because its essential oil is toxic, so avoid this form. To slow milk production, steep 1 tablespoon of fresh whole sage leaf or dried herb in one cup (0.25 L) of boiling water for 10 to 15 minutes. Drink 3 to 6 cups per day until milk production has slowed enough to resolve parent's and baby's symptoms, then discontinue. If sage extract is used, take one dose and wait 8 to 12 hours for any side effects (nausea, vomiting, dizziness). If no side effects, consider taking a stronger dose.

- *Other herbs*, like jasmine flowers or peppermint tea can be applied topically. Parsley can be eaten with meals. Or take 1 or 2 strong, sugarless mint candies (like Altoids™) with each nursing or milk expression.

Homeopathic remedies to slow milk production include Lac caninum 30C, Pulsatilla 30C, and Ricinus communis 30C. Trained homeopathic medicine specialists choose among these treatments based on the parent's symptoms. Purchased in pellet form, these remedies are taken 5 pellets under the tongue 2 or 3 times per day and stopped when there is a noticeable decrease in milk production.

Medications to slow milk production include both prescribed and over-the-counter medications.

- *Pseudoephedrine* (Sudafed™) taken as a single 60-mg dose reduces milk production by a mean of 24%. Some respond best when taking one 60 mg dose before bedtime and others have better results when the 60 mg is spread evenly throughout the day. It passes into milk in very low levels (0.4-0.6% of the parental dose), with no side effects reported in nursing babies.

- *Oral contraceptives containing estrogen* taken to reduce overabundant milk production are usually started no earlier than 3 weeks after birth. They may be prescribed in a 4- to 7-day course of low-dose oral contraceptive pills with estrogen and progesterone once per day.

- *Cabergoline* can be taken as a last resort for parent planning to wean. Prescribed as 0.25 twice per day for 1 day, this "dry-up" medicine has fewer side effects than bromocriptine. With its half-life of 63 to 69 hours, parents should "pump and dump" for 5 days after taking it.

DIGITAL RESOURCES

bfmed.org/protocols—Download the Academy of Breastfeeding Medicine Clinical Protocols:

- #9 Galactogogues
- #32 Hyperlactation
- #33 Lactation Care for LGBTQ Patients

bit.ly/BA2-Transmasculine—Open access 2016 survey of 22 transmasculine individuals who gave birth, 16 of whom nursed

firstdroplets.com—Videos by Dr. Jane Morton for parents of term and preterm babies show how to maximize milk production by learning hand expression before birth and using it after birth.

lowmilksupply.org—An online resource created by the authors of the book, *Making More Milk*, it includes strategies for boosting low milk production, including galactogogues.

MobiMotherhood.org—A website for parents experiencing nursing challenges such as low milk production. MOBI stands for "mothers overcoming breastfeeding issues."

CHAPTER 12 MILK EXPRESSION AND STORAGE

MILK EXPRESSION BASICS

How often lactating parents express milk and their reasons for doing so affect nursing outcomes in different ways. For example, learning to hand express during the last month of a low-risk pregnancy is linked to greater breastfeeding self-confidence and fewer formula supplements in the hospital. Occasional pumping at home increases nursing duration. But pumping often or exclusively shortens it. In many parts of the world, nearly all nursing parents plan to pump after birth, even in countries with paid parental leave.

The most common reasons parents give for expressing milk is to provide feeds for their baby when they're apart or having latching struggles, to boost milk production, and to keep themselves comfortable.

HOW MUCH MILK TO EXPECT when expressing depends on the following factors.

- Practice time with the method, because milk expression is a learned skill that involves conditioning the parent's body to respond to the expression method like a nursing baby. The response is as much psychological as it is physical. At first, expect to express drops.

- Baby's age, because the volume of milk available to express varies by stage of lactation. The first month milk production ramps up from very little to full production. Between 1 and 6 months, production stays fairly stable. When solids are started around 6 months, it decreases.

- Exclusively nursing or not, because when a baby receives other foods or drinks, less milk is produced, so less is available to express. If about half of baby's milk intake comes from nursing, expect to express about half the milk of an exclusively nursing parent.

- Time elapsed since the last milk removal affects volume expressed, because the longer the parent waits to express milk, the greater the milk yield—to a point. On average, if parents whose baby is exclusively nursing express between regular nursing sessions, expect to express about half a feed. If parents express for a missed feed, expect to express a full feed. See Table 12.1 for average feeding volumes by age.

- Storage capacity affects the volume of milk available. Parents with a larger storage capacity usually express more milk at a session than those with a smaller storage capacity (p. 18).

- Time of day matters. Most parents express more milk in the morning than later in the day.

- Pump settings and fit affect milk yields. In general, pumps that offer more combinations of vacuum and speed pump more milk, because users can tailor their setting to their body's response. A good pump fit (p. 326) is vital when pumping often. A too-small nipple tunnel can damage nipples and slow milk flow. A too-large nipple tunnel can cause discomfort. Unlike nursing and hand expression, with regular pumping, nipple size increases, so pump fit can change over time.

- Emotional state, such as upset, frustration, and anger blocks milk ejection. If milk yields go down when a parent feels emotional, take a break and try expressing later.

- Whether or not hands-on pumping techniques are used affects milk yield. The use of compression and massage boost milk yields by nearly 50%. For details, see p. 211.

Table 12.1. Average Feeding Volume by Age

Baby's Age	Average Milk Per Feed	Average Milk Intake Per Day
First week after Day 4	1-2 oz. (30-59 mL)	10-20 oz. (300-600 mL)
Weeks 2 and 3	2-3 oz. (59-89 mL)	15-25 oz. (450-750 mL)
Month 1-6	3-4 oz. (89-118 mL)	25-30 oz. (750-887 mL)

Adapted from Kent, J. C., Gardner, H., & Geddes, D. T. (2016). Breastmilk production in the first 4 weeks after birth of term infants. *Nutrients, 8*(12) and Kent, J. C., Hepworth, A. R., Sherriff, J. L., et al. (2013). Longitudinal changes in breastfeeding patterns from 1 to 6 months of lactation. *Breastfeeding Medicine, 8*, 401-407.

VOLUME OF MILK EXPRESSED AND BOTTLE-FEEDING
If a baby takes more milk from a bottle than a parent can express at a session, this is not necessarily a sign of low milk production. Many babies take more milk from a bottle than during a nursing session. Unless paced bottle-feeding techniques are used (p. 312), this may be in part because the bottle provides a more consistent milk flow, which can override a baby's appetite control mechanism and lead to overfeeding. During nursing, milk flow varies with milk ejection, and babies typically consume less milk during direct nursing. Unless there are other signs of low milk production, taking more milk from the bottle does not necessarily indicate a problem.

UNEVEN MILK YIELDS It is more common for one side to yield more milk than the other, and these differences are often significant. Before assuming this is normal, first check the pump fit, as one nipple may be larger and need a different size nipple tunnel. But what matters to the baby is getting enough milk overall, not whether she gets the same volume from both sides. Some differences in milk output and production may be due to usage (if baby or parent favors one side during nursing). Or one side may simply be a naturally larger milk producer. If parents are concerned about appearing lopsided, both sides will likely return to their original size after weaning.

MILK EJECTION DURING EXPRESSION is critical for effective milk removal. Without milk ejection, at most only about a half ounce (15mL) can be expressed, with most milk staying in the gland. On average, during nursing it takes about a minute for milk ejection to occur, but during the first few times milk is expressed, it may take longer as parents condition their body to the feel of the method. Most parents average 3 to 4 milk ejections per nursing session., and they should have a comparable number while pumping. With more milk ejections come higher milk yields. But the law of diminishing returns applies. On average, during the first milk ejection parents express a little less than half of their available milk. As the volume of milk in the gland decreases, milk flow slows, and less milk is expressed with each subsequent milk ejection (Table 12.2).

Table 12.2. Average Volume of Milk Expressed During Each Milk Ejection

Milk ejection	Average volume of milk expressed
1st	54 mL (1.8 oz.)
2nd	37 mL (1.3 oz.)
3rd	16 mL (0.5 oz.)
4th	13 mL (0.4 oz.)
5th	7 mL (0.2 oz.)
6th	7 mL (0.2 oz.)
7th	2 mL (0.1 oz.)

Adapted from Kent, J. C., Mitoulas, L. R., Cregan, M. D., et al. (2008). Importance of vacuum for breastmilk expression. *Breastfeeding Medicine, 3*(1), 11-19.

STRATEGIES FOR TRIGGERING MILK EJECTIONS A parent's body can become conditioned to the feel of the baby nursing or a specific pump and may benefit from the following tips to trigger milk ejections when starting to express or when changing methods.

- **Environment:** Express in a comfortable place with good arm and back support for complete relaxation and minimal distraction. For some, a pre-expression ritual—such as massage, breathing exercises, using a blanket or sweater for warmth—may help.

- **Senses, mind, and feelings:** Use no more than two of the following: touch (dry warmth, massage, compression), sight (photo or video of baby), smell (baby's blanket, clothing), taste (sip a favorite beverage), hearing (listen to a recording of baby cooing or crying, call and check on baby), mind/feelings (close the eyes, relax, and imagine the feel of skin-to-skin contact with baby or the baby nursing, think loving thoughts about the baby).

Whether hand-expressing or using a breast pump, try different speeds and rhythms to trigger more milk ejections and higher milk yields. For example, if the parent's body is conditioned to the baby's sucking patterns during nursing, try to mimic it with the pump. Try this as an experiment:

- Begin at a fast speed to trigger milk ejection more quickly.

- At milk ejection—when milk starts flowing faster—slow the speed to drain the milk faster.

- When the milk slows to a trickle, return to a fast speed to trigger the next milk ejection faster, repeating until done, using milk flow as a guide.

Use whatever expression rhythm produces faster milk flow.

If milk ejection is delayed or inhibited, as a starting point, suggest expressing from one side while the baby nurses on the other side, so baby can trigger milk ejection. If milk ejection is inhibited by stress or upset, suggest taking a break and trying again later.

MILK EXPRESSION METHODS

The choice of expression method will depend in part on how often parents plan to express, their familiarity with the methods, and their preferences. For most, the highest milk yields come from a combination of pumping and hand expression (p. 211).

MILK EXPRESSION STRATEGIES

HAND EXPRESSING IN THE LAST MONTH OF A HEALTHY PREGNANCY teaches parents a skill that increases confidence they can exclusively nurse and reduces supplementation after delivery. For those at risk of low milk production, their colostrum can be stored and used as a supplement during the hospital stay, if needed. Hand expression once or twice per day during the last month of a low-risk pregnancy does not increase risk of early labor.

Begin hand-expressing at around 36 weeks of pregnancy. Often the easiest place is in the shower. Using a 3 mL syringe, draw up the drops as they are expressed and keep the syringe in the refrigerator between expressions. Reuse the same syringe, freezing it either when it is full or after 2 days. If a large volume of colostrum is expressed, collect it in a clean spoon or medicine cup, and draw it up into the syringe for storage.

BOOSTING MILK YIELDS can be done in several ways.

EXPRESSSING COLOSTRUM within an hour of delivery usually yields much more milk than if the first expression occurs later. To help trigger milk ejections for effective colostrum expression, create a relaxed environment, spend time in parent-baby skin-to-skin contact, and apply warm compresses. Reverse pressure softening (p. 333) may yield more colostrum.

PUMPING AFTER MILK INCREASE (after Day 3 to 5)   If milk yields are lower than expected, first review these basics.

- How many times per day do parents pump? Ignore time intervals (e.g., every 3 hours). Instead, note the times of each pump session on a typical day and then add them together for the daily total. If <8, suggest more pump sessions.

- How long is each pump session? Single- or double-pumping? Using hands-on pumping techniques (p. 211)? If so, go over what they are doing step by step. If they are missing a step or two, it may be possible to improve their routine and their results.

- What is the longest stretch between pump sessions? Stretches longer than about 6 to 8 hours can slow milk production for some. Plan to pump at least once during the night.

- Which pump(s) are they using? Which brands and models? Is it possible to upgrade?

- When was the pump fit last checked? Fit can change over time (p. 326).

- How much time is spent in skin-to-skin contact? More time can improve milk yields.

- What is their goal? Those wanting to lactate long term spend more time pumping.

HANDS-ON PUMPING increases milk yields by an average of nearly 50%. Start it after milk increase on Day 3 or 4 post-delivery by following these steps.

1. Massage both mammary glands for about a minute or so to enhance milk flow.

2. Double pump while compressing and massaging, which can be done one-handed (Figure 12.1) or with both hands when wearing a hands-free pumping band or bra.
3. Massage again. After pumping 15 minutes, remove the pump parts and massage both sides again for a minute, focusing on areas that still feel hard or full.
4. Finish with either hand expression or single pumping, whichever yields more milk. Focus on one side at a time, go back and forth using compression and massage until well drained.

Share hands-on pumping with links to demo videos at **bit.ly/BA2-HandsOnPumpNM**.

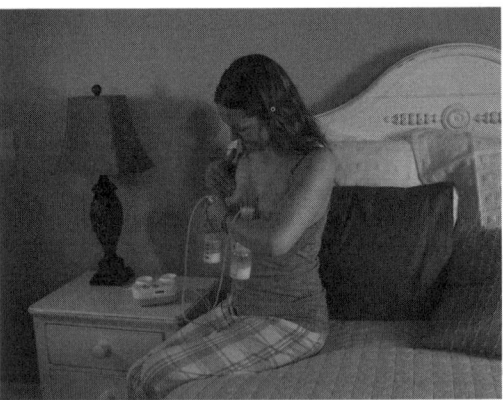

Figure 12.1 This mother supports her double-pump parts with one hand and arm while using her free hand to compress and massage.

OTHER STRATEGIES TO BOOST MILK YIELDS include applying warmth to the glands before expressing, acupuncture and acupressure, and the use of audio-assisted relaxation techniques or music therapy. Any strategy that boosts milk production (Chapter 11) usually boosts milk yields.

STORING MILK WHILE EXCLUSIVELY NURSING can be done without affecting the next nursing session with the following strategies:

- Express both sides about 30 to 60 minutes after a morning nursing.
- Express milk from one side during or between feeds, leaving the other side fuller.

If an hour passes between a milk expression and the next nursing, the baby's feeding pattern will not usually be affected. But if the baby wants to feed sooner than an hour, it's fine to nurse anyway. Most babies will be patient with the slower milk flow. Baby may simply feed longer, take each side more than once, or want to nurse again sooner than usual at the next feed.

EXCLUSIVE PUMPING is linked to shorter duration of lactation, but it gives families the option of partial or exclusive human-milk-feeding when direct nursing is not an option. Parents who learn about exclusive pumping before their baby's birth consider it a more positive experience. When milk expression must take the baby's place in establishing or maintaining milk production, some basic knowledge and effective expression techniques are vital.

ESTABLISHING FULL MILK PRODUCTION WITH PUMPING
Milk-expression strategies for exclusive pumping vary by stage of lactation. The goal is to reach full milk production of about 750 mL (25 oz.) per day per baby by Day 10 to 14. Intensive milk expression during the first weeks is key to adequate long-term milk production

Stage 1: The First Few Days

- Start expressing within an hour of birth. If a pump isn't available, hand express.
- Use massage and compression while double-pumping for 15 minutes, followed by hand expression at least 5 times per day for the first 5 days.
- Express ≥ 8 to 10 times per 24 hours, expecting only drops of milk.
- Express at least once at night, going no longer than 5 to 6 hours between sessions.

Stage 2: From Milk Increase (Days 3 to 5) to Full Milk Production

Begin when the parent can express about 1 oz. (30 mL) from both sides combined:

- Use hands-on pumping techniques (p. 211), which takes on average 25 minutes per session.
- Express ≥8 to 10 times per 24 hours, focusing on daily total, not intervals between.
- Express at least once at night, going no longer than 5 to 6 hours between sessions.

Stage 3: At Full Milk Production (750 mL [25 oz.] per day per baby)

- Decrease the number of pump sessions to 6 or 7 (see next section) and shorten pump times to 10 to 15 minutes, monitoring 24-hour milk yields once per week.

- Try sleeping for 7 to 8 hours at night, expressing right before bed and immediately upon waking. If parents wake in great discomfort, continue one pump session at night.

MAINTAINING FULL MILK PRODUCTION WITH PUMPING requires less milk expression than increasing milk production. When parents with full milk production cannot nurse for any reason, help them individualize their expression plan by adjusting these factors.

- Number of daily expressions needed to maintain production (their "magic number") will vary among parents by storage capacity. For most, this number will be 5 to 7 sessions per day. For those with a very small storage capacity, it may be more; if very large, it may be less. Parents can determine this number by experimenting. They will know they have found it when their milk production stays steady over time without dropping.
- Length of expression sessions also matter. For some, after the first 2 weeks, longer milk expressions that drain the glands more fully may offset fewer sessions.
- Longest stretch between milk removals is also key, as very long stretches may slow milk-making. Parents with a medium storage capacity may stay stable with a longest stretch of 7 or 8 hours. But with a small storage capacity milk-making may slow with stretches longer than 5 or 6 hours. Sometimes, milk yields can be boosted simply by decreasing the longest stretch.

At least once a week record 24-hour milk yields and respond quickly if they dip. The faster parents respond by increased milk expression, the sooner production will rebound.

TROUBLESHOOTING FALLING MILK YIELDS involves first reviewing the basics (the bulleted list on p. 211). Also discuss health-related factors that affect milk production, such as taking a medication that affects lactation, a history of breast or chest surgery, thyroid problems, or other issues that can affect milk production. See Chapter 11 for a more complete list.

Strategies to boost milk production include:

- Begin or refine hands-on pumping. If parents say they are doing hands-on pumping, ask them to describe step-by-step what they are doing to see if improvement is possible.
- Pump more times per day. If their number of pump sessions dropped below their magic number, for most, >8 expressions per day will speed milk-making. Going from 6 to 7 sessions per day is unlikely to boost yields. The sessions don't have to be at regular time intervals. Parents can bunch them together every hour when it's more convenient.

- Consider other options, such as the use of galactogogues (p. 196), acupuncture and acupressure, chiropractic, and the use of music therapy or relaxation techniques.

AFTER REACHING FULL PRODUCTION, WHAT'S NEXT? Parents need to know their options. Human milk is recommended for baby's first full year, but even motivated families find it difficult to make exclusive pumping work long-term because it takes so much more time and effort.

Transitioning Baby to Direct Nursing is possible at any age, because babies are hardwired to nurse (Chapter 1). This transition is a learning process that requires time and patience. Strategies include:

- Keep all interactions on the parent's body positive. Never let nursing attempts become a battle. While near the nipple, give the baby skin-to-skin and eye contact. Smile, talk, and enjoy each other. Let the baby move away if she wants. When she fusses or cries, stop and comfort her.
- Begin with the starter positions (p. 6), which trigger babies' innate feeding behaviors.
- Try nursing while she's in a light sleep or drowsy state.

Approach this transition in the same way as a nursing strike (p. 71 and 72).

One emotional barrier that prevents many families from transitioning from exclusive pumping to direct nursing is their worry about accurately gauging their baby's milk intake. Direct nursing may feel risky, even after the baby is not at risk and is fully capable of nursing effectively. Suggest families think of nursing as a normal behavior (like walking and talking) that babies are hardwired to do.

Describe the expected weight gain, and arrange for regular weight checks during the transition. Suggest families take note of their baby's diaper output and post-feeding behavior before transitioning to nursing, so that they will be more aware of what to look for afterward.

Weaning from Exclusive Pumping is another option if a parent decides not to transition the baby to direct nursing. The following approaches can be used individually or in combination to make weaning from the pump safer and comfortable. If parents feel full, encourage them to pump to comfort (not a full pumping). Remaining too full for too long increases the risk of pain and mastitis.

- Eliminate one daily pump session every 3 days or so, leaving for last the first morning and last evening pump sessions. This gives milk production time to adjust downward before dropping another pumping. When a pump session is dropped, adjust the timing so all sessions are about the same time interval apart. Repeat until fully weaned from pumping.

- Gradually increase the intervals between pump sessions. If parents previously pumped every 3 hours during the day, delay it to 4 to 5 hours, and wait 3 days or so to increase the time intervals again. Repeat until the parent no longer feels the need to pump.
- Keep the number of pump sessions per day the same, but stop sooner. If parents were pumping 120 mL (4 oz.) per session, stop pumping after 90 mL (3 oz.). Give their body 3 days or so to adjust, and repeat until they no longer feel the need to pump.

Pumping to comfort as needed will not prolong the process. It simply makes it safer, more comfortable, and prevents painful fullness from developing into mastitis.

If parents already have a blocked duct (a hardened or tender area in the mammary gland), another option is to fully drain that side with the pump and then go for longer and longer stretches without pumping. Encourage parents to use whichever of these strategies works best for them.

MILK STORAGE AND HANDLING

Milk storage guidelines for healthy, term babies are listed in Table 12.3.

Current guidelines recommend against storing milk that collects in breast shells ("drip milk") and refreezing thawed human milk. Partially thawed milk should be evaluated on a case-by-case basis.

The smell and taste of refrigerated and frozen milk changes over time. Soapy and rancid smelling milk are in the normal range, as the enzyme lipase breaks down fat in the stored milk. If the milk-storage guidelines are followed, it is safe to feed babies stored milk that smells or tastes soapy or rancid. If the baby won't take it, parents can try mixing it with fresh milk or donate it to a milk bank. In some cases, this change in smell and taste may be prevented by scalding the milk before cooling and storing it. To scald milk, put it in a pan on the stove and heat it to about 180° F (82° C) or until bubbles form around the edges but before boiling. Then cool it quickly and refrigerate or freeze it.

After feeding expressed milk, if some is left in a container, the Academy of Breastfeeding Medicine (ABM) recommends discarding any remaining milk within 1 to 2 hours after the feed.

No compelling evidence exists that milk stored during a candida infection should be discarded.

Table 12.3. Mature Milk Storage Times for Healthy Term Babies at Home

Milk Storage/ Handling	Deep Freeze (0°F/ -18°C)	Refrigerator/ Freezer (variable 0°F/-18°C)	Refrigerator (39°F/4°C)	Room Temperature (50°F-85°F/ 10°C-29°C)
Fresh	Optimal: ≤6 mo. Okay: ≤12 mo.	Ideal: ≤3 mo. Okay: ≤6 mo.	Ideal: 4 days Okay if very clean conditions: 5-8 days	Ideal: ≤4 hr. Okay if very clean conditions: 6-8 hr.
Frozen, Thawed in Fridge	Do not refreeze	Do not refreeze	≤24 hr.	≤4 hr.
Thawed, Warmed, Not Fed	Do not refreeze	Do not refreeze	≤4 hr.	Until feed ends
Fed	Discard	Discard	Discard	Until feed ends

Adapted from CDC. (2019). Storage and preparation of breast milk. From **https://www.cdc.gov/breastfeeding/pdf/preparation-of-breast-milk_H.pdf**

Eglash, A., Simon, L., & Academy of Breastfeeding, M. (2017). ABM Clinical Protocol #8: Human milk storage information for home use for full-term infants, revised 2017. *Breastfeeding Medicine, 12*(7), 390-395.

Jones, F. (2019). *Best Practice for Expressing, Storing, and Handling Human Milk in Hospitals, Homes, and Child Care Settings* (4th ed.). Fort Worth, TX: Human Milk Banking Association of North America.

HANDLING AND PREPARING EXPRESSED MILK After milk is expressed, to improve safety and prevent waste:

- Label each batch with the date and time it was expressed, and if needed, the baby's name.

- Store milk in volumes no larger than the baby is likely to take at a feed.

- When combining batches of milk expressed at different times, cool the milk first, and label it with the date of the oldest milk. Start a new container every 24 hours.

- If the baby is fed expressed milk exclusively or primarily, to provide the most nutrients and bioactive components, first feed fresh milk, second refrigerated milk, and third frozen milk.

- When storing milk in reusable containers, before use, make sure they are washed in hot, soapy water, rinsed well, and air dried. Regular sterilization of milk storage containers and pump parts is not currently recommended, because no benefits were found.

Human milk is not a biohazardous substance, so no gloves or other special precautions are needed when handling it. It can be safely poured down the drain when discarded.

THE APPEARANCE OF EXPRESSED MILK can vary greatly. For realistic expectations, parents need to know that expressed milk:

- Separates into layers, like any milk that is not homogenized. Before feeding the separated milk to the baby, suggest swirling it gently to mix the layers.
- Comes in a variety of colors, such as bluish, yellowish, or even brownish. Consuming some foods, food dyes, and medications, can change milk's color to pink-orange, green, and black. Frozen milk may take on a yellowish color, which is not a sign of spoilage.

FOR HOSPITALIZED BABIES, parents need to use the hospital's milk-storage guidelines, which vary by institution. Preterm and sick babies are at greater risk for serious and life-threatening health problems, so stricter hygiene precautions are needed. Simple steps like handwashing before expressing milk can be critical in preventing contamination of the milk. But some previously recommended procedures—such as cleaning the nipples before expressing and discarding the first drops of milk—are no longer done, because they were not beneficial.

THAWING FROZEN MILK AND WARMING MILK FOR FEEDS is best done gently and gradually, keep heat low. To thaw frozen milk, use one of the following methods:

- Thaw milk in the refrigerator overnight, which causes less fat loss than thawing in warm water. Thawed milk can be refrigerated for up to 24 hours.
- Thaw at room temperature, making sure to refrigerate it as soon as it is completely thawed.
- Hold the container under warm running water for a few minutes.
- Hold the container in water that was previously heated on the stove to ideally no more than body temperature (98° F/37° C). If the water cools and the milk is not yet thawed, remove the container of milk and reheat the water. Do not heat the milk on the stove burner directly.
- Thaw in a waterless warming device.

If using water to thaw or warm milk, tilt or hold the container, so the water cannot seep under the lid. Thawed milk should be either fed immediately or refrigerated.

Warming milk for feeds is important for preterm babies, as cold milk may lower their body temperature. To warm milk, allow about 20 minutes and hold the container under lukewarm running water or hold it in a pan of lukewarm water that was previously heated to no more than about body temperature (98° F/37° C) on the stove. Too much heat during warming can cause dangerous hot spots in the milk, and higher heat deactivates the milk's bioactive proteins and decreases its fat content. Healthy term and older babies can drink chilled milk directly from the refrigerator.

Caution parents against using a microwave to thaw or warm human milk. Warming it in a microwave reduces bacterial levels but also reduces its anti-infective factors. Also, microwaves heat liquids unevenly. Even if swirled or shaken, hot spots remain that can burn the baby's throat.

STORAGE CONTAINERS   Glass and most solid food-grade plastic containers without BPA and with solid, tight-fitting lids are recommended for both hospital and home use. The effects of glass and polypropylene plastic containers on stored milk are similar. Avoid storing expressed milk in specimen cups and containers made from polycarbonate plastic and stainless steel.

Polyethylene milk bags are acceptable for home use. However, milk stored in bags lose significant amounts of the milk's IgA and its bacteria-fighting capability. Even so, these bags have practical benefits. They take up less storage space than hard-sided containers and can be attached to breast pump parts in place of a bottle, reducing risk of contamination when transferring milk to another container. Because they are not reused, there is less to wash, but this makes them less eco-friendly than reusable containers. Avoid the thinner "disposable bottle liners," which tear easily. If this type of bag is used, suggest first inserting the bag of milk inside another bag before sealing and storing it.

Milk storage bags are not recommended for hospitalized babies because they are not airtight, and may leak. When storing milk in bags, suggest parents leave space for milk expansion during freezing, close the bag tightly, and lay each bag flat during freezing. After the milk freezes, provide extra protection by inserting the bags into a bin with a lid or into a disposable freezer bag and seal it.

REDUCING THE RISKS OF MILK SHARING   A growing number of nursing families either donate or receive expressed milk from other families. The grass-roots growth of milk sharing reflects a widespread belief among parents in the importance of human milk to their babies. Milk sharing is usually done without guidance from healthcare providers or lactation supporters, but when working with families, lactation providers and supporters can encourage an open discussion of the pros and cons of milk sharing, with a focus on safety and reducing risk.

In 2012, the milk-sharing organization Eats on Feets' founder Shell Walker published its "four pillars of breast milk sharing," which is available on its website at **bit.ly/BA2-FourPillars**.

As a result of these recommendations, studies found nearly all milk-sharing families use safe practices, but reinforcing this information has value. When in discussion with milk-sharing families:

- Offer to provide the latest milk-storage guidelines.
- Suggest avoiding milk for sale, which is more likely to be diluted with other milks and be shipped under unsafe conditions. Very few milk sharing transactions involve financial compensation.

DIGITAL RESOURCES

bit.ly/BA2-BolmanMassage—A 4.5-minute video showing some of the techniques described in the article Bolman, M., Saju, L, Oganesyan, K., et al. (2013). Recapturing the art of therapeutic breast massage during breastfeeding. Journal of Human Lactation, 28(3):328-331.

bit.ly/BA2-HandsOnPumpingDemo—A 9.5-minute video by Dr. Jane Morton demonstrating hands-on pumping techniques, which incorporates manual expression and massage.

bit.ly/BA2-HandsOnPumpNM—Blog post summary from this author about how to do hands-on pumping with links to the Stanford videos.

bit.ly/BA2-PumpingPretermHandout—"Pumping Milk for Your Preterm Baby" (English and Spanish) by Kay Hoover and Barbara Wilson-Clay. A 4-page booklet with full-color photos, a weekly pumping log, and low-literacy text with instructions for those exclusively pumping from birth.

bit.ly/BA2-StanfordHandExpress—A 7.5-minute video by Dr. Jane Morton demonstrating the manual expression technique used at Stanford University Hospital.

CHAPTER 13 NIPPLE ISSUES

NIPPLE PAIN

Nipple pain is usually a solvable problem. If left unaddressed, it can contribute to depression.

WHAT'S NORMAL AFTER BIRTH Mild nipple pain is considered normal during the first 2 weeks of nursing if it resolves with milk ejection and there is no skin damage. This normal early pain usually peaks around the fourth day of nursing and is mostly gone by Day 10. Suggest seeking help if the pain is moderate to severe or skin trauma develops. If there is no skin trauma, shooting pains between feeds may be due to vasospasm or Raynaud's phenomenon. Increasing pain with skin trauma may be a sign of mastitis, or a bacterial or yeast infection.

The nursing parent's perception of nipple pain (mild or severe) is partly determined by the degree of skin trauma, but other factors affect it, too. Hunger, fatigue anxiety, and lack of social support may raise pain levels, as well as the use of inflammatory medications and a history of pain disorders. The presence or absence of these and other factors explain why two parents with the same degree of nipple trauma may perceive their pain level very differently.

NIPPLE PAIN DURING THE FIRST WEEK

One or more of the following factors may contribute to early nipple pain.

Interactive Factors

- Shallow latch—Nipple may look pinched after feeds, the areola may appear bruised
- Suction—Baby pulled off without first breaking the suction
- Fit—With a small mouth/large nipple, baby can fit only the nipple in his mouth

Baby Factors

- Variations in oral anatomy—Tongue-tie, lip-tie, unusual palate shape, short or recessed jaw
- Strong or unusual sucking, clamping, biting, or clenching.

Parent Factors

- Engorgement—Shallow latch due to taut mammary tissue
- Vasospasm or Raynaud's phenomenon—Nipple changes color after feed
- Nipple anatomical variations—Nipple appears inverted or dimpled

- Use or misuse of pumps or products—Check pump fit, level of suction, use of teats/dummies; poorly fitting bras; wet breast pads, irritating creams/ointments

NIPPLE PAIN AT ANY TIME

More than one of these factors may contribute to nipple pain at any stage of lactation.

Interactive Factors

- Shallow latch—Older babies/toddlers may nurse acrobatically
- Candida/thrush—Diagnosis/treatment needed

Baby Factors

- Teething and biting
- Pulling off the nipple without first breaking the suction.
- Unusual feeding positions—Usually an older baby or toddler

Parent Factors

- Overabundant milk production—Baby may clamp or clench to slow flow
- Blebs, blisters
- Skin problems—Dermatitis, impetigo, eczema, psoriasis, poison ivy/oak
- Sores—Herpes, infected Montgomery glands
- Pregnancy—Hormonal changes may cause nipple discomfort
- Referred pain—From mastitis, fibromyalgia, pulled muscle, pinched nerve
- Use or misuse of pumps or products—Check pump fit and suction level, use of teats/dummies; wet nursing pads, creams/ointments

Complications of Nipple Trauma

- Mastitis
- Bacterial or fungal infection
- Mammary dysbiosis (p. 30) or lactiferous duct infection (p. 36)

TEETHING AND BITING do not have to lead to weaning. Use the following strategies to reduce nursing pain from teething and to prevent biting.

NIPPLE PAIN FROM TEETHING When a baby's teeth are about to erupt, his gums feel sore, and applying pressure feels soothing. But when a nursing baby bears down with his gums to apply pressure during feeds, this may temporarily cause nipple pain. To prevent painful nursing until teeth erupt, before nursing, give baby a cold, wet washcloth or teething toy to chew on to numb sore gums. If baby is on solid foods, a frozen bagel, peas, or berries are soothing and may make nursing more comfortable. Avoid numbing products that may also numb baby's tongue and the nipple.

STRATEGIES FOR THE NURSING BABY WHO BITES Most nursing babies do not bite after their teeth erupt. But when they do, it is not necessary to stop nursing. While a baby is actively nursing, his tongue covers his teeth and he can't bite. Biting usually occurs at the end of a feed.

If a baby bites, stay calm and first break the suction with a finger to prevent further damage. To prevent future biting:

- Give baby complete attention while nursing.
- Learn to recognize the end of a feed. Notice if tension develops in baby's jaw before he bites. If it happens, break the suction and take him off.
- Don't pressure a disinterested baby to nurse. If the baby pushes away, offer to nurse later.
- Make sure baby latches deeply, which triggers active sucking, lessening the odds of biting.
- Remove a sleeping baby who is not actively sucking. Gently insert a finger between baby's gums to release the nipple. If baby bites, he'll bite the finger instead.
- Keep milk production abundant. Some babies bite when frustrated by slow milk flow.
- Note behaviors that lead to biting. Some babies bite when teased, pressured to nurse, or when someone is yelling nearby. Notice what happened before the bite and avoid it.
- Keep nursing relaxed and positive. Some babies bite when the parent is tense. If frazzled, try deep breathing or nursing lying down or in a darkened room.
- Give praise when baby doesn't bite. Say "good baby" when he is gentle.

To discourage a persistent biter, try:

- Stop the feed. Remove the temptation for baby to make the parent jump or startle again.
- Offer a teether or anything else acceptable to bite.
- Set baby quickly on the floor to give the message that biting brings negative results. After a few seconds of distress, comfort baby.

- Keep a finger near the baby's mouth ready to break the suction, if needed. Some distractible babies try to turn and look with the nipple still in their mouth. If the parent responds consistently by breaking the suction, baby will learn that turning away means losing the nipple.

Babies don't understand that biting causes pain. They learn to associate their parent with feelings of comfort and relief from hunger. These positive associations help baby learn quickly not to bite.

COMFORT MEASURES may help reduce nipple pain from most causes:

- Take an analgesia compatible with nursing.
- Stimulate a milk ejection before latching by expressing milk.
- Nurse first on the least sore side until the milk ejection occurs, then switch sides.
- Try varying positions at each nursing session.
- Wear breast shells between feeds to reduce clothing friction and pressure.

Use the type of breast shells with large nipple openings (not the smaller ones to draw out inverted nipples). Red circles on the skin when the breast shells are removed indicate a larger size bra cup is needed.

If the pain is severe enough that the parent wants to take a break from direct nursing, suggest expressing milk while the nipples heal.

Comfort measures for vasospasm and Raynaud's phonenomon include gentle massage and applying dry heat after nursing to more quickly return blood flow to the nipple.

TREATMENTS FOR NIPPLE TRAUMA Due to the poor quality of much of the research on nipple treatments, it is not known if one treatment is more effective than another. A randomized controlled trial found that all-purpose nipple ointment (APNO)—a mixture prepared by the pharmacist that contains an antibiotic, antifungal and anti-inflammatory—was found no more effective at reducing pain than ultra-purified lanolin. Another randomized controlled trial found ultra-purified lanolin no more effective at reducing pain than no treatment at all in terms of nursing exclusivity and duration. Even so, the use of topical treatments for nipple pain is nearly universal in some countries.

Drawbacks of using topical treatments include the following.

- An unfamiliar taste on the nipple may cause fussiness or distress during latch.

- If the product is unsafe for baby to ingest, removing it before nursing may cause more skin damage.
- Clogging nipple pores or reducing oxygen to the wound may occur, slowing healing.
- Dry skin can occur if alcohol is one of the ingredients.
- If numbing agents are included, they may numb baby's mouth or delay milk ejection.

Even the use of natural substances like virgin olive oil and virgin coconut oil (both are inexpensive and have anti-inflammatory properties) may cause skin reactions like dermatitis in sensitive users.

Vitamin E is no longer recommended to treat nipple trauma due to skin reactions in some users and elevated vitamin E levels in nursing babies.

Nipple treatments that may be soothing and are available to everyone include expressed milk and warm water compresses.

Newer nipple-pain treatments that are being studied but do not yet have enough evidence to be recommended are silver nipple cups and low-level laser and LED phototherapies.

Nipple shields, in unusual cases, may be used to help reduce nipple pain, but they are not the best first choice. If pain is caused by a shallow latch and the baby's jaws close on the tip of the shield, rather than its soft brim, this compresses the nipple and pain continues. However, if the cause of the nipple pain cannot be corrected quickly, a nipple shield may decrease the pain enough to make direct nursing tolerable until the problem is corrected.

Blood swallowed from traumatized nipples is not harmful to the nursing baby.

PREVENTING INFECTION Broken skin on the nipple increases risk of nipple infection, mastitis, and other complications. When there is skin damage, to prevent infection:

- Wash daily with warm soapy water and a warm water rinse in a bath or shower.
- After nursing, rinse with tap or saline water to prevent organisms in baby's mouth from colonizing the wound.
- After rinsing, apply a thin layer of mupirocin ointment, which does not have to be removed and is compatible with nursing.

BACTERIAL, FUNGAL AND VIRAL NIPPLE INFECTIONS

After correcting the cause of nipple trauma, if the skin damage does not heal quickly or nipple pain does not diminish or even intensifies, a bacterial or fungal infection may be present. In some cases, both bacterial and fungal infections may be present and need to be treated. Symptoms common to both bacterial and fungal infection are slow or no healing and continuing or intensifying pain. But other symptoms set them apart.

BACTERIAL INFECTIONS, which are more common than fungal infections, often feature visible yellow pus in the traumatized area or yellow scabs or crusty areas on the nipple. But even if no yellow is visible, a bacterial infection is still possible.

TREATMENTS FOR BACTERIAL INFECTIONS Use of a topical antibiotic ointment on traumatized nipples may help prevent a bacterial infection from developing, but once a bacterial infection is present, topical treatments are less effective than a 14-day course of oral antibiotics.

IMPETIGO is a type of bacterial infection that may cause nipple pain. It appears as honey-crusted cracks and reddened nipples. The colonizing staph crusting may also block nipple pores, causing mastitis. To treat it, clean the nipple with a washcloth containing soap and water to remove the crusting, rinse, then apply prescribed mupirocin antibiotic ointment. Topical ointment may clear the impetigo, but oral antibiotics may be necessary.

CANDIDIASIS OR THRUSH is an overgrowth of the fungus *Candida albicans*, the one-celled organism involved with most cases of thrush and vaginal yeast infections. It thrives in moist, dark environments, such as on the nipples, in the vagina, the mouth, and baby's diaper area. This fungus normally lives in our body in balance with other organisms, but illness, pregnancy, antibiotic use, and anything else that throws the body out of balance can cause an unhealthy overgrowth.

A lot is still unknown about the prevalence of candida infections among nursing parents. Its prevalence may vary in part by climate, with more cases occurring in warmer areas.

THRUSH SYMPTOMS The existence of burning or shooting pain alone is not enough to confirm the presence of a yeast infection. A combination of symptoms, such as shooting pain with shiny skin on the nipple and areola or flaky nipples and areolae, is more reliable. If these symptoms appear alone, they are much less likely to indicate candida. Other possible candida symptoms include white plaques on the nipples and areolae or red or inflamed-looking nipples and areolae.

In the baby, possible thrush symptoms include white patches on the baby's gums, cheeks, palate, tonsils, and/or tongue (if wiped off, they may look red or bleed), diaper rash (may be simply red or red with raised dots). Most nursing babies have a white, milky coating on their tongue, which is not a sign of thrush unless white patches spread to the baby's cheeks and gums. Some babies have a yeast rash on their bottom but no symptoms in their mouth.

Before a nursing parent is treated for candida —especially if the baby has no symptoms—rule out other possible causes of nipple pain. When the parent has shooting or burning deep mammary pain, first consider causes other than yeast (p. 35).

THRUSH TREATMENTS   If thrush is diagnosed by a healthcare provider, to prevent a recurrence, discuss treating both parent and baby, even if one has no symptoms. If after treatment, thrush persists, treating the nursing couple at the same time may be more effective. Over-the-counter and prescribed treatments are available for yeast infections

Thrush Treatment Options for the Baby

Over-the-counter treatments:

- **Gentian violet** was once recommended as a thrush treatment for parents and babies, but because it is a carcinogen, some health organizations now advise against its use.

Treatments requiring a prescription

- **Nystatin suspension.**   Apply 1 dropperful in each cheek 4 to 8 times daily for at least 2 weeks. It is most effective if used after every feed. One study found nystatin effective in only 32% of cases, while oral fluconazole suspension was effective in 100%.

- **Miconazole gel.**   Apply the 25 mg gel (not available in the U.S.) 4 times daily.

- **Clotrimazole gel.**   Pharmacists make this oral gel by crushing a 10 mg clotrimazole lozenge, mixing it with 5 mL of glycerin or 3 mL of methylcellulose. Apply to baby's mouth every 3 hours for five applications.

- **Fluconazole.**   Give 6 mg/kg oral suspension via dropper as a first dose followed by 3 mg/kg/day once daily for 2 weeks.

Thrush Treatment Options for the Parent

Over-the-counter treatments:

- **Gentian violet** was once recommended as a treatment for thrush in parents and babies, but because it is a carcinogen, some health organizations now advise against its use.
- **Miconazole.** Apply cream or lotion (2%) to nipples/areolae 2 to 4 times daily for 7 days.
- **Ketoconazole.** Apply cream (2%) to nipples/areolae 2 to 4 times daily until at least 2 days after symptoms disappear.

Treatments requiring a prescription

- **Clotrimazole.** Over-the-counter (OTC) and prescription versions are available. Apply OTC version to nipples/areolae after feeds 2 to 4 times daily until at least 2 days after symptoms disappear. Pharmacists make prescribed version a gel by crushing a 10 mg clotrimazole lozenge and mixing it with 5 mL of glycerin or 3 mL of methylcellulose. Apply to nipples/areolae every 3 hours for five applications.
- **Nystatin cream or ointment.** Apply 4 times per day for 14 days. Note: Nystatin is much less effective than other treatment options (see "Baby" on previous page).
- **Nystatin with triamcinolone (corticosteroid).** Apply cream or ointment to nipples/areolae 4 times daily until at least 2 days after symptoms resolve.
- **Oral fluconazole.** Used when topical treatments are ineffective. Take either a 200 mg or 400 mg loading dose, then 100 mg 2 times daily for at least 2 weeks. Continue for 1 week after pain resolves. The single-dose treatment for vaginal yeast infections is not usually effective.

Nursing parents who prefer a more "natural" treatment can mix 1 teaspoon (5 mL) of vinegar with 1 cup (236 mL) of water and apply after each nursing session to nipple and allow to air dry.

Continue nursing during thrush treatment. Rinse the nipples with clear water and air dry after each nursing session. In some cases, the parent may first feel worse for a day or two before feeling better.

RECURRING THRUSH after treatment indicates the need to take the following precautions.

- Treat the partner and, if nursing more than one child, the other sibling.
- Wash hands often, especially after changing diapers and using the toilet.
- Wash baby's hands often if he sucks thumb or fingers.

- Wash toys that baby puts in his mouth in hot, soapy water and rinse well.
- Use paper towels for hand drying. Discard after use.

If pacifiers, bottle nipples/teats, or teethers are used, boil them daily for 20 minutes to kill the yeast. After 1 week of treatment, discard them and buy new ones. If breast pumps are used, boil daily for 20 minutes all parts that touch the milk. Use only disposable nursing pads and discard after each feed.

VIRAL HERPES INFECTIONS Herpes simplex 1 (cold sores or fever blisters) and 2 (genital herpes) are two different herpes viruses spread by contact with the sores. They are small, painful, fluid-filled, red-rimmed blisters that dry after a few days and form a scab. Genital herpes sores can be spread to other body parts, including the nipple, by touch.

These herpes viruses are often fatal to newborns when contracted during the first 3 weeks after birth. If a sore on the nipple or mammary gland could be herpes, it should be cultured. If the sores can be covered so the baby cannot touch them, nursing can continue. But if the sores are on the nipple, areola, or anywhere else the baby might touch while nursing, express milk from that side until the sores heal. Until then, baby can nurse on the unaffected side. If the parent's hand or pump parts touch the sores while expressing milk, the milk may be contaminated with the virus and it should be discarded. If the hands or pump parts do not touch the sores, the newborn may be fed the milk.

Serious complications from contracting herpes are much less likely in babies older than 1 month.

Although herpes is not life-threatening in an older baby, take steps to avoid spreading it to the child. The sores can be very painful for a week or more and may make eating and drinking difficult.

When a nursing parent contracts other herpes infections, such as shingles and chickenpox, contagious sores may erupt on the nipple and mammary gland (see p. 140).

OTHER SKIN PROBLEMS

Skin problems that occur anywhere else on the body can also occur on the nipple and mammary gland and may be entirely unrelated to nursing. Hives, for example, can occur as an allergic reaction to a substance touched or consumed.

QUESTIONS TO ASK include what the skin problem looks like and the following:

- Have they recently used any cream, ointment, pads, or other product on or near their nipples? Eczema and other types of dermatitis sometimes develop when topical cortisone, antifungals, and mupirocin are used.

- Have they used a new laundry product or toiletry product, like cologne, deodorant, or powder near their mammary glands? In some parents, these products cause irritation.

- Have they used any tools or devices on their nipples, like a breast pump, breast shells, nipple shields, or nipple everters? Too-high suction levels sometimes cause skin damage. Exposure to plastics may cause a reaction in some sensitive parents.

- Do they have a health problem? Are they taking any medications? Skin problems may be a sign of an allergic reaction or sensitivity to a medication. Health problems like celiac disease increase the risk of skin reactions.

- Is the baby eating solid foods, teething, or taking a medication? Parents can react to foods, medications, and teething gels in a baby's mouth. Rinsing the baby's mouth with water before nursing or eliminating the irritating food for a while may help.

- Do parent and child have a similar skin problem anywhere else on their bodies, or do they have a history of allergic skin reactions? Skin problems unrelated to nursing can spread to the nipple area. If so, parents may be familiar with it and the treatments that work for them.

BASIC STRATEGIES for unexplained skin problems are: stop using suspected product, take showers often, wear all-cotton bras, expose the nipple to sunlight and air for 15 minutes, and after nursing, rinse the affected nipple with warm water, pat dry, and dry with a hair dryer on low setting.

Continued pain and slow or stalled healing are signs it's time to consult a healthcare provider, preferably a dermatologist.

RULE OUT PAGET'S DISEASE If nipple eczema does not improve within 3 weeks of treatment, see immediately a healthcare provider to rule out Paget's disease, an unusual form of breast cancer. Paget's disease is sometimes mistaken for nipple eczema. It usually appears on one nipple, comes on gradually, has an irregular but distinct edge, and the nipple is almost always affected, sometimes disappearing. Because its symptoms seem minor, the average wait before being seen is 30 weeks. Waiting this long decreases the odds of survival. Early detection is vital.

NIPPLE BLISTERS AND BLEBS

BLISTERS on the nipple that are clear are usually caused by friction and/or high vacuum. They may form on the tip of the nipple if the baby is latched shallowly and putting undue pressure on it. In this case, try a deeper latch. Starter positions (p. 6) may help a young baby latch deeper if baby is allowed to self-attach. A deeper latch may be all that's needed to reduce pain and prevent a blister from recurring.

To open a blister, first apply warm, wet compresses before nursing. The moisture will soften the nipple skin, and the heat will thin it, causing some blisters to open. If not, see opening a bleb in the next section.

BLEBS OR MILK BLISTERS look like a white spot on the nipple. The cause is not fully understood. A bleb could indicate a plug caused by a granule of thickened milk blocking the milk from flowing at the nipple, or its cause may be a thin layer of skin blocking the nipple pore from the outside. Some think it is a small pressure cyst that forms at the end of a milk duct.

Blebs sometimes coincide with bouts of mastitis, but whether it's the cause or effect is unclear.

Blebs may or may not be painful. If not, no treatment is needed. It will likely resolve on its own.

OTHER CAUSES OF A WHITE SPOT ON THE NIPPLE that is not a bleb (which may or may not be painful) include:

- A build-up of dead skin, like cradle cap, which can be removed by rubbing it with a lubricating oil like lecithin.
- After the baby bites the nipple, a white spot may form from an accumulation of saliva and milk moisture under skin edges. To treat this, clean the area with soap and water like any bite wound and apply topical antibiotic ointment to prevent infection (p. 225).
- Thrush may cause a small blister-like sore to form on the nipple. See p. 227 for treatments.

TREATING BLEBS If a bleb is painful, there are several home treatments that may help resolve it. First, apply wet heat to the bleb, either with warm compresses or by soaking the nipple in warm water (side-lying in a bathtub or leaning forward into a basin of warm water). Then rub the nipple with a damp cloth to remove any excess skin. It may also help to lubricate the nipple with olive oil. After this, express milk from that duct by compressing at the edge of the areola behind the plug. Expressing a thickened string of milk may help open the duct and keep it open.

If the bleb is painful and persists despite these treatments, see a healthcare provider to open it with a sterile needle. In many cases, when the duct is opened, milk from behind the plug flows and brings relief. After the bleb is opened, to prevent infection, wash it daily with a mild soap and water and rinse well with water. To prevent infection, apply a thin layer of a topical mupirocin antibiotic to the affected nipple after feeds.

If the bleb is dry, it may have formed as an inflammatory tissue reaction to nipple trauma. A healthcare provider can treat this by prescribing a mid-potency steroid ointment, which is applied in a thin layer after nursing and covered with plastic wrap until the next feed. Within days, the dry bleb should heal.

TO PREVENT RECURRING BLEBS, try reducing saturated fats in the diet and taking a lecithin supplement. Suggested dosages of lecithin range from 1 tablespoon per day to 1 tablespoon 3 to 4 times a day or one to two 1,200 mg capsules 3 or 4 times per day.

NIPPLE TYPES AND PROCEDURES

It is not unusual for the left and right nipples to vary. One nipple may protrude while the other is flat or inverted. Both nipples may be flat, but one may protrude more than the other. Both nipples may be inverted but one may be more inverted than the other. The baby may show a preference for the nipple that is less inverted or more protruding.

FLAT NIPPLES do not protrude or become erect when stimulated by touch or cold. Protruding (everted) nipples are not necessary for effective nursing. Most babies suck on anything, including adult arms, shoulders, and necks, none of which have protruding nipples.

INVERTED NIPPLES retract rather than protrude when the areola is compressed.

A nipple may appear everted at rest but retract when stimulated. If a nipple appears inverted at rest, but when the areola is compressed, it everts, then this is not a true inverted nipple.

The classification system used for inverted nipples is based on the amount of connective tissue the nipple contains (its degree of fibrosis) and how easily the nipple can be made to protrude.

- Grade I inverted nipples can be easily everted manually and may stay everted after nursing. A nursing baby who sucks normally will easily draw them out.
- Grade II inverted nipples are moderately inverted. A term baby may draw them out, but they will retract again after feeds. At first, some preterm or sick babies may find them challenging.

- Grade III are severely inverted and can barely be pulled out. Rare, they may make drawing the nipple out during nursing difficult or in extreme cases impossible.

DIMPLED NIPPLES (folded nipples) are a type of inverted nipple in which only a part of the nipple is inverted. It will not protrude or harden when stimulated, but it can be manually opened or drawn out during nursing or pumping. It does not, however, stay open afterwards.

INVERTED NIPPLE TREATMENTS DURING PREGNANCY Wearing breast shells during pregnancy, one common treatment, is associated with poorer nursing outcomes. Perhaps telling parent their nipples are problematic reduces confidence in their ability to nurse.

EARLY NURSING STRATEGIES FOR FLAT AND INVERTED NIPPLES involve following these best practices to minimize feeding problems.

- Immediate and uninterrupted skin-to-skin contact during the first 2 hours after birth
- Encourage the baby to do the breast crawl for the first feed.
- Suggest early and frequent nursing.
- Provide a private, comfortable, and supportive environment.
- Keep nursing couples together and in body contact as much as possible day and night.
- Try the starter positions (p. 6) during the early learning period to take advantage of babies' inborn feeding behaviors to make early nursing easier.
- Avoid artificial nipples during the early weeks, until baby has lots of practice nursing.

IF BABY DOESN'T LATCH OR LATCHES TO ONLY ONE SIDE, feed often from that side, express milk often from the unused side, and continue trying both sides. Most nursing parents have one nipple that is easier for the baby to take. When offering the unused side, start first by expressing some milk on the nipple or in baby's mouth to entice him. A helper can drip milk near the nipple with a spoon while the parent helps baby attach to that side.

Draw Out the Nipple Before Latch Attempts to help baby take the unused side. Do this by:

- **Pulling back slightly on the tissue near the edge of the areola** to help the nipple protrude
- **Roll the nipple** between thumb and index finger for a minute or two and then quickly touch it with a moist, cold cloth.

- **Shape or support the gland** with the breast sandwich, nipple tilting, and other techniques to help the baby latch deeper and trigger active sucking (p. 321).
- **Wear breast shells** (hard plastic, worn before feeds) no more than 30 minutes before a feed.
- **Use a breast pump** before nursing to soften the areola and pull out the nipple uniformly.
- **Use a commercial or homemade nipple everter** for 30 to 60 seconds several times per day to draw out inverted nipples for easier latching. A modified 10 or 20 mL disposable syringe (depending on nipple size), can be converted to a small suction device.

Nipple Shields may help a non-latching baby nurse directly. For details on fit, application, latching, and weaning from the shield, see p. 329.

Milk Expression can be used when none of the above strategies result in direct nursing. Use of a breast pump may help draw out the nipple. How long exclusive milk expression is necessary will depend on the type of inverted nipple and the degree of inversion. For some, one pump session is enough for the nipple to stay out. If so, the parent can start nursing on that side immediately. But more pumping may be needed. Rarely, exclusive pumping may be needed.

If the nipple is drawn out by the pump but inverts again when the baby pauses during nursing, try a short pump session to draw out the nipple and use a nursing supplementer (see p. 315) to encourage more continuous sucking as a temporary transition to exclusive nursing.

If it's necessary to pump exclusively—either for a time or indefinitely, see p. 214.

PAIN AND INVERTED NIPPLES Depending on the type and degree of nipple inversion, some parents experience persistent nipple pain with direct nursing. With some types of inverted nipples, normal nursing may even cause trauma. If the nipple retracts between feeds, the skin may stay moist, contributing to chapping. If so, it may help to dry the nipple after feeds with a hair dryer set on low.

Some nursing parents experience nipple pain for about 2 weeks, as their baby's sucking gradually draws out their nipples. Others have persistent sore nipples for a longer time. Sometimes, instead of stretching, the fibrous tissue that inverts the nipple remains tight, creating a point of stress that can cause cracks or blisters. When the nipple can be drawn into the back of the baby's mouth and the baby begins nursing effectively, many are able to nurse without discomfort.

LESS COMMON NIPPLE TYPES may or may not affect nursing.

ACCESSORY NIPPLES are extra nipples, some with and some without milk-making glands attached. Up to 6% of peoplehave extra mammary tissue and/or nipples (also called **supernumerary nipples**). These extra glands and nipples are remnants from the embryonic development of the mammary ridge. Some have ducts that leak milk through the skin without a nipple. For details on keeping these parents comfortable after birth, see p. 40.

DOUBLE OR BIFURCATED NIPPLES occur when two nipples emerge from one areola. This should not affect nursing, as long as they are close enough together that the baby can latch to both nipples at the same time. Positioning adjustments may make this easier. When pumping, the nipple tunnel should be large enough to comfortably accommodate both nipples.

BLIND NIPPLES are those with no nipple pores, making milk flow impossible. This is very rare, and may occur in just one gland, with the other side forming normally. In these cases, ultrasound will reveal missing ducts and pores

PIERCED NIPPLES are more common in recent years and may or may not cause nursing problems. Several published case reports exist of successful direct nursing in parents with pierced nipples.

POSSIBLE LACTATION COMPLICATIONS OF PIERCED NIPPLES include altered nipple sensation, milk flow problems, and mastitis. After a nipple piercing, healing usually takes 6 to 12 months, with a 10% to 20% increased risk of mastitis unrelated to lactation. Among nursing parents, three cases of low milk production were reported in women with a history of nipple piercing. The researchers attributed their low milk production to scar tissue blocking the milk ducts.

QUESTIONS TO ASK when helping nursing parents with pierced nipples include:

- Were there any complications from the nipple piercing?
- Do they remove the nipple jewelry before nursing?
- Do their nipples feel numb or hypersensitive?
- Is there any obvious scarring on the nipples? If so, where?
- Has their nursing baby been gaining weight in the expected range?
- Have they seen any nipple discharge other than milk?

Numbness of the nipples may be a sign of nerve damage, which may affect milk ejection. The nursing baby's healthy weight gain rules out most potential problems. Hypersensitivity could make nursing painful. Scarring could affect milk flow. Encourage all parents to remove their nipple jewelry before nursing to prevent choking. If parents are concerned about their nipple piercing closing before the baby weans, suggest using temporary jewelry to keep it open.

DIGITAL RESOURCES

bfmed.org/protocols—Free, downloadable fully referenced protocols are ideal for sharing with healthcare providers from the Academy of Breastfeeding Medicine:

- #26 Persistent pain with breastfeeding

CHAPTER 14 NUTRITION, EXERCISE, AND LIFESTYLE ISSUES

NUTRITION FOR NURSING PARENTS

NUTRITION BASICS are the same for nursing parents as for the rest of the family. Suggest eating a nutrient-dense diet, choosing fresh foods in as close to their natural state as possible. Rather than counting calories, suggest using appetite as a guide or "eat to hunger." Choose fresh fruits and vegetables, whole grains, and foods rich in calcium and protein. The specific foods will vary by personal preference, culture, climate, and family finances.

The types of fatty acids in a nursing parent's diet will vary with the types of fats they eat.

Even when food is scarce, most nursing parents make ample milk, but when unexplained low milk production is an issue, focus on lactation-critical nutrients, such as protein, calcium, omega-3 fatty acids, and fiber, as well as any potential deficiencies of vitamin B_{12}, iodine, zinc, and iron.

When nursing parents fast, any changes in the baby's nursing pattern or behavior are temporary.

FLUIDS Suggest nursing parents "drink to thirst" and expect they will feel thirstier while nursing. Drink more fluids if they are constipated or their urine is concentrated. Contrary to popular belief, drinking more fluids is not associated with increased milk production.

It is not necessary for nursing parents to "drink milk to make milk."

SUPPLEMENTS: VITAMINS, MINERALS, OMEGA-3S, AND PROBIOTICS may not benefit well-nourished nursing parents with healthy vitamin D levels. But in those who are undernourished or nutrient-deficient, supplements may improve parent's and baby's health.

FOODS TO EAT OR AVOID No specific foods should be consumed or avoided during lactation. Most nursing parents can eat anything in moderation without any effect on their baby.

When nursing parents eat foods with different flavors, these flavors pass into their milk, giving the baby a preview of the tastes she will experience later from solid foods she eats at the family table.

REACTIONS TO A FOOD IN THE PARENT'S DIET Fussiness and gassiness are normal during the newborn period and are unlikely to be a reaction to something in the parent's diet. During the first year, only about 5% of nursing babies react to a food their parent consumes.

When a baby does react to a food in the parent's diet, the specific food that causes a reaction will vary from baby to baby. It is far more likely a baby will react to a food she is fed directly, such as formula or solids, rather than to a food in her parent's diet. A reaction is more likely if there is a family history of allergy and is accompanied by physical symptoms, such as:

- Skin reactions: eczema, dermatitis, hives, rash, dry skin
- Gastrointestinal reactions: vomiting, diarrhea, pain, blood or mucus in stools
- Respiratory reactions: congestion, runny nose, wheezing, coughing

If a baby has an acute reaction to a new food in the parent's diet, it may appear as soon as 1 hour after ingestion and usually resolves within 24 hours.

In Western countries, the most common food to cause a reaction in babies through mother's milk is dairy, followed by other mostly protein foods, such as eggs, corn, soy, citrus fruits, nuts, peanuts, and wheat. Nursing babies who are fed formula during the first 24 hours of life are 7 times more likely than other nursing babies to develop a cow-milk protein allergy.

When parents eliminate from their diet a food they eat regularly, some babies improve within a few days. But it often takes 3 to 4 weeks before cow-milk protein clears fully from their system and the baby's reaction resolves completely.

Elimination of dairy for a few months is not associated with greater-than-normal loss of bone mineral density. If there is a concern, the nursing parent can take calcium supplements.

If parents plan to make any major changes in their diet, suggest eliminating no more than one or two foods at a time, so they can more easily pinpoint the cause and get skilled help in evaluating their diet. After an elimination diet, if the baby's symptoms continue and other causes are ruled out, another option is for the nursing parent to go on a low-allergen diet consisting of lamb, rice, squash, and pears.

After an offending food is eliminated, the nursing parent can re-introduce it within 6 months or so.

If a baby's stools contain blood and/or mucus and eliminating dairy does not resolve it, rule out other causes, such as anal fissure, antibiotic use, GI infection, and a family history of inflammatory bowel disease. In most cases, it will clear in time with continued nursing.

CAFFEINE, CHOCOLATE, AND HERBAL TEAS Moderate caffeine intake by the nursing parent (2 to 3 cups of coffee per day) is not a problem for most nursing babies.

Chocolate contains theobromine, a substance similar to caffeine, but in much smaller amounts. Moderate consumption of chocolate does not cause a reaction in most nursing babies.

Regarding herbs, many modern medications are derived from the herbs used in teas and home remedies. Like drugs, herbs can affect lactation and the nursing baby. In large amounts, herbal teas made from sage, peppermint, and parsley can slow milk production. Major brands of herbal teas are safe for nursing parents. But use with caution "private" brand teas and teas from single herbs.

BONE HEALTH Some bone loss occurs during lactation, but by 6 months or so after weaning, bone density is back to prepregnancy levels. Longer lifetime nursing is associated with improved bone health.

Calcium intake from foods or supplements does not appear to affect calcium levels in milk or the nursing parent's bone density.

VEGETARIAN AND VEGAN FAMILIES Nursing parents who consume no animal products (vegans) need a reliable source of vitamin B_{12} to prevent a vitamin B_{12} deficiency in themselves and their nursing baby. Suggest they either take vitamin B_{12} supplements or eat foods fortified with vitamin B_{12}. In babies, if this deficiency is caught early and treated with vitamin B_{12}, it can be reversed. If left untreated, it may cause irreversible neurological problems.

WEIGHT AND WEIGHT LOSS Many—but not all—nursing parents lose weight gradually during the first 6 months after birth. Gradual weight loss is more likely in parents who nurse exclusively. After 6 months, weight is usually more stable. If nursing parents want to lose weight faster, suggest eating less and exercising more, avoiding extreme weight loss programs. When eating less to lose weight, eat nutrient-dense foods and consider a vitamin-and-mineral supplement. A minimum of 1800 calories per day is recommended during lactation, but 1500 calories per day does not affect milk production or composition in previously well-nourished parents. Encourage parents to eat a healthy diet for their own sake to boost their energy level and resistance to illness.

Extremely low carb diets are not recommended during lactation. If parents want to try a low-carb diet, suggest a moderate version that includes some carbohydrates.

UNDERWEIGHT AND EATING DISORDERS put nursing parents at risk for vitamin deficiencies. If they become deficient in vitamin A, D, B_6, or B_{12}, this may affect milk composition. But even if undernourished nursing parents are not vitamin deficient, consuming too few calories may lower their energy level and resistance to illness. With extreme malnutrition lasting for weeks, milk production may eventually decrease. When nursing parents are malnourished, the most cost- and resource-effective strategy is to supplement nursing parents rather than their babies.

Eating disorders, such as anorexia and bulimia nervosa, increase the risk of preterm birth and pregnancy and birth complications, as well as reduced length at birth. A healthy weight gain during pregnancy, however, offsets these risks.

Regarding lactation, exclusively nursing babies of parents with eating disorders gain weight within the normal range. Some parents with eating disorders embrace nursing; others reject it. Parents with a current or past eating disorder are more likely to nurse on a schedule and be less aware of their baby's hunger and satiety cues.

OBESITY before and during pregnancy is linked to lower rates of nursing initiation. For those who do nurse, does obesity have a physical effect on lactation? Possibly. Excess body fat releases hormones like estrogen and male hormones (androgens) that affect metabolism (increasing risk of insulin resistance and heart disease). During puberty, these hormones may disrupt normal development of the mammary glands. After birth, they may alter the body's response to sucking. Research found a link between prepregnancy obesity and a delay in milk increase after birth. But this delay may be due in part to delays in early nursing among overweight and obese parents, who are less likely to nurse their newborns within the first 2 hours after birth, a variable also associated with a delay in milk increase. Rat studies found a link between obesity and prolactin resistance.

Overweight and obese parents are also more likely to suffer from medical conditions that may affect early milk production, such as diabetes and polycystic ovary syndrome (PCOS).

Newborns of obese nursing parents are more likely to receive formula supplements during their hospital stay than newborns of normal-weight parents. Physical factors may have some effect on this, but after birth, obese parents are also more likely to receive a lower quality of lactation care than other parents.

Low self-esteem, shaming, and cultural discrimination may affect nursing outcomes in obese parents. Nursing parents with high BMIs report a reluctance to nurse in front of others—

even in their own home—and consider that one major barrier to meeting their feeding goals.

Cultural beliefs play a role, too. In areas where virtually all families nurse, obese parents begin nursing at the same rate as normal-weight parents. But even there, obese parents stop nursing earlier. If a culture does not consider obesity a negative, its nursing parents may be less likely to feel embarrassed or self-conscious about exposing their bodies around others.

Even with larger mammary glands and larger nipples, obese parents do not have more latching struggles than in normal-weight families.

Strategies to provide a better quality of care and better nursing outcomes for obese parents include:

During pregnancy:

- Provide nutritional counseling to keep pregnancy weight gain in the recommended range by putting the focus on consuming nutrient-rich foods and avoiding non-nutritious choices, such as soda and candy.
- Learn the basics of how milk production works.
- During the last month of pregnancy, learn and practice hand expression, demonstrated on the website **firstdroplets.com**.
- Arrange for labor support and learn non-drug pain management techniques to help reduce the odds of a cesarean delivery.

After birth, emphasize nursing early, often, and effectively to promote healthy milk production.

- Plan to keep the newborn in skin-to-skin contact during the first 1 to 2 hours and nurse within the first 2 hours after birth.
- Limit separation and encourage the nursing couple to share lots of skin-to-skin and body contact as well as frequent feeds, ideally at least 8 to 12 feeds per 24 hours.
- During the first few days, several times each day after nursing, express extra colostrum into a spoon to feed the baby some "dessert."
- Find a comfortable feeding position that allows the parent to relax and avoids resting a heavy gland on the baby's chest.

Targeted efforts are needed to provide the support obese parents need to meet their feeding goals.

A nursing parent with a high BMI may have an unrealistic view of the baby's weight, leading to early weaning or negative assumptions about the baby's weight gain.

WEIGHT-LOSS SURGERY Depending on the specific procedure used, many parents with a history of weight-loss surgery need to take vitamin and mineral supplements to avoid deficiencies. These procedures limit the amount of food the digestive system can hold and may affect the body's ability to absorb nutrients from food. Regular blood tests post-surgery can check for nutritional deficiencies. A vitamin B_{12} deficiency, for example may cause a deficiency in the nursing baby..

Milk composition is the same in those with a history of weight-loss surgery as in those without.

Encourage nursing families to learn the basics of milk production, take regular supplements as directed, share their history with the baby's healthcare provider, and regularly monitor their own health and their baby's weight gain and health.

EXERCISE

Moderate exercise improves cardiovascular fitness, blood lipid profiles, and insulin response. Exercise also relieves stress and improves mood.

Even when nursing parents exercise moderately and eat less to lose weight, milk production and composition appear unaffected. Exercise has no effect on baby's weight gain and growth or nursing outcomes.

Exercising to exhaustion increases levels of lactic acid in the milk, but there is no benefit to postponing nursing.

When nursing parents are ready to start exercising after birth, suggest they first talk to their healthcare provider and then start gradually. It may be easier for a new parent to exercise more often if the baby is included by combining exercise with other activities, like walking with the baby in a stroller or carrier or doing exercise routines that include the baby.

Little specific information is available to guide elite athletes during lactation.

GROOMING: HAIR CARE, TANNING, AND PIERCINGS

No evidence exists that nursing parents' use of hair-care products or tanning beds affect their nursing baby.

Some parents with pierced nipples have successfully nursed, but some have experienced feeding problems related to their piercing (p. 235).

SUBSTANCE USE DURING LACTATION

ALCOHOL Recommendations on how much alcohol consumption is compatible with nursing vary by country and organization. It was once thought that drinking alcohol in moderation is compatible with nursing. Now most agree that alcohol consumption should be minimized during lactation, due to concerns about impaired motor development and growth in the baby and possible decreased milk consumption and sleep disturbances. Some experts conclude that there is no known safe amount of alcohol in human milk, especially during the first month, and recommend nursing parents refrain from nursing after any amount of drinking until the alcohol is out of their milk. After the first month, they suggest limiting alcohol intake to one to two standard drinks per day and drink them just after nursing to limit the amount of alcohol the baby receives.

The alcohol in one drink clears the blood and milk quickly without the need for pumping and dumping. In a 120-pound parent, it takes 2 to 3 hours for the alcohol in one glass of beer or wine to leave the milk. When alcohol is consumed without food, blood alcohol levels peak about 20 to 40 minutes after the drink. When consumed with a meal, their peak blood alcohol levels occur about 60 to 90 minutes later.

The more alcohol consumed, the longer it takes for it to clear the blood and milk. To calculate the clearance of more than one alcoholic drink in parents of different weights, see **bit.ly/BA2-AlcoholCalculator.**

Nursing or expressing milk before drinking alcohol reduces alcohol availability in the nursing parent's body. Both eating a meal and expressing milk within the hour before drinking reduces the total availability of alcohol in their system by 58%.

Alcohol disrupts a nursing parent's hormonal balance and decreases the volume of milk the baby takes at a nursing session. Exposure to alcohol in the milk causes nursing babies to sleep less.

Drinking large amounts of alcohol or drinking regularly over time, may harm the nursing baby by causing some of the same symptoms as fetal alcohol syndrome, with these babies being smaller in size and having lower verbal IQ scores than the children whose nursing parent did not drink.

TOBACCO Many parents who smoke cigarettes believe wrongly that formula is "safer" for babies than nursing. But the opposite is true. When parents smoke and don't nurse, it not only increases their own health risks, it increases their baby's risk of infection, respiratory illness, respiratory allergy, asthma, and SIDS. Encourage parents to nurse and, if possible, quit smoking. If they can't quit, suggest they smoke as little as possible and smoke outdoors away from baby.

Smoking during pregnancy increases risk of lower birth weight and preterm birth. The more cigarettes smoked, the greater the risk to the baby.

PHYSICAL OR PSYCHOLOGICAL EFFECTS Parents who smoke are less likely to initiate nursing, and those who do nurse are more likely to wean earlier than nonsmoking parents. But physical effects of smoking may only play a partial role in these differences. Smoking reduces fat levels in milk, but oddly, smoking was linked to a greater weight gain in nursing babies. Studies examining the neurological effects of smoking during pregnancy and lactation find babies of smokers have lower LATCH assessment scores and have more feeding problems. After birth, babies of smokers experienced withdrawal symptoms.

But earlier weaning in smoking parents has more to do with parents' anxiety about how smoking affects their milk and their baby. Most smoking parents wean to formula earlier because they think it is safer than nursing. This is due in part to misinformed advice from healthcare providers who discourage smoking parents from nursing.

STRATEGIES TO MINIMIZE NURSING BABIES' EXPOSURE to nicotine and secondhand smoke include:

- Smoke fewer cigarettes per day or quit entirely.

- Smoke after nursing. Waiting a couple of hours allows milk nicotine levels to fall significantly before the baby nurses again. But nursing sooner is better than giving formula.

- Smoke outside or in a separate room. No matter how a baby is fed, breathing cigarette smoke poses health risks for everyone in the family.

NICOTINE REPLACEMENT PRODUCTS used to quit smoking are compatible with nursing. Gums, lozenges, tablets, inhalers, and nasal sprays are used intermittently over the day. Suggest parents use them after nursing. On average, with recommended use, these replacement products provide about as much nicotine per day as less than one pack of cigarettes.

Transdermal nicotine patches provide a steady level of nicotine in the user's blood and milk, which is lower than smoking. Suggest removing the patch at bedtime for lower nicotine levels at night. While the patch is used, babies receive 70% less nicotine and its metabolite cotinine than while parent smoked.

Some use e-cigarettes (aka vaping) to quit smoking. Battery powered, they look like a regular cigarette and mimic the smoking experience without the harmful compounds released during smoking. The amount of nicotine delivered by vaping is minimal and comparable to a nicotine inhaler.

CANNABIS, legal in some places and not in others, is used for medical and recreational purposes. Derived from the *Cannabis sativa* or hemp plant, its forms include marijuana from its dried leaves, stems, and flower buds, hashish from the resin in its flower buds, and oils from extracted cannabidiol (CBD) diluted with a carrier oil. Its psychoactive ingredient is delta-9-tetrahydrocannabinol (THC). Today's cannabis products contain much higher THC levels than those of decades ago. CBD oils, used to treat pain and nausea, have very low THC levels, so they do not have the psychoactive effect of other cannabis products.

SMOKED OR EATEN When smoked, about 25% of the THC is absorbed, while only about 12% is absorbed when it is eaten.

THC enters the fatty tissues and is stored, so urine screens may be positive several weeks after the last use. Even where cannabis is legal for medical and recreational use, a positive urine screen may require medical staff to contact child protective services for an evaluation.

THC PASSES INTO HUMAN MILK, with peak levels occurring at 1 hour after exposure and the relative infant dose at 2.5% of the nursing parent's dose. THC can be detected in milk for up to 6 days after the last cannabis use. In heavy cannabis users, the level of THC in milk and blood are up to 8 times higher than the levels in occasional users. When cannabis is used regularly, THC is stored in body fat, increasing its half-life (normally 25 to 35 hours) to 4 days. After a nursing parent uses cannabis, THC can be detected in the baby's urine for up to 3 weeks.

EFFECTS OF CANNABIS ON THE NURSING BABY The most significant concern is the possible effect of THC on the baby's rapidly developing brain. THC is quickly absorbed by both the milk and the brain. Repeated cannabis exposure can disrupt neurological development, with the potential to cause permanent neurobehavioral and cognitive impairment. Exposure of the nursing baby during the first month of life may decrease motor development at 1 year.

EFFECTS OF CANNABIS ON LACTATION Cannabis use may lower prolactin and oxytocin levels in nursing parents and may reduce sucking in babies, both of which could reduce milk removal and production.

RECOMMENDATIONS ABOUT CANNABIS USE DURING LACTATION vary because research is scant and conflicting. The central messages include:

- Much is unknown about cannabis' effects on the baby's brain, and just because it may be legal and "natural," that does not make it safe to use during pregnancy and lactation.

- After birth, if a urine screen for cannabis is positive—possible for weeks after the last use—child protective services may be contacted.

- Keep the baby away from any contact with secondhand cannabis smoke.

- If cannabis is used for medical reasons, discuss possible alternative treatments, and if none exist, weigh the risks and benefits of continuing to nurse while using cannabis.

- If possible, stop using cannabis during pregnancy and lactation. If stopping its use is not an option, reduce it as much as possible.

For more, see the Academy of Breastfeeding Medicine's Clinical Protocol #21 at **bfmed.org/protocols**.

OPIOIDS, NAS, AND TREATMENTS In recent decades, the use of opioids—both legal and illicit—skyrocketed. Prescription opioids are among the most commonly used narcotic pain relievers and include codeine, morphine, oxycodone, fentanyl, and hydrocodone. Morphine is often given for pain relief after a cesarean delivery due to its short half-life—1.5 to 2 hours—it leaves the body quickly, which is an advantage in nursing parents.

Opioid drugs can be an appropriate choice when taken short term but are often overprescribed for longer periods, which leads to drug dependence known as ***opioid use disorder***. Some who develop this disorder switch to illicit and highly addictive opioids such as heroin due to lower costs.

NEONATAL ABSTINENCE SYNDROME (NAS) is the withdrawal process that occurs when a baby is born to a parent regularly using opioids, including opioid-substitute drugs like methadone, which treats opioid dependence.

NAS occurs in the majority of opioid exposed newborns. Its symptoms occur where the opiate receptors are located, such as the central nervous system and the digestive tract. Digestive symptoms include vomiting, diarrhea, poor weight gain, and poor feeding, which may include uncoordinated sucking that may contribute to nursing challenges.

Lactation Eases NAS Symptoms Newborns with NAS who nurse or receive expressed human milk have better outcomes than those exclusively formula-fed, needing less drug treatment for a shorter time. Rooming-in during the hospital stay also leads to better NAS outcomes.

Lactation and Treatment for Adult Opioid Dependence The medications used to treat adults for opioid dependence, such as methadone and buprenorphine, are compatible with nursing. But nursing initiation and duration vary greatly among birthing parents in treatment for opioid-use disorder. Factors that affect nursing outcomes include the model of care used, whether consistent lactation advice is given, and how much lactation support is available.

METHAMPHETAMINE, or meth, is a stimulant drug that affects the central nervous system and is highly addictive. Meth is used as a powder, a pill, or as crystal meth, which looks like glass fragments or rocks. It can be smoked, snorted, injected, or ingested orally or anally. Meth is contraindicated during nursing, and if used, the lactating parent needs to pump and dump for at least 100 hours after use or until their urine screen is negative. If parents use meth regularly, assume they lack the good judgment needed to avoid nursing while under the influence and need treatment.

COCAINE is a central nervous system stimulant that can be smoked, snorted, or injected. With repeated use, tolerance can develop. Cocaine passes into milk in significant amounts and can cause cocaine intoxication in the nursing baby. Reported symptoms in the baby include irritability, vomiting, dilated pupils, tremors, and increased heart and respiratory rates. After cocaine use, the nursing parent needs to pump and dump for at least 24 hours. Although the effects of cocaine on the nursing parent can fade within 20 to 30 minutes, cocaine is metabolized slowly and is found in adults' urine for up to 7 days and even longer in babies' urine.

Because illicit drugs are rarely pure, cocaine may also contain other drugs that may be harmful to the nursing baby. Cocaine use is contraindicated during lactation. Topical cocaine can also be hazardous.

HALLUCINOGENIC DRUGS, include PCP (angel dust), gamma hydroxybutyric acid (ecstasy), and LSD (acid). Significant amounts of these drugs pass easily through the blood-brain barrier, which make them very likely to transfer quickly into human milk. Their use is contraindicated during lactation.

- **PCP** (half-life of 24 to 51 hours)—Because it is stored in fatty tissue, PCP can be detected in the user's urine for 14 to 30 days.

- **Ecstasy** (half-life of 20 to 60 minutes)—Depending on dose, after use the lactating parent needs to pump and dump for at least 12 to 24 hours.

- **LSD** (half-life of 3 hours)—This very potent drug crosses the blood-brain barrier and may cause hallucinations in the baby. LSD is found in the parent's urine for 34 to 120 hours.

NURSING AND THE USE OF ILLICIT SUBSTANCES In most cases, untreated mental-health issues lead to regular use of illicit substances as a type of self-medication. Termed ***substance use disorder*** (SUD), more than 75% of those diagnosed with SUD suffer from depressive disorders and 25% have four or more different mental-health diagnoses. Illicit substance use can occur in any family, but it is more likely in those who are poor, unemployed, lack safe housing and social support, and who have a history of trauma. Using illicit substances during pregnancy increases risk for birth defects, fetal growth restrictions, preterm birth, impaired neurological development, and after birth, signs of toxicity or withdrawal.

In families with a history of illicit drug use, nursing may be risky. The nursing baby may be exposed to dangerous substances through the milk. In those who use illicit drugs, use of multiple drugs is the norm, in part because illicit drugs are often cut with other substances. Because psychiatric disorders are so common in these individuals, the nursing parent may also be taking psychiatric medications. Infection, such as HIV (p. 142) and hepatitis B and C (p. 138) are also more common in illicit drug users. Yet in spite of the risks, these parents and babies stand to benefit significantly from nursing.

This picture is complicated even more because it can be difficult to separate a baby's exposure to a drug during pregnancy from exposure through the milk. Unfortunately, the decision to nurse after birth does not decrease the odds that a previous illicit drug user will use again. See the ABM's Clinical Protocol #21 for specific topics to discuss with families with a history of illicit drug use to determine if nursing should be considered (free and downloadable at **bfmed.org/protocols**).

It is difficult for any lactation supporter to discourage a parent from nursing. But where the nursing parent is using dangerous substances that could harm the baby, the risks of nursing sometimes outweighs its benefits.

When nursing parents are under the influence of illicit drugs, no matter how the baby is fed, their ability to provide adequate care is impaired.

DIGITAL RESOURCES

bfmed.org/protocols—Free and downloadable, fully referenced protocols available in multiple languages, suitable for sharing with healthcare providers:

- #21: Guidelines for breastfeeding and substance use or substance use disorder
- #24: Allergic proctocolitis in the exclusively breastfed infant
- #29: Iron, zinc, and vitamin D supplementation during breastfeeding

bit.ly/BA2-AlcoholCalculator—From Canadian scientists, created for parents and professionals to determine—based on parent weight and number of alcoholic drinks—the length of time needed for alcohol to completely clear the milk

CHAPTER 15   PREGNANCY AND TANDEM NURSING

NURSING DURING PREGNANCY

Many parents have mixed feelings about nursing during pregnancy, and the following are common concerns.

CONCERNS ABOUT THE UNBORN BABY   Nursing during pregnancy should not negatively affect the unborn baby if the birthing parent is well-nourished and the older sibling consumes other foods and drinks.

CONCERNS ABOUT THE EFFECTS ON THE PREGNANCY The uterine contractions that occur during nursing are similar to those occurring during sexual relations. During a high-risk pregnancy, unless the couple is advised to avoid sexual relations due to potential preterm labor, nursing should not be contraindicated.

CONCERNS ABOUT THE NURSING PARENT'S NUTRITION, HEALTH, AND COMFORT   Staying well-nourished promotes healthy pregnancy weight gain, which lowers risk of birth complications. If a parent is malnourished during pregnancy, improving nutrition or providing nutritional supplements eliminates the health risks.

Managing an active child can be difficult when early-pregnancy nausea strikes. For some, nursing does not increase feelings of nausea but holding a squirming child does. For others, increased nausea occurs during nursing, whether or not their child is active. This may be due in part to an increased body awareness during nursing. Try sharing frequent small meals with the child to reduce both nausea and the child's hunger, one motivation to nurse. Try limiting nursing to a shorter time, such as the length of a favorite song. During pregnancy, as well as afterward, setting limits on nursing with the older child—such as night weaning--is a workable alternative to full weaning.

With any kind of discomfort associated with nursing, let the child know that this discomfort is not the child's fault and avoid blaming the unborn baby. If nursing during pregnancy is uncomfortable, try these strategies.

- Vary nursing positions, ensuring a deep latch, with the nipple as far back in his mouth as possible.
- Use childbirth breathing techniques while nursing.
- Ask the child to be gentler or limit nursing to a shorter time, assuring the child that the pain is not his fault.

- Hand-express until milk ejection occurs, as pain decreases when milk is flowing.

When nursing during pregnancy, many parents feel restless, irritable, or have other strong negative feelings. If so, while nursing, suggest using distraction, such as putting their focus on an electronic device or using visualization. Some families find taking orally 250 mg to 500 mg of magnesium supplements per day during pregnancy helps alleviate these feelings. Knowing they are not alone with these negative feelings can be tremendously reassuring. Many online groups offer peer support for those experiencing these challenges.

One possible advantage of continued nursing is that it may simplify managing pregnancy-related fatigue by making it easier to convince the nursing child to lie down and nurse when it's time to rest.

MILK PRODUCTION DURING PREGNANCY About midway through pregnancy, milk production decreases markedly as milk turns to colostrum. Some nursing children respond to this change in milk volume and taste by nursing less or weaning. Some suddenly begin eating and drinking more of other foods and beverages. The nursing child who is old enough to talk may comment on the change in flavor. Some children who wean want to resume nursing after the baby is born. Others continue to nurse during the pregnancy despite these changes.

Age alone does not predict whether a child will wean during pregnancy. But babies younger than 12 months are unlikely to be physically ready to wean. If pregnancy occurs prior to 1 year, suggest monitoring baby's weight gain to make sure he stays well-nourished. The natural pregnancy-related decrease in milk production could compromise baby's nutritional needs. If weight gain falters, consult baby's healthcare provider about appropriate supplements. The baby with a faltering weight gain may need more solid foods or donor milk and/or infant formula.

As the milk changes to colostrum in preparation for the birth, the nursing child will not "use up" all the colostrum. No matter how often or long he nurses, colostrum will still be available after birth for the newborn.

TANDEM NURSING

DEFINITIONS "Tandem nursing" and "co-nursing" are not the same. Tandem nursing refers to "nursing siblings who are not twins." Tandem nursing may happen by design or by default and can be both joyful and stressful. "Co-nursing," on the other hand, refers to adult partners who both nurse one or more children (p. 280).

PRACTICAL DETAILS During the first few days after birth, make it a priority to nurse the newborn often (a minimum of 8 feeds/day). If the older sibling has an intense desire to nurse, consider arranging special outings for him, where he receives extra attention. After the first few days, encourage each family to manage nursing both children in whatever way works best for them.

Tandem nursing can help minimize engorgement and ensure abundant milk production. If the older sibling nurses often in the early weeks, this may cause changes in his stools, making them less formed, as colostrum and transitional milk can have a laxative effect.

Normal hygiene, such as a daily shower, is usually enough while tandem nursing, even in case of illness. It is not necessary to limit each child to one side or to wash the nipples between children, because the children have already been exposed to any illness.

While tandem nursing, suggest the parent eat well, drink enough fluids, and get enough rest. Help from the partner or support person can make it easier to meet both children's needs.

EMOTIONAL ADJUSTMENTS For the older sibling, continuing to nurse after the new baby is born may help ease his emotional adjustment. From the adult perspective, nursing parents react differently to tandem nursing. Some enjoy it; others do not. Parents may decide during pregnancy to tandem nurse because they are focused on the older sibling's needs. After birth, feelings may shift dramatically. Opposing feelings are also common.

If the parent's feelings about tandem nursing are negative or uncomfortable, suggest possible adjustments. Try varying the older child's feeding positions or nursing the siblings separately rather than together. Some find they can better handle these difficult feelings by reducing their older child's time nursing, keeping each feed short but not eliminating or postponing them. Others nurse less often by distracting their older child with other activities, postponing feeds, or offering substitutions, such as snacks or drinks before the older child asks to nurse. Some parents find that taking oral magnesium supplements (250 mg to 500 mg per day) helps reduce feelings of agitation or aversion that arise during nursing.

When a nursing parent is consistently unhappy with tandem nursing, using weaning strategies to reduce the number of nursing sessions per day may help. A partial weaning and/or night weaning may make it easier for the parent to continue. If not, see Chapter 19 for tips on weaning.

CHAPTER 16 PRETERM BABY

Being born preterm covers a broad spectrum of gestational ages, feeding abilities, and health issues, from tiny, fragile infants born months early to healthy, robust late preterm babies.

PARENTS' ROLE IN THE PREEMIE'S CARE

After a preterm birth, grief may affect parents' ability to process and remember information and affect their intention to nurse. They may be even more motivated to nurse due to their baby's physical vulnerabilities. Or their fragile emotional state may make nursing feel like an intrusion.

Even if nursing was not the original plan, the family needs to know the importance of expressed milk to their preterm baby's health. Taking an active role in the baby's care can reduce parents' anxiety and feelings of helplessness and over time help them form a closer bond with their baby.

MILK EXPRESSION can be lifesaving for very preterm babies, so parents need to know about best practices, even if it feels overwhelming at times. Encourage them to seek support.

When pumping exclusively for a preterm baby, parents want to know what to expect and how to handle common problems, such as nipple pain, engorgement, and struggles with milk production.

Even if donor milk is available, infant health outcomes are better when parents' own expressed milk is provided.

SKIN-TO-SKIN CONTACT (SSC) is sometimes referred to as kangaroo care or kangaroo mother care. Providing preemies with SSC as soon after birth as possible for as long as possible improves infant stability, reduces stress, promotes growth, and enhances the parent-child bond.

Any parent can provide their preemie with SSC. Wearing only a diaper and a hat, hold the preemie chest-to-chest against parents' bare skin, covered by a shirt, a blanket, or a binder tight enough to support the baby in the kangaroo position. Support the baby with her head turned to one side, her chin slightly raised, and arms and legs flexed.

Nearly all preterm babies benefit from SSC, but in the following cases, it may need to be delayed: in babies born <28 weeks gestation or <750 g, when the baby is unstable or very sick, is on mechanical ventilation for a serious illness, on certain drugs, or had recent surgery.

NURSING THE PRETERM BABY

Human milk is important for preemies, but so is direct nursing. Preemies who nurse in the NICU are more likely to be nursing at discharge and to receive human milk at and after discharge. Direct nursing benefits preemies by enhancing neurological development and bonding. It also benefits parents, because intensive pumping is time-consuming and challenging to maintain.

WHAT TO EXPECT Preterm babies are different from term babies. Preemies may nurse less effectively because they have low muscle tone, small mouths without fat pads in their cheeks, less body fat, which increases temperature instability, and less stable heart rate and breathing. Because preemies' brains are smaller and less developed than term newborns, they have less control over their head and limbs and spend more time asleep or drowsy.

PREDICTABLE PHASES OF PRETERM NURSING Swedish researcher Kerstin Hedberg Nyqvist developed a road map of the predictable phases preemies experience as they move to effective direct nursing (Box 16.1). This road map provides realistic expectations and the positive perspective that nursing will improve with time, practice, and maturity.

Box 16.1. The Road Map: Phases of Preterm Nursing

Babies born closer to term or healthier may start at a later phase.

1. Frequent milk expression, baby is tube-fed, lots of skin-to-skin contact
2. Nursing begins: rooting, licking, or mouthing the nipple with no milk intake yet
3. Single sucks, short bursts, long pauses, baby stays latched for short time, some milk intake
4. Longer sucking bursts, baby stays latched longer, milk intake variable but baby takes more milk more often, need to plan supplementation strategy
5. Milk intake increases with occasional larger volumes
6. More milk intake with immature sucking pattern, short bursts, long pauses, full nursing possible with semi-demand feeding
7. Effective, mature sucking pattern of a term baby, can now nurse on cue

WHEN TO START NURSING Rather than thinking in terms of "readiness" for direct nursing, think of it as a normal behavior to be facilitated as early as possible, like walking or talking. In some places, gestational age and weight are not considered. Nursing begins when baby is off the ventilator and continuous positive airway (CPAP) machine and has no severe instability. Some babies latch and nurse as early as 28 weeks gestation.

Direct nursing is less physically stressful for preterm babies than bottle-feeding, which due to its fast flow causes more heart rate and breathing irregularities and lower oxygen blood levels. Direct nursing should ideally be baby's first oral feed.

HOW TO START NURSING The recommendation to start on a "emptied" gland is based on research done with bottle-feeding preemies and does not apply to nursing. Right before nursing sessions, avoid stressful medical procedures or stimulating events like diaper changes.

REALISTIC EXPECTATIONS Suggest families think of early nursing as a learning process. The baby may begin by licking or mouthing the nipple. She may suck in short bursts and fall asleep quickly (see Box 16.1). It is okay if the baby does not take milk during the first few nursing sessions. If needed, she will be supplemented with milk afterwards.

PRIVACY is ideal, preferably a separate room with a door. If the baby is on a monitor, oxygen, and an IV, a private room may not be possible. But even in a busy NICU, a private area can be created with a curtain or screen. If that's impossible, position the parent's chair with its back to the room.

COMFORT A comfortable chair that reclines with good back and arm support is ideal, but even in a straight-backed chair, the parent can move their hips forward for a body slope used with starter positions (p. 6). Extra pillows may help. Choose clothing that gives baby easy access to the nipple. Make sure the baby is not too warm or overheated, which can make her drowsy. Close contact with the parent's body will provide warmth, and a hat and a blanket over her may be all that's needed.

SOUND AND LIGHT A calm, quiet environment helps keep stimulation manageable for baby, so encourage others to talk quietly. Try to position the nursing couple away from flashing lights and, if possible, dim the room lights and protect the baby's eyes from direct light.

RELAXED TIME TOGETHER To reduce stress, ask not to be rushed or interrupted.

MAKE SKILLED LACTATION HELP AVAILABLE during the first few nursing sessions. Parents will gain confidence while they learn baby's cues. If needed, offer practical suggestions for helping baby latch deeply and comfortable positions. Demonstrate with a doll unless parents ask for hands-on help.

If the baby had previous breathing or heartbeat irregularities, suggest a healthcare provider monitor the baby during early feeds. If the baby remains stable during the first few feeds, the nursing parent can learn how to observe the baby's breathing and skin color and when to ask for help if needed

HELPING BABY LATCH AND FEED   Before nursing attempts, start with unrestricted skin-to-skin contact. When baby is snuggled under the nursing parent's clothing, it is easy to tell from the baby's movements when she is arousing and ready to feed. Other cues include changes in her breathing, sounds, eyes opening, and sucking movements.

Use whatever feeding positions work best. To latch deeply and feed well, good body and head support are vital. One option is the starter positions (p. 6), in which baby lies tummy down on the parent's body, with the baby's head supported by the parent's arm. After latching, gravity helps keep the nipple deeply in baby's mouth. Babies have better oxygenation, exert more sucking pressure, and take more milk when they feed prone.

If upright feeding positions are used, the parent needs to provide baby with body and head support.

- Ensure good back, neck, and arm support for the parent.
- Hold the baby with her entire front facing and touching the parent.
- When guiding the baby to the nipple, suggest parents put their palm on baby's back, thumb and index finger supporting the base of her head.
- Align the baby nose to nipple (p. 319), so she can approach the gland chin first, with a wide-open mouth and head slightly tilted back to make swallowing easier.
- Apply gentle pressure on the baby's shoulders as she latches to ensure she takes a big mouthful and throughout the feed, so she stays deeply latched.
- If needed, put a pillow under baby to support her at nipple height.

After latching, avoid extra movements or touching. Because preterm babies are easily overstimulated, even normal patting and rocking may be too much and cause baby to tune out.

In upright feeding positions, try with and without mammary support to see which works better.

After a period of exclusive pumping, at first, milk ejection may take some time, as the parent's body adjusts to the feel of baby nursing. The baby may suck for several minutes before the milk starts to flow. Soon, though, the parent's body will become conditioned to the feel of the baby nursing and the milk will flow more quickly. In the meantime, to speed milk flow, before nursing spend time in skin-to-skin contact. If this doesn't help, before latching, stimulate milk ejection with a pump or by hand. Or after latch, pump the opposite side to trigger milk ejection sooner.

Parents can learn to recognize the signs it is safe for the baby to continue nursing and the signs baby needs to stop. Signs the baby can continue nursing include regular heartbeat and breathing, unchanging skin color, stable muscle tone, movements showing baby wants more (snuggling closer, hand to face, smiles), calm state, and looking at the parent. Signs it's time to stop nursing include changes in heartbeat and breathing, skin color changes, spitting up or gagging, low muscle tone, sticking out tongue, flexing or extending arms and legs, arching away, finger splaying, low alertness or fast shifts between states, looking tense, surprised, or scared, difficulty calming, looking away, eyes float from side to side, fussiness and crying.

GAUGING NURSING EFFECTIVENESS may involve using rough indicators of milk transfer, such as audible swallowing, milk around the baby's mouth, and fresh milk when the feeding tube is aspirated. A more accurate way to measure milk intake during nursing is weighing baby before and after feeds with a baby scale accurate to 2 g.

Knowing how much milk a baby consumes during nursing can prevent over-supplementation, which can delay the transition to full nursing. It can also prevent delays in initiating direct nursing. If healthcare providers need to accurately chart baby's milk intake, this provides evidence of feeding competence, which may determine length of hospital stay and discharge plans.

EARLY NURSING PATTERNS When a preterm baby starts nursing, ideally, she should nurse often and without time restrictions. No evidence supports limiting the number of nursing sessions or arbitrarily cutting feeds short. During nursing, a preterm baby has periods of rest and activity, and restricting the time may reduce the volume of milk consumed. If baby falls asleep early in the feed, hold her while she sleeps, keeping her close to the nipple and offer it when she is in a light sleep (eyes moving under eyelids, body movement). If needed, gavage- or tube-feeding can be done while baby nurses to provide positive reinforcement for her efforts.

There is no need to offer both sides at feeds unless the baby wants both.

When a preemie begins direct nursing, nurse when baby shows feeding cues and nurse at least every 2 hours or even more often during the day. Frequent feeds are closer to a typical newborn nursing rhythm and are part of ensuring adequate milk intake in preemies who have reached the sixth phase of preterm nursing (Box 16.1). With time and maturity, their nursing frequency decreases.

In most cases, before a preterm baby is ready for exclusive nursing, she will need to be supplemented. The volume given and the feeding pattern should be based on each baby's individual needs, so that she gets enough milk each day to gain weight in the expected range as she learns to nurse.

Once the baby is taking significant milk volumes during nursing, if the family is not rooming in at the hospital, encourage them to work out a schedule with the hospital staff, so they can nurse freely when they are with their baby. When they are not there, the hospital staff will use other feeding methods.

Using a nipple shield may help if the preterm baby has trouble staying latched or is not taking much milk. In these situations, the nipple shield may increase milk intake. If it eliminates the need to supplement or shortens the time to exclusive nursing, it may be a useful tool. But nipple shields should not be used with all preterm babies. In some studies, nipple shield use is linked to failure to exclusively nurse and earlier use of formula.

Continue milk expression until the baby is exclusively nursing.

WEIGHT GAIN AND SUPPLEMENTATION In most cases, after nursing begins, the preterm baby will both nurse and receive supplements. Being well fed is vital to healthy growth and feeding effectiveness.

HOW SHOULD PRETERM BABIES GROW? Experts are uncertain about what is optimal weight gain for preemies. The idea that preterm babies should gain and grow at about the same rate expected in utero began many decades ago and was based on the growth patterns of the larger preterm babies of that time. But because preemies today are being saved much earlier and have different nutritional needs, this benchmark no longer makes sense.

Reaching intrauterine growth rates is challenging because a tiny preemie's digestive system cannot absorb and digest food like a term newborn. And any extra nutrients must be given in a digestible and absorbable form in just the right balance, so the baby's kidneys and other organs are not stressed.

The primary focus for a preterm baby is both a healthy weight gain and positive long-term health outcomes. The Academy of Breastfeeding Medicine (ABM) Clinical Protocol #12 (at **bfmed.org/protocols**) recommends a daily weight gain of 15 g to 30 g (0.5 to 1 oz.). Adequate nourishment is vital for healthy neurological development and to prevent newborn hypoglycemia and jaundice. Poor long-term outcomes can occur when preemies gain either too much or too little weight.

If the healthcare provider is concerned that the baby is gaining too slowly on expressed milk alone, ask about the target weight gain and compare it to the 15 to 30 g (0.5 to 1 oz.) per day ABM recommendation. If the weight gain is slow and the baby is receiving mostly expressed milk, ask first if the baby could be fed more milk per feed or the same volume more times per day.

Some approaches to milk expression, storage, and handling can inadvertently reduce the calories consumed by preemies and slow weight gain:

- Not draining the mammary gland as fully as possible. To remedy this, use hands-on pumping techniques (p. 211).

- Changing containers during a pump session and providing the first, low-fat milk for the baby. To remedy this, ask for larger containers.

- Not realizing the layer of fat on top of expressed milk is normal and discarding it. Explain to parents its impact on weight gain.

- Transferring the milk into another container and leaving milk fat behind in the original container's crevices. Review mixing and transferring instructions.

- Baby is fed with a slow, continuous gavage tube system that traps the milk fat in the tubing. Suggest switching to intermittent feeds.

- Infusion syringes used to tube-feed the baby are positioned so the fat rises away from the tubing. Suggest changing the syringe position so that the milk fat rises to the tubing.

If the baby is exclusively nursing and gaining weight slowly despite taking significant milk volumes, avoid switching sides often during nursing and supplement baby with milk expressed after nursing.

SUPPLEMENTING NURSING will likely be necessary until a preemie reaches phase 6 or 7 of the phases of preterm nursing (Box 16.1 on p. 256).

Milk Issues can occur in a variety of forms when parents provide expressed milk to preemies.

Milk production challenges are common, because exclusive pumping is stressful and time-consuming. Many parents find it difficult to meet their daily pumping goals. Parents working hard to provide milk may also find fortification of their milk upsetting. Families cope more easily with milk expression when they know what to expect at each stage of lactation, how to handle common problems, and how their actions affect their ability to meet their long-term goals. Emphasize that during the first 2 weeks (a critical period, see p. 183), what's most important is expressing milk 8 or more times per day and removing the milk as fully as possible. Less important are the intervals between milk expressions. Some find it easier to meet their daily milk-expression totals if they express once during the night and fit in the rest of their pump sessions during their waking hours. Some schedule a time to pump every hour for the part of the day they are more available or have help. To drain the glands most fully, hands-on pumping techniques (p. 211) yield on average 50% more milk than the pump alone.

It is common for milk volumes to fluctuate with the baby's condition. Times of crisis may cause a temporary decrease in milk expressed, which can also affect production. But if parents continue expressing milk often, milk production will rebound.

Health risks of non-human milks are significant for tiny preterm babies. Formula contains inflammatory factors that may damage their fragile organs. Preemies fed formula are at higher risk for necrotizing enterocolitis (NEC), one of the most serious and life-threatening complications of prematurity. Formula use in preemies is also linked to lower IQ scores, more vision and respiratory problems, and a greater risk of all types of infections.

The Use of Donor Milk from milk banks is more commonly used in NICUs internationally than in the past. In most cases, donor milk consists of term human milk (lower than preterm milk in many nutrients preemie's need) pooled from many carefully screened donors. Pasteurizing reduces some of the protective components of human milk, but also kills any viruses and bacteria.

Expressed milk from the preemie's parent leads to better health outcomes, in part because baby receives colostrum and transitional milk, which contain unique components that prepare their digestive and immune systems. But donor human milk is a good second choice. On the negative side, weight gain and growth may be slower when donor milk comprises a large part of baby's milk intake.

Fortification and hindmilk feeding are sometimes used for faster growth of very early and small preemies. Parents who give birth prematurely produce milk higher in several key nutrients, but within a month after delivery, their preterm milk gradually changes to term milk, even though their babies' need for extra nutrients remains high. Some preterm babies grow and develop well when fed exclusively human milk. But even with low quality evidence, it has become standard practice in some places to add extra protein, calcium, phosphorus, and sometimes other nutrients to expressed milk for extremely early and small preemies. Adding these extra nutrients increases only short-term weight gain, length, and head growth during the NICU stay, but was found to have no long-term benefits. Some companies produce human-milk-based fortifiers for the NICU.

Some slow-gaining preterm babies gain weight faster with hindmilk feeding, which involves adding extra high-fat hindmilk. This can be done by storing the first milk expressed for future use and using the milk from the second half of the expression session to feed the baby now. Hindmilk averages double or triple the fat content of foremilk and can boost the calories consumed.

Hindmilk feeding is practical only for parents expressing more milk than their baby is consuming. Foremilk and hindmilk contain about the same amount of protein, so if extra protein is recommended, hindmilk will not provide it. In some cases, fortifiers may be used with hindmilk feeding.

Milk handling and safety are vital for the preterm baby. Share the following with parents.

- Ideally, colostrum and mature milk should be fed in the order they were expressed.

- Guidelines for milk collection and storage for hospitalized babies may differ from those used for healthy term babies at home.

- If fortifier is added to expressed milk, it should be used within 24 hours.

- Routinely culturing expressed milk has no benefit, because acceptable bacterial levels for expressed human milk have not yet been determined.

Cytomegalovirus (CMV)   The risk is low, but when preterm babies are born CMV-negative at less than 1,000 g and to a CMV-positive birthing parent, it is possible for their exposure to CMV in the milk may cause them to develop a serious illness.

The American Academy of Pediatrics (AAP) considers the value to preterm babies of routinely feeding human milk from CMV positive parents to outweigh the risk of clinical disease.

According to the AAP, fresh mother's own milk is preferred in this situation.

Another option is to process expressed milk to kill or reduce CMV levels before feeding the milk to tiny preemies. Holder pasteurization (heated to 62.5°C [145°F] for 30 minutes) kills the virus but also reduces some protective components. Heating it to 72°C [162°F] for 10 to 15 seconds kills CMV and preserves more protective components. Freezing reduces CMV levels but does not eliminate it. Families and providers must weigh the risk of active CMV with the risks of processing the milk.

Other Parental Illnesses. Few parental illnesses contraindicate feeding expressed milk to a preterm baby. The few that do include HIV (only in developed countries), HTLV-1 and 2, and active tuberculosis before treatment begins. For details, see p. 142. Those that require parents temporarily express and discard milk include varicella-zoster (chickenpox), measles, and herpes sores on or near the nipple. If a herpes sore comes in contact with the nursing parent's hands or pump parts, the milk should be discarded until the herpes sore heals.

Nursing Parent's Diet and Medications Diet does not usually affect the quality or quantity of mother's milk, unless it is so restricted that parents develop vitamin deficiencies (p. 240).

Before the nursing parent takes any prescribed or over-the-counter medications, discuss this with the baby's healthcare provider. A preterm baby is more vulnerable than a term baby to drugs that pass into the milk. A drug's compatibility with lactation needs to be evaluated in light of the baby's size and condition before it is taken. When a drug is problematic, a substitute compatible with continued nursing and/or expressed milk feedings can usually be found.

Any use of cigarettes, alcohol, and/or other legal or illicit substances by the nursing parent should be discussed with the preemie's healthcare provider.

FEEDING METHODS chosen for supplementing the preterm baby will depend in part on her gestational age and condition. At first, a tiny preemie may be fed intravenously or by tube. When milk feeds by mouth begin, they may be given continuously by tube or a bolus fed every couple of hours through a nasogastric tube, called "gavage feeding." Skin-to-skin contact during these feeds helps baby better digest the milk, increases expressed milk volumes, and leads to earlier nursing.

Other options for supplementing baby by mouth include cup, bottle, and nursing supplementer. Due to its fast, consistent flow, bottle-feeding can be physically stressful for preemies and may make the transition to nursing more difficult

TRANSITIONING TO FULL NURSING usually takes time. How much time depends on how early the baby was born, the baby's health, the level of milk production, how much time the baby spends nursing, and the cultural norms. This transition may happen in the NICU or at home.

SIGNS BABY MAY BE READY   The seven phases of preterm nursing (Box 16.1, p. 256) provide a road map for parents to chart their preemie's nursing progress. When a preemie begins taking large volumes of milk during nursing, it is a good time to begin the transition to full nursing.

Nursing experience has a greater impact on nursing effectiveness than gestational age alone. Baby's health is also a factor. Preemies with health problems nurse less effectively than healthy preemies.

PREEMIES SUCK DIFFERENTLY than term babies, but this does not necessarily make them less effective. Preemies' nursing effectiveness should not be gauged by how closely their sucking pattern resembles that of a term baby. Nursing success in preterm babies is defined as the ability to nurse well enough to take enough milk each day for adequate weight gain and growth. In Sweden, with lots of nursing practice, 85% of preemies exclusively nurse at 36 weeks gestation, with some fully nursing as young as 32 weeks gestation.

LOGISTICS   Spending lots of time nursing a preterm baby in the NICU may be easy or difficult, depending on the cultural climate. In some countries, parents are encouraged to stay at the hospital to feed and care for their preemies. In other countries, nursing may be delayed and parental availability for feeds limited. In situations like this, the parent may nurse only once or twice a day. Ask if on some days parents can stay at the hospital, keep the baby in skin-to-skin contact, and nurse often. If that's not possible, make sure the hospital staff knows when parents will be there so they won't arrive to find the baby was just fed.

Use these aspects of baby's nursing to gauge nursing effectiveness and progress.

- **Rooting.**   If no rooting, trigger it by touching baby's lips with the nipple or a finger.
- **Amount of the nipple/areola in the baby's mouth.**   If baby does not latch, takes part of the nipple, or the nipple without any areola, help baby get a bigger mouthful.
- **Staying latched.**   If the baby does not stay on or only stays on for a short time, try pulling baby's body in closer.
- **Sucking.**   If the baby does not start sucking or takes very long pauses while awake and breathing calmly, talk to the baby or touch her feet or palm.

STRATEGIES TO EASE THE TRANSITION As the preemie becomes more adept at nursing, the following strategies may help ease the transition to full nursing.

Transitioning from Scheduled to Semi-demand Feedings When test-weights show the baby takes about half a feed, start a **semi-demand feeding** plan. This involves parents initiating nursing if 3 hours pass since the last feed. During waking hours, baby is nursed sooner if she shows subtle feeding cues (body movements, eyes moving under eyelids). At 3 hours, if the baby is asleep, touch her mouth to the nipple. If possible, do test-weights at each feed and total milk volumes during nursing. If not possible, gradually reduce the supplement, monitoring baby's weight gain. Baby's provider determines daily milk volumes needed by baby's weight. Parents and provider choose feeding method and how often supplements are given. Semi-demand feeding continues until term corrected age.

Transitioning from semi-demand to feeding on cue When the baby's sucking pattern becomes more mature—long, rhythmic sucking bursts interspersed with breathing—she has matured enough to regulate her own feeds and move to cue-based feeding. A baby fed on cue determines when to feed and for how long. Test-weighing is stopped, and for a time the baby is weighed every 1 to 3 days to make sure she gains weight in the expected range.

Another possible strategy In some areas, this transition happens differently. As the baby gets more adept at nursing, the parent begins nursing more times per day. An individual plan may be created in consult with baby's healthcare provider. For example, if a 1700 g baby needs 300 mL of milk in 24 hours, the baby's intake is monitored by test weighing to ensure the baby gets at least 100 mL (3.3 oz) every 8 hours from all sources. With test-weighing, families can accurately measure how much milk the baby takes while nursing and feed her on cue. At the end of each 8-hour period, if baby did not take 100 mL, she can be supplemented with what's needed. The baby begins to set the pace and gains nursing experience even before she is exclusively nursing, while parents learn their baby's cues.

MONITORING BABY'S MILK INTAKE AND WEIGHT GAIN can make this transition less worrisome. While changing baby's feeding routine, parents need to be sure the baby is getting enough milk. If the parents have access to a scale accurate to 2 g for test weights, they can monitor how much milk the baby takes during nursing and use this information to gauge how much supplement is needed. If not, frequent weight checks are needed to make sure the baby is gaining daily at least 0.5 to 1 ounce (15 g to 30 g).

Until the baby can exclusively nurse on cue, suggest the family continue milk expression.

MAKING BOTTLE-FEEDING MORE LIKE NURSING   If the baby is supplemented by bottle and is not nursing well, for an easier transition, suggest these strategies to make bottle-feeding more like nursing.

- **Latching to the bottle teat with a wide-open mouth.**   Hold the baby in a semi-upright position, touch her lips with the teat, and wait until she opens wide, allowing her to draw the teat deeply into her mouth, rather than pushing it in. Hold the bottle horizontally to keep the flow slow, and keep the baby semi-upright. Avoid letting baby take just the teat tip.
- **Bait and switch** involves bottle-feeding in a nursing position, with the baby's cheek touching the exposed gland. As the baby begins sucking-and-swallowing, quickly remove the bottle teat and insert the nipple.
- **Firmer feel and/or faster flow.**   When baby prefers the bottle, assume there is something she is looking for during nursing that she is not finding—most likely the firm feel of the teat or the immediate fast flow of the bottle. To provide one or both during nursing, try having a helper drip milk for an instant flow or using a nipple shield for a firmer feel.
- **Keep nursing attempts positive.**   Don't allow nursing to become a battleground. If a baby is fussing or crying during attempts, stop and comfort her, so that the baby does not associate nursing with frustration and unhappiness. Relaxed skin-to-skin time near the nipple will help the baby develop positive associations and make her more open to nursing.

GOING HOME   Before hospital discharge, suggest parents get actively involved in their baby's care and check on any available post-discharge services. The more time parents spend with their baby before discharge, the easier the transition to home will be. If parents have not yet spent time with baby in skin-to-skin contact, start now.

If the baby is not nursing well and the parents have not cared for their baby during most of her hospitalization, they may experience a second crisis at hospital discharge. During the first week at home, accept all offers of help and plan to spend the first weeks at home with their baby doing nothing but nursing and caring for her. Ask friends and family to spend time with any older children.

MONITORING MILK INTAKE   After discharge, parents need to know how to make sure their preemie is getting enough milk. The most reliable sign of good milk intake is a daily weight gain of at least 0.5 to 1 ounce (15 g to 30 g). Scheduling frequent weight checks provides parents with the information they need about whether baby is feeding well. Knowing that the baby's weight gain is within the expected range can ease any worries. If it's not in the expected range, parents will know they need to adjust their routine.

Another way to monitor milk intake after discharge is to rent an accurate (to 2 g) electronic scale for short-term home use, which can either be used to monitor the baby's weight gain from day to day or do pre- and post-feed test weights to determine whether supplements are needed.

TAKE THE LEAD WITH NURSING While transitioning from NICU to home, encourage parents to keep the baby on their bodies as much as possible and take the lead by offering to nurse often. Create a comfortable nursing area at home, away from activity and overstimulation, with plenty of pillows for support.

Keep baby nearby for night feeds. If the parent is not comfortable nursing lying down, try starter positions in bed (p. 6), with extra pillows for back and elbow support, and baby lying tummy down on their body. After nursing, parents can return baby to her bed or keep her next to them.

If fortification of mother's own milk is recommended after discharge, at some feeds the fortified milk can be given during nursing with a nursing supplementer or via another feeding method.

THE LATE-PRETERM AND EARLY-TERM BABY

Late-preterm babies are those born between 34 and 36 completed weeks gestation. Early-term babies (one third of all births) are those born at 37 or 38 weeks gestation.

THE LATE-PRETERM BABY may look healthy but not yet be ready to nurse on cue. Depending on the baby's gestational age at birth, her brain may be only 60% to 80% the size and maturity of a term baby. Brain immaturity affects her arousal, sleep-wake cycles, breathing, and ability to self-regulate feeding. Prematurity is significantly linked to suboptimal early nursing.

STRATEGIES FOR THE HOSPITAL STAY that help late-preterm babies master nursing include semi-demand feeding (see previous section), in which the parent initiates frequent feeds, skin-to-skin contact, keeping the nursing couple together, close monitoring of the baby, and parental education and support. To trigger inborn feeding behaviors more often, keep baby tummy down on parents' body as much as they are comfortable, helping baby latch and feed even in light sleep.

If the baby's weight loss indicates she is nursing ineffectively, see if a nipple shield helps.

IF SUPPLEMENTS ARE NEEDED, avoid overfeeding. During the hospital stay, use the feeding-volume guidelines in the ABM's Clinical Protocol #4 at **bfmed.org/protocols.**

First choice is expressed milk, then donor milk, then formula.

Late-preterm babies need careful monitoring and their parents need consistent, ongoing lactation help and support in the hospital and after discharge. Just a few weeks of maturity and growth can turn an ineffective late-preterm baby into an effective nurser. But until then, families need help and encouragement to meet their nursing goals.

THE EARLY-TERM BABY is born at 37 or 38 weeks gestation, which encompasses one-third of all births. Being born just 2 or 3 weeks early decreases the number of babies who nurse during the first hour after birth, any nursing, as well as nursing intensity and exclusivity. These families need extra lactation support.

PRETERM TWINS, TRIPLETS, AND MORE

Multiples—twins, triplets, and more—are often born preterm, so during pregnancy suggest parents prepare for this possibility in the following ways.

- Take an early lactation class.
- Spend time with nursing families, either in person or online.
- Meet the hospital lactation staff, the lactation consultants on the perinatal unit, and those in the special-care nursery. Discuss lactation services (hours and days of availability) and options that promote nursing.
- Learn how milk production works.
- Learn about milk expression before the babies are born. View the videos on **firstdroplets.com**
- Discuss the benefits of skin-to-skin contact.
- Plan to begin nursing as soon as possible after delivery.
- Arrange for help at home for at least the first month, but ideally for the first 3 months.

If milk expression is needed, set a goal of bringing in full milk production (750 mL [25 oz.] per baby per day), ideally within the first 2 weeks (see p. 214).

One baby often nurses more effectively than another. It may help to nurse two babies together (p. 15), so the more effective baby can trigger milk ejection for the less effective baby.

Some families of multiples bring one baby home before the others are discharged. This may involve nursing at home and continuing to express milk for one or more babies in the hospital.

DIGITAL RESOURCES

bfmed.org/protocols—To download the Academy of Breastfeeding Medicine Clinical Protocols:

- #10 Breastfeeding the late preterm baby
- #12 NICU graduate going home

bit.ly/BA2-VLBW—Wight, N., Kim, J., Rhine, W. Mayer, O., Morris, M., Sey, R., Nisher,C. (2018). *Nutritional Support of the Very Low Birth Weight Infant (VLBW): A Quality Improvement Toolkit.* Stanford, CA: California Perinatal Quality Carae Collaborative.

CHAPTER 17 RELACTATION AND INDUCED LACTATION

DEFINITIONS AND GOALS

DEFINITIONS *Relactation* is the process of increasing milk production in someone who was previously pregnant. The decision to relactate is often made when there is some milk production, but it may also be made many years after the last nursing. The difference between relactation and increasing low milk production is one of degree. Usually, relactation occurs after nursing parents spent weeks or months nursing very little or not at all. They may or may not have nursed after birth. Unlike those inducing lactation, those relactating experienced the development of milk-making tissue during pregnancy. If relactating parents can transition the baby to direct nursing, feed 10 to 12 times per day, spend lots of time daily touching and holding the baby, and there are no physical obstacles to making milk, over several weeks the odds are good of measurable milk production.

Induced lactation is the process of stimulating milk production in someone with no history of pregnancy. Induced lactation was once referred to as "adoptive nursing," but with modern reproductive technologies, this term may not apply. A parent may adopt a baby or surrogacy may be involved. The nursing parent may be a transgender man or woman. Or the parents may co-nurse, with one female partner of a same-sex couple giving birth while the other induces lactation, or both may induce lactation for an adopted baby.

Parents inducing lactation begin without the mammary development that occurs during pregnancy. Some liken induced lactation to building a house by hand with bricks and mortar rather than with construction equipment. It is a much slower process.

DISCUSS GOALS AND GATHER INFORMATION Different families have different goals for relactation and induced lactation. Some parents' primary motivation is for greater emotional closeness with their biological or adopted child. Milk production may be the top priority when the baby has an intolerance or allergy to human-milk substitutes or a medical condition for which human milk is recommended. Some relactate or induce lactation to help provide human milk as a treatment for a sick friend or relative. In the developing world, infant survival is closely linked to breastfeeding, so when milk production is low, mothers and babies are hospitalized together to ensure successful relactation.

THE LONG-TERM PERSPECTIVE When relactating or inducing lactation, if parents nurse long enough, eventually their baby's need for milk and their milk production will match. Some parents bring in enough milk before the baby arrives so they never need to use formula or donor milk. Some families discontinue supplements during the early months. Some discontinue supplements after 6 months, when solid foods take their place in baby's diet. For some, it may be closer to 12 months, when their child is eating more solids and drinking other liquids. But all nursing parents and babies eventually reach the point when extra milk is unnecessary.

FACTORS TO CONSIDER when creating a plan for families include:

- The baby's age, which may affect his willingness to nurse, with younger babies generally more willing to nurse than older babies
- Baby's current response to nursing
- Nursing history, with some past nursing increasing the odds of baby transitioning more easily to nursing
- Health, medication, or anatomy issues in parent or baby that may affect nursing, such as infertility issues, hormonal contraception, unusual breast or nipple anatomy, or tongue-tie
- Parent's availability for nursing, which may be affected by job or household workloads
- Available support from partner, family, and friends

If nursing parents are relactating for a baby they recently birthed, ask what happened with nursing. The dynamics that caused milk production to decrease may still exist and need to be addressed.

STRATEGIES TO INCREASE MILK PRODUCTION

The process of relactating and inducing lactation are similar and involve these basic strategies.

- Frequent mammary stimulation by nursing or expressing milk
- Lots of parent-baby body contact (skin-to-skin and/or dressed)
- Optional use of galactogogues (milk-boosting substances)

With any plan, incorporate only those strategies parents feel comfortable using. With induced lactation, if the goal is greater intimacy, the plan may be to wait until the baby arrives and simply nurse often (perhaps with a nursing supplementer) with lots of body contact day and night. But if milk production is a high priority and the family knows ahead of time when the baby will arrive, one option is the induced lactation protocols described on p. 275. Even with little lead time, induced lactation is definitely possible. If the family is adopting, the type of adoption may affect how far in advance they know for certain the baby's arrival date. If surrogacy is involved, there may be more time and greater certainty about when the baby will be in their arms.

MAMMARY STIMULATION AND BODY CONTACT are the most effective strategy for stimulating milk production, especially if they are done often and around-the-clock. Suggest parents:

- Nurse at least 10 to 12 times per day. Before milk production begins, nipple stimulation releases the hormone prolactin, which stimulates milk production and the growth of milk-making tissue.
- Make sure baby latches deeply, which triggers more active sucking and greater milk removal.
- Offer each side more than once at each nursing session for more stimulation.
- Use compression or massage to increase time spent actively sucking.
- Keep baby close at night and guide the sleeping baby to latch in a light sleep to increase the number of nursing sessions each day.
- Avoid soothers (pacifiers, swings) and limit all sucking to the nursing parent to increase the time spent stimulating milk production.

As much as it is possible and they are comfortable with it, suggest parents keep baby on their body (in a soft carrier or in arms) whenever they can to trigger feeding behaviors and enhance milk production.

Milk expression can speed the rate of milk production. If the baby is nursing effectively, make nursing a higher priority than milk expression. But if the nursing parent is away from the baby regularly or the baby is not yet nursing effectively, milk expression can be vital to meeting goals.

The first choice of method if milk expression will be done often is a rental-grade pump with a double-pump kit, because it may be more effective than other pumps at stimulating milk production. However, many parents inducing lactation find the first milk produced is easier to express by hand. If parents plan to express milk regularly, try double pumping at least once in the middle of the night, when prolactin levels are naturally higher. Where pumps are not available or are outside a family's means, suggest hand expression. Milk expression is most effective when both pumps, mammary compression, and hand expression are used together.

Pumping strategies to boost milk production include:

- Massage and compress while pumping and hand express after. See p. 211 for details on hands-on pumping, a strategy proven to boost milk-making.

- Express milk long enough per session to remove the milk as fully as possible. Hands-on pumping takes on average 25 minutes per session. At some sessions, keep going until 2 minutes after the last drop of milk.

- Double pumping (pumping both sides at once) can be a huge time saver, and may boost milk production faster.

If regular milk expression is part of a family's plan, consider these strategies.

- Express milk after or between feeds for more mammary stimulation. After baby arrives, most parents stop expressing and nurse instead. But if they want to also express milk, suggest hand-expressing whenever practical, such as for a few minutes whenever they use the toilet. Even if little or no milk is expressed, its main purpose is to speed milk production.

- Now and then, express intensively to give milk production a quick boost. See p. 196 for details on "power pumping" and other strategies.

- Keep the longest stretch between milk removals shorter than 8 hours, because "full glands make milk slower."

- Keep a digital or written record of milk volume expressed to help gauge progress.

GALACTOGOGUES, milk-boosting substances, speed milk production in some parents. They include prescribed medications and/or herbal preparations. For details, see p. 196. Any parents interested in using galactogogues should discuss them with their healthcare provider in light of their health history. In many parts of the world, galactogogues are not used to reach full milk production.

INDUCED LACTATION PROTOCOLS If a family knows in advance when the baby is expected, they may decide to spend time before the baby comes stimulating milk production. Making milk without pregnancy may involve preparing the mammary glands to make milk, stimulating milk production, and nursing to make milk. Parents may choose to work on the first two steps before the baby arrives. They can be skipped if there is no time before baby joins the family or the parents prefer to wait until baby arrives to begin bringing in milk.

Some lactation consultants create a customized personal protocol for inducing lactation or relactation based on the family's specific needs and preferences. Some families use the Newman-Goldfarb induced lactation protocols available online at **asklenore.info**. These protocols were developed by Canadian pediatrician Jack Newman and Canadian lactation consultant Lenore Goldfarb. At this writing, the effectiveness of these protocols has not yet been studied. These online protocols are:

- **Regular Protocol** for those with at least 6 months before their baby's arrival
- **Accelerated Protocol** for those with less than 6 months
- **Menopause Protocol** for those whose reproductive organs were surgically removed or who experienced a naturally occurring menopause

With all three protocols, parents take daily without interruption one active oral contraceptive pill (containing 1 to 2 mg of progesterone and no more than 0.035 mg of estrogen). They also take daily domperidone, a prescribed galactogogue. Before the baby arrives, the oral contraceptive is stopped (the timing varies among the protocols), which is intended to cause a drop in the user's progesterone level, while the domperidone continues to be taken to stimulate an increase in blood prolactin levels, ideally causing milk to increase. This process is intended to mimic (at much lower levels) the hormonal changes that naturally occur after birth. After the oral contraceptive is stopped, to further stimulate milk production, herbs are started and the parent inducing lactation begins pumping every 3 hours with an automatic double pump. Possible side effects of these protocols include prolonged breakthrough menstrual bleeding, increased blood pressure, and weight gain.

Anyone considering a protocol involving drugs or herbs needs to consult their healthcare provider to review these options in light of their health history. These protocols are not intended to be used after the baby arrives.

CULTURAL DIFFERENCES AND MILK PRODUCTION

In developing countries, there is a long history of successful relactation and induced lactation. But in many developed countries, even parents who birth their babies doubt their ability to make enough milk, and parents relactating and inducing lactation are less likely to reach full milk production. This may be because parents in the developing world are more knowledgeable about nursing, nurse frequently, keep their babies close, and have cultural support for breastfeeding. They also may have reproductive and lactation histories that may make nursing easier, even though they are less likely to have access to prescribed galactogogues. Parents in the West can maximize milk production by emulating the parenting styles of developing countries and by creating a strong lactation support network.

Another difference is that in developing countries, most parents relactating or inducing lactation supplement their babies with easy-to-clean, temporary feeding methods, such as spoons and cups. Feeding bottles—a long-term feeding method—are rarely used due to contamination risks. In developed countries, however, feeding bottles are common, and due to their fast flow, the baby is more likely to take more supplement than needed.

PHYSICAL AND EMOTIONAL CHANGES may occur as milk production increases, and parents should know to expect some or all of the following:

- Menstrual changes, such as menstruating irregularly or cessation of menstruation for a time
- Changes in mammary tissue, such as darkening of the areolae, an increase in size, and feelings of tissue fullness, tenderness, and/or heaviness
- Mood changes from variations in levels of lactation-related hormones, which may improve mood or trigger feelings of anxiety, nervousness, depression, fear, or anger

Feeling overwhelmed or like giving up may be a sign of impending milk increase.

Getting more rest, eating a more nutritious diet, and drinking more fluids are not likely to boost milk production, but they can boost morale and the ability to cope.

TRANSITIONING BABY TO NURSING

HELPING BABY LATCH AND FEED Some babies latch and feed easily and enthusiastically. Others nurse only with patience and encouragement. Babies fed for long periods with feeding bottles may at first be more reluctant to nurse than babies fed other ways. But because babies are hardwired to nurse, most will eventually get there. Inborn feeding behaviors have been reported from all over the world in adopted children as old as school age.

THE FIRST FOCUS FOR ADOPTIVE PARENTS is their developing relationship with the child. Because nursing is an intimate act, children are more likely to latch and feed when they trust and feel close to their new parent. When adoptive parents welcome the child to the family, at first, they are strangers to the child. Before offering to nurse, suggest finding ways to become emotionally closer, such as holding, carrying, co-sleeping, co-bathing, and being responsive to the child's needs.

For the first few weeks, it may help to make their relationship exclusive, which may mean others do not hold the child. The child's personality and past experiences with feeding will also affect his response to nursing. If the child is used to being fed quickly with a fast-flow bottle, it may help to transition gradually by first shifting to a medium-flow teat and then a slow-flow teat. Gradual steps—such as bottle-feeding in a nursing position—can allow baby to experience feeding as something that is less overwhelming and more pleasurable before offering to nurse. Patience and persistence are key.

For the older adopted baby or toddler, it may help to spend time with other nursing families, such as at lactation support group meetings, where the child can see other babies and children nursing.

STRATEGIES FOR ANY PARENT are listed below. If after several feeding attempts, the baby continues to balk at nursing:

- Keep the parent's body a pleasant place to be, not a battleground. If nursing feels stressful, feed another way and give baby lots of cuddle time on the parent's chest, especially while asleep.
- Spend time touching and in skin-to-skin contact. When not feeding, hold the baby and—if baby likes it, give skin-to-skin contact, perhaps by taking warm baths together.
- Try nursing while baby is drowsy or in a light sleep. Some babies nurse more easily when in a relaxed, sleepy state.
- Use feeding positions baby likes best and experiment, starting first with a semi-reclined position with baby tummy down and supported on the parent's body (p. 6).
- Try nursing in a private place without distractions. This could be a quiet, darkened room or an area with dim lighting.
- Trigger a milk ejection before baby latches to give an instant reward or try expressing milk first onto baby's lips.
- Try shaping and/or supporting the mammary tissue. Using the sandwich technique, nipple tilting, and other techniques may help the baby latch deeper and better trigger active sucking. For details, see p. 321.
- Try nursing in motion, while walking or rocking.
- When baby nurses well, spend lots of time nursing.
- Nurse for comfort, not just for food. Nurse rather than using a pacifier.
- Offer to nurse when baby is not too hungry or too full.
- Make nursing a time of closeness when baby gets special attention.
- Supplement as needed to make sure the baby gets the milk he needs to feel strong, calm, and open to nursing.

TOOLS AND OTHER STRATEGIES may help make the transition to nursing go more smoothly in some situations.

- Have a helper drip expressed milk with a spoon near the nipple during latch. Swallowing triggers sucking.
- Feed a little milk first. Some babies will try nursing if they are not very hungry.
- Try a nursing supplementer. If slow milk flow is an issue, it may help the baby stay active longer.

If the baby is used to bottle-feeding, try these strategies.

- Switch to a slower-flow bottle teat.
- Make taking the bottle more like latching. Brush the bottle teat lightly against the baby's lips and wait for him to open wide before allowing him to draw it in.
- Hold the bottle against the mammary tissue so baby gets used to feeding there.
- Wrap the bottle in a cloth and feed it against the exposed nipple, so the baby cannot touch the hard plastic of the bottle while feeding but can feel the parent's skin.
- Try "bait and switch." Begin bottle-feeding in a nursing position. While the baby actively sucks and swallows, pull out the bottle teat and insert the parent's nipple. (Try also with a pacifier/dummy.)
- Try using a silicone nipple shield, which mimics the feel of a bottle teat.

GAUGING ADEQUATE MILK INTAKE As the young baby begins swallowing more milk and nursing longer, parents can start the process of gradually decreasing the volume of supplement. Before doing so, though, have the baby weighed by his healthcare provider and schedule weight checks at least weekly on the same scale. If the baby is younger than 3 months and his weight gain slips below about 30 g (about 1 oz.) per day or about 200 g. (7 oz.) per week, this is a sign the baby needs more supplement.

During this transition, the goal is to feed the young baby the smallest volume of supplement needed while actively nursing as much as possible to stimulate faster milk production. Babies need to stay well nourished. If the supplement is reduced too quickly and the baby becomes weak from low milk intake, this can compromise baby's ability to nurse. On the other hand, if baby receives too much supplement, he will be too full to nurse often or long enough to stimulate faster milk production.

BABY'S WEIGHT GAIN is the most reliable indicator of how close the milk production is to meeting his needs. Regular weight checks will help parents keep the baby's milk intake in the right range. If needed, test-weighing, using a scale accurate to 2 g, can measure milk intake during nursing to provides more information. But keep in mind that milk intake varies during the day.

Milk expression can provide clues to milk production, but it is less reliable than baby's weight, because not all lactating parents—even those with excellent milk production—can express milk effectively, especially at first.

OTHER SIGNS OF MILK INTAKE, such as audible swallowing and diaper output, are not completely reliable but can provide clues on a daily basis. Between regular weight checks, suggest parents make note every day of the following.

- Number of baby's stools
- Number of nursing sessions per day and baby's response
- Volume of supplement given over 24 hours and when it is given

Parents may find it reassuring as they decrease the supplement to see baby's stooling stay stable.

Knowing the signs of dehydration can be helpful, especially if baby is obviously well hydrated. If not, these signs can serve as a warning to increase the supplement.

- Two or fewer wet diapers in 24 hours
- When skin is pinched, it stays pinched looking
- Extreme sleepiness or lethargy
- Dry mouth and eyes

Signs that the baby's milk intake during nursing is increasing include:

- Less supplement taken and greater interest in nursing may mean it's time to reduce the supplement. If using a nursing supplementer, try starting the feed without it and end with it.
- Milder-smelling stools in a baby taking formula may indicate greater intake of human milk.
- Better health and temperament. A diaper rash or skin condition may improve. A baby who was lethargic may become more active or if tense, more relaxed.

WHEN DECREASING THE SUPPLEMENT, if the baby continues to gain at least 7 oz. (200 g) per week, it means human-milk intake is filling the gap. Other signs that it's time to decrease the supplement include:

- Baby wants to spend more time nursing or seems full faster.
- Baby lets milk dribble out while sucking or shows other signs of satiety.
- Baby leaves supplement in the container several feedings in a row

Unless it is obvious the supplement needs to be decreased faster, cutting back by a half-ounce (15 mL) per feed works well for many families, allowing a day or two in between reductions. An alternative to cutting back the same volume at every feed is to handle feeds differently at different times of day. Begin reducing supplements by offering less at the first morning feed and more in the evening. As milk production continues to increase, the first morning feed is usually the best time to eliminate the supplement completely. If the baby seems comfortable after receiving less supplement than usual, continue to gradually reduce the volume offered without leaving the baby hungry. Avoid giving baby more supplement than he wants.

Milk production may dip slightly as menstruation starts, but with a few days of increased nursing, milk production usually quickly rebounds.

CO-NURSING WITH PARTNERS

In some families, both parents nurse the baby, known as co-nursing, which has several advantages.

- Sharing nursing makes life with a newborn easier and less intense.
- Sharing night feeds means both parents get more sleep.
- The birthing parent can go out more easily without worry about the baby being unhappy.
- Nursing affirms a transgender woman's status as a woman by confirming her ability to nurture the baby at her breast and stimulating more mature breast development.
- Co-nursing reduces feelings of jealousy that are common in non-nursing partners.

Co-nursing may occur in several different types of families.

CISGENDER FEMALE COUPLES, in which both women were assigned as female at birth and both identify as female (cisgender). In some of these families, only the birthing parent breastfeeds or only the non-gestational parent breastfeeds by relactating or inducing lactation. In other families, both women co-nurse in one of several different ways.

- Both women give birth within a short time of each other and breastfeed both babies.

- One woman gives birth and the other relactates or induces lactation.
- Neither woman gives birth, and the couple adopts a baby or the baby is born via surrogacy, with both women relactating or inducing lactation.

TRANSGENDER WOMEN AND THEIR PARTNERS In this situation, transgender women—those assigned as male at birth who identify as female and transitioned to female—induce lactation. In one case report, a transgender woman who received hormone therapy for 6 years before her adopted baby was born, produced enough milk to fully sustain the baby for the first 6 weeks. Estrogen therapy grows mammary tissue. In another case, a transgender woman induced lactation and shared breastfeeding with her female partner, who was also the baby's birth mother.

TRANSGENDER MEN AND THEIR PARTNERS Transgender men are those assigned as female at birth but identify as male and transitioned to male. Transgender men may become pregnant, give birth, and nurse their babies, which some refer to as "chestfeeding." Their partners may be anywhere on the gender spectrum and may choose to nurse, too. Some transgender men have surgery to reduce their mammary tissue, which may affect milk production (see p. 49).

BIRTHING MOTHERS AND FATHERS Male lactation is known in other species, and there are some anecdotal accounts of cisgender men producing milk. If a father wants to experience nursing, consider "dry nursing," which means nursing to feel the emotional closeness but not to produce milk. In general, any parent who has not experienced a female puberty or estrogen therapy is likely to have much less mammary tissue than those who have, which decreases the odds of producing much milk.

BALANCING MILK PRODUCTION between partners requires an understanding of each family's goals and priorities as they sort out for themselves how best to manage the logistics of co-nursing. In some families, one partner may co-nurse mainly to experience the emotional closeness of nursing. Milk production may be a higher priority for one partner than the other. Or they may decide that sharing feeds and parenting equally is their top priority. The following are strategies for different priorities and goals.

THE BIRTHING PARENT'S MILK PRODUCTION IS THE PRIORITY Due to the hormonal effects of pregnancy, the birthing parent is likely to have a natural milk-production advantage. For this reason, some couples decide the birthing parent should primarily or exclusively nurse during the early weeks, to allow the birthing parent to establish full milk production, even if they plan to co-nurse later.

THE STAY-AT-HOME PARTNER'S MILK PRODUCTION IS THE PRIORITY   In some families, deciding how often each partner nurses may be influenced by the couple's employment plans. If one partner plans to care for the baby while the other works outside the home, that couple may put a higher priority on the stay-at-home partner's milk production.

DIGITAL RESOURCES

asklenore.info—Location of the Protocols for Induced Lactation created by Lenore Goldfarb and Canadian pediatrician Jack Newman.

sweetpeabreastfeeding.com—Website of U.S. lactation consultant Alyssa Schnell, author of *Breastfeeding Without Birthing*, which includes free webinars, podcasts, and articles for parents and professionals on relactation and inducing lactation.

CHAPTER 18 VACCINES, VITAMINS, AND OTHER SUPPLEMENTS

VACCINES

VACCINES IN THE NURSING BABY The same immunization schedule is recommended for all babies, nursing or not. Nursing does not need to be delayed before, during, or after immunization.

Nursing enhances a baby's immune response to vaccinations. Some immunizations produce a more active immune response, and therefore offer more protection from disease in nursing babies as compared with formula-fed babies.

While a baby is receiving an immunization, nursing is an effective way to soothe babies and reduce pain. The Academy of Breastfeeding Medicine (ABM) states in its Clinical Protocol #23 on nonpharmacological pain relief for nursing babies that nursing should be the first choice to alleviate procedural pain in newborns. This file is free and downloadable at **bfmed.org/protocols**.

VACCINES IN THE NURSING PARENT With the exception of the smallpox and yellow-fever vaccines, all vaccines given to parents are compatible with nursing. Neither inactivated nor live virus vaccines administered to lactating parents affect the safety of nursing.

When nursing parents are immunized, their baby receives temporary protection from that illness in the same way as when they are exposed to an illness. Their body produces antibodies to the illness that pass into the milk. For example, when mothers were immunized with a rotavirus vaccine during the first month after birth, this provided their breastfeeding babies with passive protection from rotavirus diarrhea for their first 4 months.

RUBELLA VACCINE is not recommended for anyone who may become pregnant within the next 28 days, as the rubella virus is associated with birth defects when contracted during pregnancy. In parents without immunity to rubella (which can be determined with a blood test), immunization immediately after birth is often recommended.

RHOGAM Nursing is not affected when an Rh-negative parent receives Rh immune globulin (RhoGAM) after birth. When an Rh-negative parent gives birth to an Rh-positive baby, an injection of RhoGAM is recommended to prevent complications in future pregnancies. Any Rh antibodies in mother's milk are inactivated in the baby's stomach, so nursing is recommended, even when high doses are given.

VITAMINS AND OTHER SUPPLEMENTS

VITAMIN SUPPLEMENTS AND THE NURSING BABY Human milk evolved over millennia to contain what our babies need, but not all babies are born full term, and due to changes over time in lifestyle and diet, in many cases, exclusively nursing babies benefit from vitamin and/or mineral supplements.

VITAMIN D SUPPLEMENTS Daily supplements of 400 IU of vitamin D are recommended for all exclusively nursing babies and in some parts of the world, for all babies. Vitamin D is made by the body when the skin is exposed to the sun's ultraviolet rays. Only about 10% to 20% of our vitamin D intake comes from food. As people spent more time indoors and used sunscreen when outside, the incidence of vitamin-D deficiency and rickets increased. During pregnancy today, widespread incidence of vitamin D deficiency can be found in most parts of the world.

Babies born to vitamin-D deficient parents are at increased risk of vitamin D deficiency, which is linked to many health problems. Parents and babies with dark skin are at greater risk of vitamin D deficiency because darker skin pigmentation acts as a natural filter of ultraviolet light.

Nursing babies can be supplemented with vitamin D drops. An alternative that benefits both parent and baby is to supplement the nursing parent. Parents' vitamin D blood levels determine the vitamin D levels in their milk. To ensure baby receives healthy levels of vitamin D via mother's milk, parents need to take higher doses than are found in prenatal vitamins. They can do this in two ways.

- Taking orally 6400 IU of vitamin D per day
- Getting vitamin-D injections, either as a one-time injection of 150,000 IU after birth, which keeps baby vitamin D sufficient for 28 days, or as one 60,000 IU injection daily on 10 consecutive days (600,000 IU total) beginning 1 to 2 days after birth, which keeps nursing babies' vitamin D sufficient for 6 months.

VITAMIN B_{12} SUPPLEMENTS (or the use of vitamin B_{12}-fortified foods) are recommended for nursing babies whose nursing parent is vitamin B_{12} deficient. Those at risk of a vitamin B_{12} deficiency include those whose diet contains no animal products (vegan) and those with a history of weight-loss surgery, Crohn's disease, or other malabsorption disorders. Nursing parents with a vitamin B_{12} deficiency produce milk low in vitamin B_{12}, so their nursing babies are also at risk of vitamin B_{12} deficiency. Symptoms in the baby (disinterest in feeding, slow weight gain, neurological problems) often develop before symptoms in the parent, appearing within the first few months or going unrecognized until later. A blood test can detect this deficiency in the parent. If deficient, both parent and baby may need to receive vitamin B_{12} supplements. For more details, see p. 239.

IRON SUPPLEMENTS Healthy iron levels are important for normal development, but routine iron supplements can be detrimental in babies with healthy iron levels. Most babies born full term at average or above average birth weight to well-nourished parents have enough iron stores to last 6 to 9 months. Iron in human milk is much better absorbed than iron from other sources, up to 50% absorption from human milk compared with 4% absorption from infant formula. But the iron level in human milk is low, which is why nursing babies benefit from solid foods high in iron beginning at around 6 months.

If blood iron levels get too low, baby is at risk for iron deficiency and anemia, which are associated with developmental delays and neurological problems. If these levels stay too low for too long, neurological problems may become irreversible.

The American Academy of Pediatrics (AAP) recommends routine iron supplements for all nursing babies starting at 4 months. But its AAP Section on Breastfeeding concluded this recommendation was based on inadequate research. Routinely supplementing iron-sufficient babies with extra iron can also lead to problems with immune function, growth, and increased risk of illness.

If there is concern about a baby's iron levels, a simple blood test in the provider's office can be done to determine iron status.

On the other hand, babies born with low iron stores at birth (usually babies born preterm, growth restricted, low birth weight, or born to iron-deficient parents) may need extra iron before 6 months. Low iron stores at birth may be depleted before 6 months. In these cases, the AAP recommends providing iron supplements along with exclusive nursing.

FLUORIDE SUPPLEMENTS are not recommended for nursing babies younger than 6 months, due to the risk of permanent discoloration of the teeth (fluorosis). Fluoride supplements are only recommended after 6 months when the fluoride level of local drinking water is less than 0.3 ppm.

VITAMIN AND OTHER SUPPLEMENTS FOR THE NURSING PARENT Well-nourished nursing parents with healthy vitamin D levels may get all the nutrients they need from their diet. The same may not be true for malnourished parents.

UNDERNOURISHED OR NUTRIENT-DEFICIENT NURSING PARENTS may benefit from supplements. Examples include parents who have limited exposure to sunlight, those on a vegan or very restricted diet, those who are chronically undernourished, those with intestinal parasites, Crohn's disease, or other malabsorption diseases, and those with a history of weight-loss surgery. Without supplements, parents in these situations may eventually develop vitamin or mineral deficiencies that can lead to a decrease in their milk levels of some nutrients, such as iodine, choline, A, D, B_1, B_2, B_6, or B_{12}, which may negatively affect the health of their nursing baby.

VITAMIN D SUPPLEMENTS   See p. 284 on vitamin D supplements in the nursing baby.

VITAMIN B_{12} SUPPLEMENTS   Vegan nursing parents consume no animal products (the only foods containing B_{12}), so to safeguard their and their baby's health, vitamin B_{12} supplements or foods fortified with B_{12} are necessary to prevent deficiency. See p. 239 for details. The same may be true for nursing parents with a history of weight-loss surgery (see p. 242) or any other health condition that interferes with nutrient absorption.

IRON SUPPLEMENTS   If a nursing parent becomes iron-deficient or anemic, iron supplements can help bring their iron levels up to normal. However, iron levels in milk are not affected by the nursing parent's blood iron levels, so taking iron supplements will not affect the iron level in the milk.

TAKING MEGA-DOSES OF VITAMINS, especially some fat-soluble vitamins, is not recommended, as this may be harmful to both nursing parent and baby.

Water-Soluble Vitamins include vitamin C and the B-complex vitamins (thiamin [B_1], riboflavin [B_2], niacin [B_3], pantothenic acid [B_5], pyridoxine [B_6], biotin [B_7], folic acid or folate [B_9], and cobalamin [B_{12}]). They are flushed through a nursing parent's system daily and do not accumulate, so if a nursing parent takes higher-than-recommended doses of these vitamins to treat a health problem (such as B_2 for migraine, B_6 for neuritis, C for the common cold), this should not affect nursing.

Fat-Soluble Vitamins are stored in fat and tissue and include vitamins A, D, E, and K and should not be taken in mega-doses unless the nursing parent is deficient and being treated to bring blood levels up to normal. Vitamin A is secreted into human milk and is stored in the liver. Doses of more than 5,000 IUs of vitamin A per day are not recommended for adults.

Vitamin D is also a fat-soluble vitamin, but it behaves more like a hormone. It is made in our bodies during skin exposure to sunlight. Due to the rise in vitamin D deficiency worldwide, larger-than-recommended doses may be beneficial to many nursing parents and babies. For details, see p. 284.

OMEGA-3 FATTY ACIDS may benefit nursing couples. The total amount of fat in human milk is stable, independent of diet. But diet plays a major role in the proportion of different types of fats in the milk, with omega-3 supplements increasing their levels in milk. For babies, more omega-3 fatty acids like DHA and ARA is associated with better psychomotor development. For nursing parents, omega-3 supplements are an effective treatment for postpartum depression.

In areas where fish consumption is common (one serving of oily fish per week), recommended levels of omega-3 fatty acids are found in mother's milk. But if a parent's diet is low in omega-3s, taking an omega-3 supplement may be beneficial. More long-term studies are needed.

PROBIOTICS The research is mixed on the benefits to babies of probiotics taken by nursing parents. According to some (but not all) studies, taking probiotics during pregnancy and lactation improved baby's health by reducing the incidence of allergy and gastrointestinal problems. Spanish research found that taking probiotics during pregnancy and lactation may prevent and/or treat mastitis in nursing parents. More research is needed.

CHAPTER 19 WEANING FROM NURSING

In the U.K., weaning refers to starting solid foods. But in this chapter, weaning is defined as the end of nursing. Weaning is not a single act but a process that begins when baby begins taking anything other than human milk and ends with the last nursing session.

RECOMMENDATIONS

The American Academy of Pediatrics (AAP) and the World Health Organization (WHO) recommend exclusive nursing for 6 months. After solid foods are started, the AAP recommends nursing continue for at least 1 year or longer, and the WHO recommends 2 years or longer. Health risks of early weaning include greater risk of maternal and infant illness and death. The vast majority of deaths occur in developing countries, where food and water may be contaminated and health care less available. But even in the developed world, early weaning carries health risks for both nursing parents and babies.

THE DECISION TO WEAN

When families ask for information on weaning, they may feel vulnerable to criticism. Before answering their questions, the first step is to affirm them.

WEANING: CULTURE AND HISTORY Every nursing child eventually weans. But in different cultures, weaning may be viewed very differently. In many parts of the world, weaning is considered a natural stage of growth, a sign that the child has had his fill and is ready to move into the wider world. In other areas, such as the U.S. and the U.K., weaning is often expected by 1 year. When viewed cross-culturally, the average age of weaning is 3 to 4 years. According to anthropologists, without the influence of culture, the "natural" age of weaning for humans is between 2.5 and 7 years.

THE NURSING PARENT'S PERSPECTIVE The decision to wean is often more influenced by a nursing parent's overall feelings about nursing than by a specific problem. Nursing is a complex social behavior, and there are often deeper issues than nipple pain or worries about milk production. Factors such as cultural norms and lack of support often play a major role.

Nursing satisfaction is determined in part by parents' interpretations of their baby's behavior. For example, unrealistic expectations of how long a newborn should be satisfied after nursing may lead to worries about milk production, which can lead to decreased enjoyment of nursing, which can lead to weaning. The parent's perception of their ability to successfully nurture their baby is a factor closely linked to their satisfaction with nursing. There is often much more going on below the surface. The decision to wean involves a convoluted interplay of factors.

THE INFLUENCE OF OTHERS Timing of weaning is influenced by others' opinions and the presence or absence of social support. In cultures where early weaning is the norm, the longer babies nurse, the less support parents receive. The less support for lactation parents receive from healthcare providers, the earlier they are likely to wean. The nursing parent's partner often has a significant effect on length of lactation, either positive or negative.

WEANING DYNAMICS

THE ROLE OF PARENT AND CHILD Children outgrow nursing as they mature, even if parents do nothing to encourage weaning. The weaning process may be driven mostly by the nursing parent, mostly by the child, or it may be mutual.

When weaning is perceived as mutual by nursing parents, their emotional adjustment tends to be easier. But weaning is not always mutual. In some cases, the child decides to wean before the parent feels ready, and the parent feels a greater sense of loss. If parents wean before the child is ready, they may worry about the child's emotional and physical adjustment to this transition.

Due to babies' biological need for human milk during the first year, babies younger than 12 months are unlikely to be developmentally ready to wean. But in areas where early weaning is the cultural norm, many families unknowingly encourage weaning by regularly substituting bottles and pacifiers for nursing. Parents may also misinterpret normal infant behavior as signs their baby is ready to wean. As babies grow and develop, it is common for them to ask to nurse less often, shorten their nursing sessions, and get distracted while nursing. These typical behaviors are not signs of weaning readiness. When a baby "weans himself" before 12 months, this is most likely a nursing strike, a solvable feeding problem described on p. 71.

WEANING BASICS The child's age and readiness to wean, as well as the approach used, will affect how easy or difficult weaning is for parent and child. If a baby is weaned before 1 year, consult the baby's healthcare provider about what to substitute for mother's milk. Powdered infant formula is not sterile, so it is not recommended for babies younger than 3 months.

Feeding method will vary by age and location. Babies older than 6 to 8 months can usually wean to a cup. In developing countries where water is unsafe and sanitation poor, infant feeding bottles are not recommended. Easy-to-clean containers without crevices, such as small cups with straight sides or spoons are safer.

APPROACHES TO WEANING fall into three general categories: gradual, partial, and abrupt.

GRADUAL WEANING allows nursing parents to avoid painful fullness and reduce risk of mastitis. It also gives parents time before their milk is gone to be sure the baby tolerates whatever alternative food is substituted.

Gradual Weaning Between Birth and 12 Months Before a baby is old enough to have strong preferences about his daily routine, weaning usually involves substituting a feeding of infant formula for a nursing session. During a gradual weaning, it may take about 2 to 3 weeks for the nursing parent to comfortably go from exclusive nursing to fully weaned. To help accomplish this, suggest the family:

- Note the times each day the baby usually nurses.
- Pick one daily feed (leave for last the first morning nursing, when most nursing parents feel fullest) and instead feed the substitute food by the chosen method.
- Allow at least 3 days before dropping another nursing to give milk production time to decrease comfortably and gradually.
- Repeat until weaning is complete.

If the weaning parent experiences any uncomfortable fullness, suggest expressing milk just to comfort or allowing the baby to nurse for a short time. While weaning, give the child extra focused attention and cuddling. Expect him to seek other sucking outlets and decide which one the parent prefers.

Gradual Weaning After 12 Months can be a positive experience if the child's preferences are respected. Try different weaning strategies and use those that work best with the child.

- Don't offer, don't refuse, which means nursing when the child asks but not offering when he doesn't ask. When used with other strategies, this can speed the process.
- Offer regular meals, snacks, and drinks to minimize his hunger and thirst and age-appropriate fun activities to avoid nursing out of boredom.
- Change daily routines. Think about the times and places he asks to nurse and how to change their routine, so he will be reminded less often.
- Get the partner or a support person involved. If the child nurses when he wakes, suggest the partner get him up

and make his breakfast. Suggest the partner handle night waking and plan special daytime outings.

- Anticipate and offer substitutes and distractions before the child asks to nurse. Once he asks, he may get upset if a substitute is offered.
- Postpone. This works for a child who nurses at irregular times and places and is old enough to accept waiting. If postponing leaves the child feeling that the nursing parent is keeping him at arm's length, he may become even more determined to nurse. If so, use other strategies.
- Shorten the length of each nursing. This is most effective with children older than 2 years and is a good beginning to the weaning process.
- Bargaining can work well with the older child. A child who is close to outgrowing nursing may give up nursing earlier by mutual agreement. But most children younger than 3 years are not mature enough to understand the meaning of a promise.

Adjust the weaning plan as needed based on the child's reactions and preferences, and be flexible when unusual situations arise. If the child becomes upset and cries or insists upon nursing even when the parent tries to distract or comfort him in other ways, this may mean weaning is going too fast or that different strategies would be better. Other signs that weaning may be moving too fast are regressions in behavior (stuttering, night-waking, clinginess), a new or increased fear of separation, biting (if he has never bitten before), stomach upsets, and constipation.

Natural Weaning is a type of gradual weaning that allows the child to outgrow nursing at his own pace.

The age that children outgrow nursing will vary. One way some families handle the social challenges of nursing an older child is to keep nursing private, which is possible because an older child does not usually nurse as often as a young baby. Time-tested strategies for avoiding nursing in less-than-friendly places include:

- Set limits on where and when the child can nurse.
- Bring snacks, drinks, toys, and/or books to distract the child when out.
- Choose a code word for nursing that isn't obvious to others.
- Find private places to nurse away from home, such as clothing fitting rooms or family lounges.
- Carefully choose clothing. Two-piece outfits and cover-ups like ponchos make nursing less obvious.

Parents who nurse longer than their cultural norm find this easier if they have support from like-minded families. Suggest connecting online or in person with groups that support nursing families.

PARTIAL WEANING involves eliminating some nursing sessions while continuing others. This can be an alternative to full weaning for employed parents who do not plan to nurse or express milk at work. It is an option for parents feeling overwhelmed by exclusive nursing or by intense cluster nursing. Some parents with a history of sexual abuse find the intimate contact of nursing difficult and limited nursing may feel more manageable.

Before beginning a partial weaning, first, decide what the baby will be fed instead of human milk.

- If baby is younger than 1 year, ask baby's healthcare provider to recommend a substitute for missed feeds.
- If baby is older than 1 year, family foods and other milks or drinks can be substituted for nursing.

Next, suggest parents take note of their usual nursing times and decide which feeds to drop. If they will be away from the baby for part of the day, suggest starting with a feed during those hours (avoid dropping the first morning feed, when parents likely feel full already). After dropping a feed, continue giving the substitute at this feed.

Before dropping another feed, wait at least 3 days for milk production to adjust downward. If uncomfortable feelings of fullness develop, express just enough milk to stay comfortable to slow milk production gradually and avoid pain and health risks.

When the desired level of nursing is reached and there is no longer uncomfortable fullness between feeds, the partial weaning is complete. Nursing can continue at this level as long as the parent wishes.

Night Weaning refers to a type of partial weaning that restricts the child's nursing to the parent's waking hours. Parents may decide to night wean when they feel overwhelmed or exhausted from frequent night feeds and the child is old enough to safely sleep for many hours at night without feeding (after 6 to 9 months). As with any weaning, night weaning is best done gradually. Possible strategies include:

- Encourage the child to cluster feeds before bedtime to reduce nursing from hunger or thirst.
- Have drinks or snacks available if the child awakens.
- Involve the partner or a support person in handling night waking.

It's important to keep expectations of night weaning realistic. Eliminating nursing at night is not the same as eliminating night waking. In other words, night weaning does not necessarily mean more sleep. Children wake at night for reasons other than hunger. And when they wake, nursing helps them return to sleep faster. Weaning does not guarantee children will sleep all night. And if they can't nurse after waking, it may take more time and effort to get them back to sleep. For this reason, night weaning can make nights more challenging for the whole family.

ABRUPT WEANING is the most difficult both physically and emotionally. It is often recommended by those unaware of other options. It can be painful and increase the risk of mastitis and other health problems. Nursing parents with nipple pain are most likely to wean abruptly. At the rare times it must be done, do it as gradually as possible, using milk expression when needed to avoid overfullness, and give the child extra focused attention.

If a baby under 1 year abruptly weans and seems distressed when nursing is offered, it may be a nursing strike (p. 71).

COMFORT MEASURES DURING WEANING The more gradual the weaning, the fewer comfort measures are needed. Very little research is available on comfort measures during weaning. Breast-binding, once recommended during weaning but never studied, has fallen out of favor. The "dry-up" medication bromocriptine is no longer recommended to suppress milk production, because of potentially life-threatening side effects.

Expressing milk while weaning can increase comfort and reduce health risks. Whether weaning is gradual or abrupt, use milk expression to stay comfortable by pumping to comfort as needed to avoid overfullness. Another milk-expression strategy that is especially recommended for those with a blocked duct is to remove the milk from both sides as fully as possible then go for longer and longer stretches without nursing or expressing.

Other possible comfort measures recommended in the popular literature include:

- Wear a firm bra for support, if needed, one size larger than usual.
- Reduce salt intake.
- Massage with warmth to prevent blockage.
- Add foods to the diet that reduce milk production (parsley, mint, and sage) and minimize foods that boost it (oats, alfalfa, barley, and sesame seeds).
- Wear chilled cabbage leaves inside the bra, replacing them every 4 to 8 hours with fresh chilled leaves.

- For no more than 1 week, every day drink 3 cups (750 mL) of sage tea, made by steeping 1½ teaspoons (6 mL) of dry sage leaves in a pint of freshly boiled water for 10 minutes.
- Take two 100 mg vitamin B_6 (pyridoxine) pills 3 times a day for the first day and one tablet daily thereafter. Possible side effects include nausea, vomiting, diarrhea, and dark yellow-colored urine.

PHYSICAL AND EMOTIONAL CHANGES WITH WEANING
Some nursing parents have no physical or emotional symptoms while weaning, others notice a change in their energy levels (higher or lower), feelings (happier or sadder), body weight (gaining or losing), hair texture or shine, and appetite.

If the nursing parent's menstrual cycles have not returned before weaning, expect them to return along with fertility after weaning.

CHAPTER 20 WEIGHT GAIN AND GROWTH

NORMAL GROWTH

AGES AND STAGES Babies grow quickly, but the rate that babies lose weight after birth, gain weight, and grow in length and head circumference changes during the first year.

WEIGHT LOSS AFTER BIRTH occurs in most newborns, no matter what and how they are fed. In exclusively nursing babies, the lowest weight is usually on the third or fourth day. Exclusively nursing babies born vaginally have a median weight loss of 7.1% compared with 8.6% for those born by cesarean. On average, nursing babies born by cesarean are still losing weight at 72 hours while those born vaginally begin gaining weight between 48 and 72 hours.

Factors other than milk intake associated with greater weight loss after birth include:

- Born in the U.S. Significantly more U.S. babies lose >10% of birth weight compared with babies born elsewhere.
- Excess IV fluids received within 2 hours of delivery inflate baby's birth weight and act as a diuretic after birth. To offset this effect and reduce unnecessary formula supplements, researchers recommend calculating baby's weight loss from their 24-hour weight rather than birth weight.
- Receiving epidural anesthesia
- Above-average birth weight
- Female gender

If a baby loses 8-10% of birth weight, take a closer look at the nursing dynamics to see if they can be improved. If a baby loses >10% of birth weight, evaluate nursing dynamics and suggest baby be checked for jaundice and dehydration. If feeding problems are not overcome quickly or if the baby shows signs of dehydration, supplements may be needed. To prevent excess weight loss, encourage families to learn hand expression before birth and use it during the early days to feed extra colostrum by spoon (see **firstdroplets.com**).

Most nursing babies begin gaining weight by about Day 4 and regain their birth weight by about Day 10 to 14. If a baby does not regain birth weight by 2 weeks, this is another red flag to take a closer look at how nursing is going and make any needed adjustments.

GROWTH FROM BIRTH TO 12 MONTHS After Day 3 or 4, an average weight gain is about 8 oz (245 g) per week for the first

3 months, with boys gaining slightly faster than girls. Weight gain after birth should always be measured from the lowest weight, which usually occurs on the third or fourth day.

Between 3 and 12 months, weight gain gradually slows as baby's growth rate slows. On average, nursing babies double their birth weights by about 5 to 6 months of age.

During the second 6 months of life, healthy, thriving babies average a month's growth in length of about 1 inch (2.5 cm) and head circumference of about 0.5 inch (1.27 cm). At 12 months, the average nursing baby weighs about 2.5 times her birth weight, has increased in length by 50%, and has increased head circumference by 33%.

Formula-fed babies average a significantly greater weight gain than nursing babies between 3 and 12 months, which increases risk of childhood overweight and obesity and increases risk of other negative health outcomes.

AFTER 12 MONTHS, nursing is still an important source of a baby's nourishment, with mother's milk providing 35% to 40% of their energy intake between 1 and 2 years.

GROWTH CHARTS can be helpful in understanding how one baby's growth compares to the growth of other babies the same age. But growth charts can also confuse parents and healthcare providers and put the focus in the wrong place. A weight that falls at a higher percentile is not "good," and a weight that falls at a lower percentile is not "bad." By definition, there will be healthy children at every percentile. Some will be chunky and some will be petite, but their percentile does not necessarily reflect their overall health or growth.

If a baby is growing consistently and well, her actual percentile is irrelevant. However, if over time her percentile drops, this is a red flag to take a closer look.

Between 3 and 12 months, a baby's percentile on the growth chart will vary depending on whether the chart is based on nursing norms. The World Health Organization's growth charts based on the growth of nursing babies are available for free download at: **who.int/childgrowth/standards/en.**

SLOW WEIGHT GAIN

When a baby is gaining weight slowly, emotions are often intense. Be prepared to listen to and acknowledge these feelings. Giving the family an outlet to express their worries may make it easier for them to discuss and evaluate their situation more objectively.

The definitions of adequate and slow weight gain have changed since the WHO growth standards were released in 2006. Previously, weight gain of 0.5 to 1 oz (14-28 g) per day during the first 3 months was considered adequate. But now, a weight gain of less than 30-40 g (1-1.3 oz) per day is considered a cause for concern.

GATHERING BASIC INFORMATION Before making suggestions, first try to determine the cause(s) of the slow weight gain, which usually fall within one of the following three areas:

- **Nursing dynamics.** Is the baby latched deeply? Is the baby nursing at least 8 times each day and nursing until done?

- **Baby's anatomy and health.** Is the baby nursing ineffectively due to anatomical variations or a health problem? Is a health problem causing slow weight gain despite a healthy milk intake?

- **Milk production.** Is the parent producing enough milk to meet the baby's needs?

Ask questions in a calm, relaxed manner and affirm whatever the nursing parent is doing right.

Be sure the baby is being regularly evaluated by a healthcare provider. If the baby's healthcare provider recommends supplementing the baby with formula and the nursing parent wants to try other alternatives first, encourage the family to contact him/her to discuss this.

WEIGHT GAIN AND LOSS should be assessed with an eye to how close it is to the expected range. Questions to ask:

- **Timing.** Was the baby's weight an issue from birth, or did the baby gain well at first?

- **Weighing issues**. Was the same scale used for each of the weight checks? Was the baby's clothing the same when she was last weighed? And when was the scale last calibrated?

- **Growth.** How much has the baby grown in length and head circumference?

- **Baby's condition**. What has the baby's healthcare provider said about the baby's overall health?

The diagnosis of failure to thrive means baby is seriously underweight and requires immediate intervention. The baby may grow little in length or head circumference, or pass concentrated urine and few stools.

A baby considered "slow-gaining," on the other hand, usually feeds well and often, has pale urine and the expected number of stools, appears alert and active, is developing normally, has good skin and muscle tone, and is gaining weight, just gaining slower than average.

OTHER SIGNS OF MILK INTAKE   Besides rate of weight gain, other factors to evaluate include:

- **Swallowing sounds** can provide clues to feeding effectiveness. After milk ejection, most babies swallow after every or every other suck with occasional pauses. Sucking many times before swallowing or no swallowing sounds at all is one possible sign of ineffective nursing.
- **Baby never seems satisfied.**   The family says the baby nurses "all the time."
- **Shallow latch**, which can contribute to slower milk flow, less milk intake, and/or difficulty staying latched.
- **Choking during nursing** can occur with very fast milk flow and also with uncoordinated sucking and swallowing or an airway abnormality.
- **Low or high muscle tone.**   "Floppy" babies with low tone include those with Down syndrome and other neurological impairments. Babies with high tone may arch away.
- **Cheek dimpling or clicking sounds** during nursing may indicate suction is being broken. If baby is gaining weight well, this is not a problem.
- **Nipple pain or trauma** can be due to shallow latch, unusual tongue movements, or anatomical variations, such as tongue-tie.
- **Unrelieved mammary fullness or recurring mastitis** may be a sign of ineffective milk removal.

If there is no audible swallowing at all, if it stops early in the feed, or if the baby usually falls asleep quickly, to encourage more active nursing, suggest trying to get a deeper latch and then using breast compression (p. 309).

Scales are available in some areas that are accurate to 2 g and can measure babies' milk intake during nursing.

Diaper output is not a reliable indicator of milk intake. If by Day 5, baby's stools are still black and tarry rather than turning yellow, suggest a weight check. At other times, at best, diaper output is a very rough indicator of milk intake, which changes over time. If slow weight gain is a concern, it may be reassuring to track diaper output on a daily basis between regular weight checks, but diaper output alone cannot substitute for an accurate weight.

A baby's temperament and sleep patterns are not reliable indicators of milk intake.

Commercial products that claim to measure milk intake during nursing may be unreliable.

BASIC NURSING DYNAMICS should be reviewed in a slow-gaining baby.

- How many times each day does the baby nurse? Most newborns nurse at least 8 times every 24 hours. If baby is nursing fewer than this, ask why. If parents nurse on a schedule or baby is sleepy, suggest increasing nursing to 10 to 12 sessions per day.

- How long does a feed usually take, does the baby take both sides, and who usually ends the feed, parent or baby? Recommend they "finish the first side first," which means the baby determines the length of the feed and feeds on the first side until she comes off on her own and then the second side is offered. If desired, the baby can go back to the first side again.

- Does the baby latch and quickly fall asleep? Does the nursing parent have nipple pain? These are both signs of a shallow latch. Nipple pain may also be a sign of anatomical variations in the baby or the nursing parent.

- What is the baby's sleep/wake pattern, and how long is baby's longest sleep stretch? If a baby does not wake to nurse at least 8 times per day, she may be unusually placid or overdressed, which can make baby sleepy. If so, unwrap the baby or dress in lighter clothes, wake baby to nurse at least once during the night, spend more time with baby resting tummy down on the parent's semi-reclined body, help baby latch during light sleep (eyes moving under eyelids), and "cluster" feeds during baby's naturally occurring alert periods.

- Is the baby regularly swaddled for long periods or using a soother, such as a pacifier or a baby swing? This may decrease the number of nursing sessions per day, which may slow weight gain.

- Is the nursing baby consuming anything other than mother's milk? If the baby younger than 6 months is fed large amounts of low-calorie liquids (such as water) or solid foods, this reduces the volume of mother's milk baby takes.

- Are they nursing with a nipple shield? If so, ask why. Shields are sometimes recommended for ineffective nursing, a possible cause of slow weight gain.

CAUSES OF SLOW WEIGHT GAIN IN THE FIRST 6 WEEKS may include one or more of the following.

Nursing Dynamics

- Shallow latch—Can decrease milk transfer and/or cause nipple pain and may be due to positioning issues or poor fit (large nipple, small mouth)
- Too little active nursing time—Scheduled, limited, or infrequent feeds, sleepy baby, overuse of swaddling or soothers (pacifier/dummy, swing), parental depression
- Less-than-optimal early nursing due to birth or hospital practices—Separation, medications, rough suctioning or rough handling during latch
- Feeding low-calorie liquids or solid foods (water, juice, cereal, etc.)—Delays/replaces nursing

Baby Factors

- Temperament—Placid/sleepy baby or fussy and difficult to settle for feeds
- Anatomy or health issues that can cause ineffective nursing—Variations in oral anatomy (tongue-tie, cleft palate, etc.), illness, airway abnormality, neurological impairment (high/low tone)
- Prematurity—Including late preterm
- Birth injury—Hematoma, broken bone, torticollis, etc.
- Health issues that can cause slow weight gain with healthy milk intake—Illness, cardiac defect, cystic fibrosis (baby tastes salty), metabolic or genetic disorder

Nursing Parent's Anatomy, Health, and Milk Production

- Mammary/nipple issues—Breast or chest surgery or injury (severed milk ducts or nerve damage preventing milk ejection), inadequate glandular tissue (hypoplasia), unusual nipple anatomy or nipple piercing (may decrease or prevent milk transfer)
- Birth-related issues—Delayed nursing, excess blood loss, retained placenta
- Health and medication issues—Serious illness, drugs/herbs that decrease milk production or are incompatible with nursing, obesity, thyroid, pituitary, or hormonal problems, birth injury that makes nursing painful, psychiatric issues, eating disorder, polycystic ovary syndrome (PCOS), gestational ovarian theca lutein cysts

CAUSES OF SLOW WEIGHT GAIN AFTER 6 WEEKS include:

Nursing Dynamics

- Too little active nursing time—Scheduled, limited, or infrequent feeds, longer nighttime sleep stretch or sleep training (depending on storage capacity), overuse of swaddling or soothers (pacifier/dummy or swing)
- Feeding baby low-calorie liquids or solid foods (water, juice, cereal, etc.)—may delay or replace nursing

Baby's Health

- Issues that can reduce baby's milk intake—Illness, allergy, reflux disease
- Issues that can cause slow weight gain with healthy milk intake—Congenital heart disease, cystic fibrosis (baby tastes salty), metabolic disorder, other metabolic and genetic disorders

Nursing Parent's Anatomy, Health, Milk Production/Transfer Issues

- Health or medications—Serious illness, drugs that decrease milk production or are incompatible with nursing, hormonal, thyroid, or pituitary problems, pregnancy, polycystic ovary syndrome, vitamin B_{12} deficiency from weight-loss surgery or a restricted diet
- Mammary/nipple issues— Nipple piercing, breast or chest surgery, injury, or insufficient glandular tissue (hypoplasia), effect on weight gain may not be obvious until baby needs full milk production to gain weight at about 5 weeks

INCREASING WEIGHT GAIN The best first strategy will depend on the baby's condition, as a seriously underfed baby may not nurse effectively. If baby shows signs of dehydration, contact her healthcare provider. If there are no signs of dehydration but baby's weight is far below what's expected, supplements may be needed right away to help boost her feeding effectiveness. If baby is healthy, alert, and her weight is not too far from healthy norms, it may make sense to start by improving nursing dynamics. Suggest the nursing parent keep a daily record of number of nursing sessions and (for the baby under 6 weeks) stools. Then review the following basic nursing dynamics to see if there is room for improvement.

- Make sure baby is latched deeply.
- If baby is nursing effectively (audible swallows after every suck or two for at least 5 minutes of active nursing) and the baby is nursing fewer than 12 times per day, increase the number of daily nursing sessions to at least 12.

- Finish the first side first, offer both sides at each feed, and use breast compression as needed to keep baby active.
- Offer both sides more than once and keep nursing for as long as the baby is willing.
- Avoid soothers (pacifiers/dummies, swings).
- Consider milk expression as many times per day as practical, using hands-on pumping techniques (p. 211).
- Limit all feeding-related activities (nursing, milk expression, supplementing) to no more than 40 minutes.
- Discuss possible use of galactogogues (p. 196).
- If a nipple shield is used, be sure baby latches deeply.
- Accept all offers of household help.

WHEN AND HOW TO SUPPLEMENT If the baby is not at risk after trying the above strategies and the baby's weight gain is improving, supplementing may not be needed. Schedule regular weight checks for the next week or two while continuing these strategies.

Before starting supplements, make sure the baby's slow weight gain is due to low milk intake by ruling out health issues that can increase baby's energy needs or prevent her from fully metabolizing the milk. Some babies gain slowly despite good milk intake due to health problems, such as a congenital heart disease, a genetic or metabolic disorder, malabsorption, intestinal blockage, parasites, or other conditions. In these cases, the best first step for a healthier weight gain—rather than supplementing—is to address the health problem.

Discuss feeding-method options and their advantages and disadvantages (p. 311). For the baby older than 6 or 8 months, a cup (either a straw or sippy cup, whichever baby masters most easily) is the logical first choice for giving extra milk. A cup will not satisfy baby's need to suck, so it is less likely than a bottle to decrease her desire to nurse. For the younger baby, discuss using a nursing supplementer, cup, feeding syringe, eyedropper, bottle. If the family is open to using a nursing supplementer, it can decrease the time spent feeding (no need to feed again after nursing), and in some cases, it may help improve the baby's effectiveness by giving positive reinforcement during nursing.

The choice of supplement is the family's to make after consulting baby's healthcare provider. This choice is also based in part on its practicality and local availability. From a health perspective, for the baby younger than 6 months, the options from most to least healthy are: 1) expressed mother's milk, 2) donor human milk, 3) non-human milks, such as infant formula. For the baby older than 6 months, high-calorie solid foods are also an option.

If there is more than enough expressed milk available, it may be possible to provide high-fat, high-calorie hindmilk by expressing milk right after the baby nurses.

The volume of extra milk a baby needs per day to gain weight varies by age (Table 20.1) and by baby. While supplementing, let baby set the pace. Babies who were underfed may start with small volumes that increase over the next day or two as their stomachs expand.

Table 20.1 Average Milk Volume by Age During the First 6 Months

Baby's Age	Average Milk Volume Per Feed	Average Milk Intake Per Day
First week (after Day 4)	1-2 oz. (30-59 mL)	10-20 oz. (300-600 mL)
Weeks 2 and 3	2-3 oz. (59-89 mL)	15-25 oz. (450-750 mL)
Months 1-6	3-4 oz. (89-118 mL)	25-30 oz. (750-887 mL)

Another approach to supplementing is suggested by Catherine Watson Genna, BS, IBCLC in Table 20.2. It involves doubling the weekly weight deficit for the volume per day. For example, if the baby should be gaining 7 oz (210 g) per week but only gained 1 oz (28 g) the previous week, start with 12 oz (360 mL) of supplement per day (7 oz target weight minus 1 oz of actual weight gain equals 6 oz x 2=12 oz/day). See how the baby responds and either increase or decrease the volume as needed.

Table 20.2 Approximate Supplmental Volume Needed Per Day to Increase Weight Gain

Weekly Weight Gain	6 oz. (170 g)	5 oz. (142 g)	4 oz. (113 g)	3 oz. (85 g)	2 oz. (57 g)	1 oz. (28 g)	0 oz. (0 g)
Weekly weight deficit	1 oz. (28 g)	2 oz. (57 g)	3 oz. (85 g)	4 oz. (113 g)	5 oz. (142 g)	6 oz. (170 g)	7 oz. (198 g)
Daily supplement needed	2 oz. (60 mL)	4 oz. (120 mL)	6 oz. (180 mL)	8 oz. (240 mL)	10 oz. (300 mL)	12 oz. (360 mL)	14 oz. (420 mL)

Begin any plan with the idea that it may need to be adjusted. Baby may or may not need a supplement at every feed. Try different approaches to see what works best.

- **Supplement only during the nursing parent's waking hours** to make the plan more manageable. Nurse exclusively during sleeping hours.

- **Supplement more or less often**. If baby's weight gain is close to borderline, try supplementing at every other feed or less often. This might work well if a baby nurses effectively and the milk production is not too low.
- **Smaller rather than larger volumes.** In general, the transition to full nursing will be easier if smaller volumes of the supplement are given more often, rather than a large volume (4 oz [118 mL] or more) once or twice a day.
- **Time of day.** Milk production is usually higher in the morning, so the baby may receive a full feed from nursing alone early in the day, with supplements needed only in afternoon and evening, as the volume of milk available at each feed decreases.
- **Effect of feeding method.** If the supplement is fed by nursing supplementer, the tubing may be clamped shut to restrict milk flow early in the feed while the baby is sucking well and getting milk. If baby begins to doze, unclamp the tubing for faster flow. If the baby is not supplemented during nursing and is sucking effectively, nurse first and give the supplement afterward. In some cases, giving the supplement first may lead to more effective nursing.

Weaning from the supplement should be done gradually as milk production and/or baby's effectiveness improves.

- **Decrease the supplement slowly.** Unless baby is obviously ready to discontinue faster, decrease the supplement by about 2 oz (59 mL) every other day while increasing time spent nursing.
- **Begin by eliminating supplements at the first morning nursing**. Many babies nurse best at this time, probably due to faster milk flow.
- **Make sure the baby is continuing to gain weight well.** Monitor the baby's weight gain at least once or twice per week using the same scale. If the baby's weight gain drops to below 5 to 6 oz (142-177 g) per week, reintroduce the supplement.
- **Expect it to take time before baby is exclusively nursing** Provide reassurance and support the family.

If it becomes clear that exclusive nursing is not an option for a family, it may help them come to terms with their disappointment if someone helps them understand what happened, sort through their feelings, and acknowledge their disappointment.

RAPID WEIGHT GAIN

If the baby's weight gain is well above average and the family expresses concern, assure them that exclusive nursing does not necessarily lead to later overweight or obesity. If a baby is at the 95th percentile in weight but also long, this does not make her overweight or obese. Overweight and obesity are determined by weight-for-length ratio. These charts for boys and girls are available free at: **who.int/childgrowth/standards/en**.

Some studies found an association between rapid early weight gain and later childhood overweight and obesity, but these studies did not control for feeding method. When fast-gaining, exclusively nursing babies reach the age when they begin rolling over, crawling and eating solid foods, their weight gain slows, and over time they slim down to a normal weight range.

Exclusive nursing is associated with reduced risk of overweight and obesity in many observational studies. Many other factors affect risk of overweight, too, such as parental obesity, which has a greater effect on a baby's risk of obesity than feeding method.

Human milk fat content is not a factor that contributes to rapid weight gain, as babies who consume higher-fat milk take less milk per day than those who consume lower-fat milk.

Trying to slow a baby's weight gain by limiting nursing time is not recommended because the young child is growing rapidly and needs the nutrients in human milk for normal development.

When baby begins eating solid foods, some feeding strategies and food choices can affect weight gain, depending on baby's age.

- **Early solid foods before 6 months** lead to more negative health outcomes, according to the World Health Organization. In some countries, babies with rapid weight gain are given solid foods early because it is believed that heavier babies "need" solid foods. When solid foods are given before baby is old enough to feed herself, parents may inadvertently overfeed their babies, establishing unhealthy eating habits. Giving large volumes of high-calorie solids may contribute to rapid weight gain. If solids are a substantial part of the baby's diet and the family wants to reduce or eliminate them, encourage them to reduce them gradually and nurse more often to boost milk production and fill the gap.

- **Food choices after 6 months** can affect a baby's weight gain. If the baby is gaining weight very rapidly, suggest avoiding "empty calories," such as sweetened foods and drinks, and offer a greater variety of fresh fruits and vegetables. Suggest nursing first, before giving solids. Encourage the family to think of mother's milk as the baby's primary food during the first year and solids as a supplement to nursing.

DIGITAL RESOURCES

firstdroplets.com-—Videos by Dr. Jane Morton for parents of term and preterm babies show how to prevent excess weight loss after birth by learning hand expression during the last month of a low-risk pregnancy and using it during the early days to increase baby's milk intake and avoid excess weight loss.

newbornweight.com—Free NEWT app for clinicians incorporates the 2015 newborn weight loss nomograms to make it easy to plot newborn weight loss by percentile, based on the data from more than 108,000 exclusively nursing U.S. babies.

who.int/childgrowth/standards/en/—World Health Organization growth standards based on breastfeeding norms. Free and downloadable charts include length/height for age, weight for age, weight for length/height, BMI for age, head circumference for age, arm circumference for age, subscapular skinfold for age, triceps skinfold for age, motor development milestones, weight velocity, length velocity, and head circumference velocity.

APPENDIX A

BREAST COMPRESSION

Breast compression is a simple technique parents can use to help keep their nursing baby actively sucking longer to increase milk intake, which also increases the milk's fat content. This technique can be useful for healthy babies who are gaining weight slowly, newborns with hypoglycemia or exaggerated jaundice, babies with cardiac problems or any other health or neurological problems that compromise baby's weight gain or growth, and parents trying to increase milk production.

This technique was popularized by Canadian pediatrician Jack Newman. Here's how he described the technique:

1. Parents need to know when the baby is getting milk (open mouth wide—pause—close mouth type of sucking.

2. When the baby is drinking milk actively, parents do not need to do any compression.

3. Once the baby is sucking, but no longer drinking, just nibbling, parents should start with the compression.

4. The baby should be sucking but not actually drinking (open mouth wide—pause—close type of sucking). As the baby sucks, parents hold their gland with one hand, the thumb on one side and the other fingers on the other side of the gland, with a good amount of gland supported by their hand. They should just bring their thumb and fingers together, compressing the tissue. This should be done firmly but not so hard it hurts.

5. The baby may start to drink again (open mouth wide—pause—close mouth type of sucking). If so, parents should keep up the pressure until the baby is back to nibbling. Once the baby is nibbling only, parents should release the pressure on the gland so their hand does not get tired, and allow milk to start flowing again.

6. When parents release the pressure, a young baby, say under 2 or 3 weeks of age, will stop sucking. She will restart sucking when she tastes milk again. An older baby may continue to suck. If the baby drinks, fine. If she sucks but does not drink, parents should restart the compression.

7. If the compression has no effect at a particular moment, this does not mean parents must immediately switch sides. Sometimes compression will work, other times not. But as the baby has nursed longer and longer, it will work less and less, as the flow of milk slows. This means not that the gland is "empty," but that the baby is getting less and less. Babies respond to flow of milk.

8. If the compression is no longer having an effect and the baby is getting sleepy, or starting to fuss because flow is slow, parents should unlatch the baby and offer the other side. Parents should then repeat the process.

9. Parents should experiment….do whatever works best for them. As long as it does not hurt to compress, and the baby gets milk, the technique is working.

APPENDIX B

FEEDING METHODS

COMPARING FEEDING METHODS Families need an alternative to nursing when parent and baby are separated at feeding times, the baby can't directly nurse or nurses ineffectively, or parents decide to feed the nursing baby in other ways. Nursing parents and their partners are the final decision-makers on feeding method, ideally after reviewing each possibility's pros and cons (Table B.1). Any feeding method should be safe, a good match for the baby's size and condition, is accessible and affordable, is easy to use and clean, is suitable for the length of time needed, and if baby will also be nursing, it promotes the transition to direct nursing. Parents and others feeding the baby also need to be comfortable using it. All methods require instruction and practice. But most are mastered quickly and get easier over time.

Table B.1 Comparing the Pros and Cons of Alternative Feeding Methods

Feeding Method	Advantages	Disadvantages
Nursing Supplementer	Reinforces direct nursing Eliminates the need to feed baby again after nursing Latching problems less likely to develop Can improve sucking skills in some babies If latched deeply, sucking stimulates milk production	Unfamiliar to many Equipment care may be stressful and time-consuming Some babies suck on tubing like a straw, which reduces stimulation If latching with tubing in place, may add stress If tape is used often, it may cause skin damage Some commercial devices are expensive
Feeding Bottles	Culturally acceptable and readily available in the West Familiar to many parents Some babies consume more milk in a shorter time Relatively inexpensive	Can replace nursing Fast flow causes more heart-rate and breathing problems in preemies May complicate transition to nursing if used for >2 feedings or after a c-section Baby uses different mouth muscles; long-term regular use increases risk of oral malformations Fast flow may cause overfeeding; long-term, regular use increases risk of obesity

Finger-Feeding	May make transition to nursing easier Can be used to improve sucking in some babies Viewed as temporary	Unfamiliar to many parents Finger-feeding equipment may not be easily available to parents Little research
Cup, spoon, or syringe	Easy to clean Readily available Inexpensive In preemies, fewer heart-rate and breathing problems than bottles and more direct nursing at discharge May make transition to nursing easier Muscles used similar to nursing	If hospital staff or parents are not well trained, can lead to feeding problems Feeding may take longer May be some milk loss from spillage

PACED BOTTLE FEEDING When a baby is bottle-fed, encourage the feeder to use techniques that reinforce nursing behaviors by making bottle-feeding more like nursing. Unlike the fast, consistent milk flow of traditional bottle-feeding, pacing provides the fast-then slow-then fast milk flow that occurs with milk ejections during nursing sessions. This pacing technique was originally used for preterm or compromised babies who struggled with fast milk flow. But many parents and lactation specialists found that it can help all bottle-feeding babies avoid overfeeding and give them more control. Here's how to do paced bottle-feeding:

- Position baby semi-upright or upright (Figure B.1).
- Touch baby's lips with the bottle teat and wait until he opens wide.
- Allow baby to draw in the teat so his lips close on the teat base, not its shaft or bottle collar, with top and bottom lips flanged out.
- Keep the end of the bottle tipped down for about a minute (the time to milk ejection), then tip it up so it is nearly horizontal. As baby starts to suck and swallow, build in pauses every few minutes by lowering the end of the bottle so milk runs out of the teat, giving baby a breathing break.
- When the baby begins sucking again, lift the end of the bottle so milk flows back into the teat.
- Repeat until baby is finished.

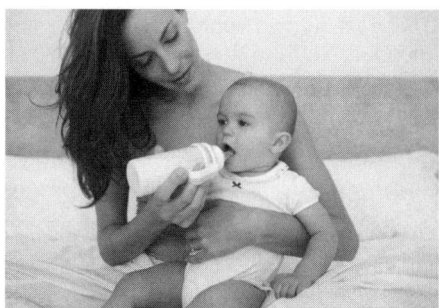

Figure B.1 Rather than pushing the bottle teat into baby's mouth, tap his lips till he opens wide and allow him to draw in the teat.

Bottle-feeds should ideally take between 15 to 30 minutes. Swallowing air is not an issue, as we all swallow air while we eat, and it is easy for baby to burp up any air after feeds. A too-fast milk flow, however, can lead to aspirating (breathing in) milk, which is a much more serious concern.

CUP, SPOON AND SYRINGE FEEDING These methods require the baby sip or lap the milk (as opposed to sucking). Technique is key. If cup-feeding, any small cup can be used, such as a shot glass or the plastic cup included with children's liquid medicines. Spoon-feeding can also be used when supplements are needed after birth. See **firstdroplets.com** for videos demonstrating spoon-feeding. Any spoon can be used. If using a syringe, remove the needle before dripping milk into baby's mouth.

While parent and baby are learning, it is best to go slowly. With practice, feeds are often quick. No matter what container is used, when starting: make sure baby is awake and alert, wrap his hands securely to prevent them from bumping the feeding container, and use a bib or cloth to protect baby's clothes from spills. Hold the baby in a sitting position (Figure B.2).

When cup-feeding:

- Raise the cup and rest its rim lightly on baby's lower lip.
- Tip the cup so the milk just touches his lips and he can sip or lap it in, but not so much that it pours into his mouth.

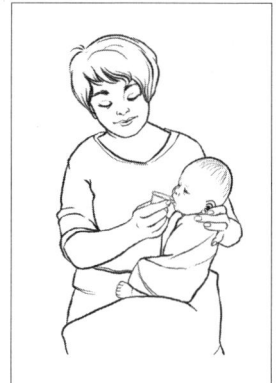

Figure B.2 Sit a baby upright when feeding by cup, spoon, or syringe. ©2021 Nancy Mohrbacher Solutions, Inc.

- Let the baby set his own sipping or lapping rhythm, pausing when needed, until he finishes. Some babies prefer the cup be tilted away between swallows, while others prefer to feed continuously. Some use their tongue to lap the milk, others sip it in.

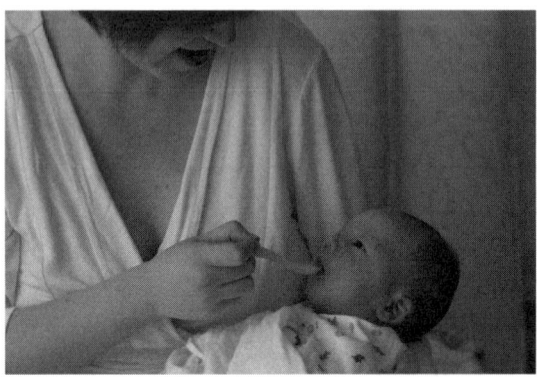

Figure B.3 Spoon-feeding is not intimidating to most parents because it is low-tech and familiar.
©2021Melanie Ham, used with permission.

When spoon-feeding:

- Fill the spoon with a mouthful of milk.
- Rest the spoon lightly on baby's lower lip (Figure B.3) and tilt it so the milk touches his lips.
- Either pour the milk into baby's mouth or allow him to sip or lap it, whichever he prefers.
- Give the baby time to swallow, refill the spoon, and repeat until baby is done.

When feeding with a syringe:

- Fill the syringe with a mouthful of milk.
- Raise it and drip the milk into baby's mouth at a slow enough pace so that he can swallow it before more is given.

FINGER-FEEDING involves feeding milk to a baby while he's sucking on the feeder's finger. It can be used with any baby to provide extra milk and can be used therapeutically to teach more normal sucking to babies with poor oral-motor skills by rewarding them with milk when they make correct feeding movements.

Whichever tool is used to finger-feed, the first step is for feeders to wash their hands well and make sure the finger used to feed the baby has a closely-trimmed nail:

- Any nursing supplementer can be used to finger-feed by placing its tubing along an adult's finger, pad side up, and extending it about a quarter-inch (6 mm) past the fingertip. If desired, the tubing can be taped to the finger, ideally lengthwise, so the baby can't suck the tape into his mouth. Tap baby's lips with the finger and wait until he opens. Allow baby to draw the finger into his mouth to the area where active sucking is triggered.

- Periodontal syringes, which typically hold 10 to 20 mL of milk each, can be used by pulling back on the plunger to draw milk into the syringe and resting the curved tip against the feeder's finger just inside the corner of the baby's mouth (about one-sixteenth of an inch or 2 mm). The plunger should be depressed slowly, only while the baby is sucking. When the baby pauses, the feeder pauses to avoid overwhelming the baby with milk.

NURSING SUPPLEMENTERS are also known as *feeding-tube devices*, *tube-feeding devices*, and *at-breast supplementers.* These devices deliver extra milk to the baby during nursing through a thin tube. The baby's natural response to a swallow is to suck. Some babies learn to suck more effectively when the steady milk flow from the tube stimulates more active and consistent sucking and swallowing. When a baby latches deeply and sucks longer or more vigorously, he also takes more milk directly from the mammary gland and stimulates faster milk production. A nursing supplementer can allow parents with low milk production to feed their baby exclusively during nursing, eliminating the need to feed him again afterwards. Unlike other feeding methods, supplementing while baby nurses provides positive reinforcement for direct nursing.

A nursing supplementer can be bought or created at home. An easy-to-make *lactation aid* functions as a siphon and consists of a bottle with a hole cut in the nipple/teat to insert one end of a feeding tube into the milk and the other end into the nursing baby's mouth. To learn more, go to **bit.ly/BA2-LactationAid**. These devices can be used alone or with a nipple shield. If used with a nipple shield, choose a device with softer tubing, so positioning the tubing inside the shield is less likely to cause the shield to shift.

INDICATIONS FOR USE   Nursing supplementers may be a good choice if milk production is low or baby is gaining weight slowly. It provides a faster, more consistent milk flow during relactation or induced lactation. Immediate milk flow may help some babies more easily transition to nursing from other feeding methods. It can provide extra milk for babies with special needs, which can sometimes help a baby learn to nurse more effectively.

TWO TYPES OF NURSING SUPPLEMENTERS fall into these general categories:

- **Suction required** These devices may be homemade or manufactured. They include a container to hold the supplement, which hangs around the user's neck, clips to clothing, or is held or set/hung from a nearby surface. When the baby latches and sucks, milk flows through the tubing. When used effectively, the nursing baby receives both the supplement through the tubing and milk directly from the mammary gland.

- **Suction not required** These homemade devices consist of either a periodontal syringe or a syringe with needle removed attached by port to a thin feeding tube. The feeder controls milk flow, and the baby does not need to generate suction.

The suction-required nursing supplementers are only a useful tool if the baby can generate enough suction to draw the supplement through the tubing. The suction-not-required supplementers can be used with babies who can't generate suction, such as those with a cleft palate or those weakened from underfeeding. The suction-not-required devices should be used with caution with babies who have cardiac defects and airway abnormalities. These babies must breathe more times per minute to maintain adequate oxygen levels. If a faster milk flow generated by the feeder forces these babies to swallow more often, this can compromise their oxygen levels.

USING A NURSING SUPPLEMENTER can be tricky. Parents may find them less intimidating if after purchase they practice assembling, using, and cleaning them before using them with the baby. Do this by first filling the container with water rather than milk and having the partner suck the water out. For podcasts and articles that feature tips and tricks for using these devices, go to **bit.ly/BA2-TipsTricks**. It also helps to know the following practical details.

Milk Type and Volume/Tubing Care If infant formula is used as a supplement, choose either the concentrate or ready-to-feed types, as powdered formula can clump and clog the thin tubing. To make sure the baby gets the milk he needs, start with enough milk in the container so that about a half-ounce (15 mL) is left after every feed. If baby takes it all, add more at that feed and start the next feed with 1 ounce (30 mL) more. If more than a half-ounce (15 mL) is left consistently, decrease the volume of milk in the supplementer at the next feed. See Table 20.2 on p. 305 for milk-volume suggestions as a starting point. Unless the parent is using disposable tubing, suggest either washing the tubing immediately after feeds or immersing it in a container of cool or warm water (not hot water, which can cook the milk), so it doesn't dry. Tubing with dried milk inside needs to be replaced.

Latching with Tubing in Place One challenge of using this device is achieving a deep latch with the tubing positioned on the nipple. Some devices include surgical tape to keep the tubing in place while baby latches. Usually, the tubing is taped just behind the areola to keep it out of baby's way, with the tape running lengthwise on the tubing and the tubing tip extending about a quarter-inch (6 mm) past the nipple tip. An alternative to using tape is to place a self-adhesive bandage at the appropriate place on the mammary gland after bathing and leave it there until the next bath or shower. At each feed, the bandage can be pinched to allow the tubing to extend under its pad. The tubing can be positioned on top of the nipple when baby latches or on the underside of the nipple so that it rests against baby's tongue during feeds. Use whichever position works better.

Latching First and Then Inserting the Tubing is only an option if the tubing is firm enough, like the tubing used with the homemade lactation aid. In this case, the baby can latch first and the tubing can be pushed into the corner of the baby's mouth until it is deep enough that milk starts to flow.

Sucking the Tubing Like a Straw can present a challenge with these devices. If baby is latched shallowly and sucks the tubing like a straw without stimulating the mammary gland, using this device will not increase milk production. If latching deeper doesn't correct this, this device will not be helpful.

Adjusting Milk Flow of a nursing supplementer can be done in several ways. Suggest the user adjust the device's milk flow so that at each nursing session, the baby sucks actively for about 10 to 20 minutes per side, switching sides about halfway through. If the milk flow is too fast, the baby may finish before 20 minutes total. If the milk flow is too slow, feeds may take more than 40 minutes, which causes the baby to quickly lose interest or it makes it difficult to fit in enough feeds per day. When using the suction-required nursing supplementers, adjust milk flow by:

- **Raising or lowering the container** Because they work like a siphon, a higher container provides faster flow and a lower container provides slower flow.

- **Increasing or decreasing tubing diameter** Some nursing supplementers include different size tubing (small, medium, large). Larger diameter tubing provides faster flow; smaller diameter tubing provides slower flow.

- **Opening or clamping one tubing** Nursing supplementers with a closed container and two tubes can be set up with either both tubes open or one or both clamped closed. Both tubes open provides faster milk flow; one tube closed provides slower milk flow.

- **Positioning one or two tubes at the nipple** When the device includes two tubes, they can either be positioned with one at each nipple to make switching sides easier, or for faster flow, both can be positioned at one nipple.

If the baby begins to nurse more effectively and/or the milk production increases, adjust the supplementer in the above ways to slow milk flow as needed to maintain ideal feeding times.

Determining Volume of Supplement Needed If baby was underfed, allow him to take as much milk as he wants to increase his energy for more effective nursing. But when a baby's weight gain is just a little slow, avoid giving so much milk that he takes less milk from the nursing parent. For the baby younger than 4 months, see Table 20.2 on p. 305 for the average recommended supplement to increase weight gain to 7 ounces (198 g.) per week.

Weaning from a Nursing Supplementer If the baby begins feeding more effectively, he may start taking all of the supplement in a shorter time. If the baby finishes feeding in less than 20 minutes, and the nursing supplementer has multiple tubing sizes, suggest switching to a smaller size tubing to slow the flow and increase feeding time for better stimulation. As the baby takes more milk from the parent, use the following strategies to gradually wean from the device:

- Lower the height of the container to slow milk flow.
- Clamp the tubing shut before baby latches and wait to unclamp it until the sound of baby's swallowing stops.
- Try nursing without the supplementer at the first morning feed, which is usually when the most milk is available.
- Use the supplementer at gradually fewer feeds each day.

As parents wean from the supplement, expect the baby will want to nurse more often. Weigh the baby regularly while weaning from the supplementer to ensure he gets enough milk. Support, encouragement, and the use of test-weighing to provide objective reassurance of baby's milk intake may be helpful in convincing parents that the nursing supplementer is no longer needed.

APPENDIX C

LATCHING TECHNIQUES

ASYMMETRICAL LATCH When baby latches deeply, on average, the nipple extends to within about 5 mm of the junction of baby's hard and soft palates. Some call this area on the roof of baby's mouth the "comfort zone," because in most cases, when the nipple reaches this area, nursing is comfortable and effective.

When upright and side-lying feeding positions are used, an *asymmetrical latch* can help achieve a deep latch. An asymmetrical latch is different from a "centered" or "bull's-eye" latch. With an asymmetrical latch, the baby latches off-center, with her lower jaw further from the nipple than her upper jaw (Figure C.1). This allows the nipple to extend deeper into the baby's mouth, which makes nursing more comfortable and effective. When babies latch shallowly, they may drain the mammary gland unevenly and may fall asleep quickly, because a shallow latch does not trigger active nursing.

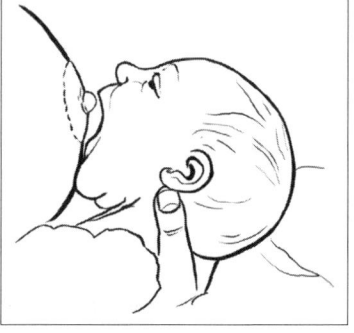

Figure C.1 During an asymmetrical latch, baby's lower jaw lands further from the nipple than her upper jaw, allowing the nipple to extend deeper in baby's mouth.

©2021, Nancy Mohrbacher Solutions, Inc.

When we drink or talk, only our lower jaw moves. The same is true during nursing, which is why some refer to the lower jaw as the "working jaw." The lower jaw does all the work of feeding, while the upper jaw simply helps keep the tissue in place. The further away from the nipple the lower jaw lands during latch, the further back in her mouth the nipple can extend.

As described in Chapter 1, a feeding position can make achieving a deep latch easier or more difficult, especially during the early weeks, when the newborn lacks much head-and-neck control. The feeding position chosen determines whether the baby or the parent controls the depth of latch. When baby rests tummy down on the parent's semi-reclined body (*starter positions*, p. 6), the baby can self-attach, automatically triggering a wide-open mouth, a relaxed jaw, and the tongue extended forward. The baby can also readjust the latch as needed until the nipple extends into the comfort zone. With baby in control of the latch (Figure C.2), there's no need for the parent to manipulate its angle.

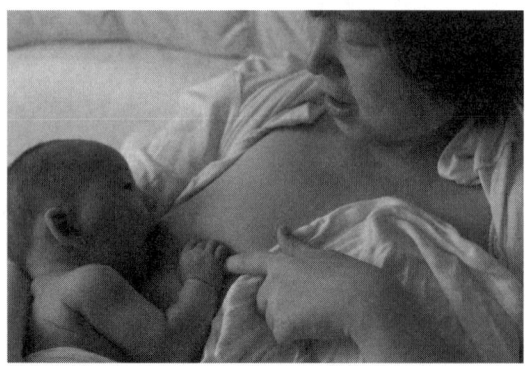

Figure C.2 Newborns can self-attach in starter positions, which simplifies early nursing.
©2021 Melanie Ham, used with permission.

During the early weeks after birth, in upright or side-lying positions, the newborn cannot self-attach as easily. Upright positions work well when baby is a little older and more coordinated, but at first, gravity pulls the newborn's body away from the nipple, so the parent must take charge of latching. During the early learning period, mastering upright or side-lying positions requires parents have normal dexterity and be able to remember many steps in the right order at a time when—due to the brain changes that occur during pregnancy and after birth—most have difficulty following instructions.

To achieve a deep latch in an upright position, suggest parents:

1. Start by aligning the baby's body so she is "nose to nipple," supporting the baby's shoulders and neck, so her head can tilt back slightly (the ***instinctive feeding position***, p. 2).

2. Make sure the baby's chin, torso, hips, legs, and feet are pulled in close with the baby's whole body touching the parent (no gaps between them).

3. Wait until the stimulation of the baby's chin and torso against the mammary gland triggers a wide-open mouth.

4. As the baby moves toward the nipple, apply gentle pressure on the baby's back and shoulders (avoid pushing on baby's head) to help her get onto the gland deeply and the nipple extend into the comfort zone.

Positioning baby nose to nipple makes an asymmetrical latch possible. During latch, if baby's lower jaw lands at the base of the nipple, a shallow latch is the result. Even when the nipple is centered in the baby's mouth, it is more difficult for it to stretch back far enough to reach the comfort zone. The baby who latches with her head tilted forward instead of slightly back is at the same disadvantage. When baby's head tilts forward, it also tilts the lower jaw (the working jaw) away from the mammary gland, resulting in a shallow latch.

MAMMARY SHAPING When a baby has trouble latching deeply, tissue-shaping techniques can sometimes make a deep latch easier. Breast sandwich and nipple tilting are two mammary-shaping techniques that can help some babies more easily take a larger mouthful of mammary tissue, which can make a huge difference, especially during the early learning period.

BREAST SANDWICH involves parents gently squeezing the mammary tissue near the areola (fingers on one side and thumb on the other) to narrow its shape and make it easier for the baby's lower jaw to land further onto the areola for a deep latch. This technique can be especially helpful for parents with firm mammary tissue, either naturally occurring or from engorgement or tissue swelling from excess IV fluids during labor. It can also be helpful during the newborn period for any nursing couple who is struggling with latch.

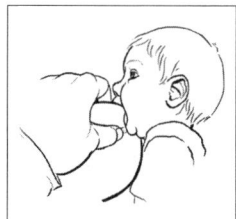

Figure C.3 The breast sandwich can help baby get a bigger mouthful and a deeper latch.
©2021, Nancy Mohrbacher Solutions, Inc.

For the breast sandwich technique to help, the oval of the compressed tissue must match the oval of the baby's mouth—wider at the corners and narrower between upper and lower lips (Figure C.3). If the directions of these two ovals do not align, mammary shaping can make latching more difficult. Two approaches can make this concept easier for parents to understand.

- **Hamburger, not taco.** Imagine taking a bite of a sandwich. First, we line it up horizontally in front of our mouth to make it easier to take a big bite. Think about how much harder it would be to take a bite if we rotated the sandwich 90°, so it was vertical rather than horizontal. Suggest when shaping the mammary tissue, the nursing parent think "hamburger," not "taco."

- **Finger moustache.** Whether parents' thumb or fingers are closest to baby's upper lip, think of them as the baby's "mustache." For the tissue and mouth ovals to align, the parents' thumb and fingers run parallel to the baby's lips.

When forming a breast sandwich, it's also important to keep fingers and thumb far enough back on the mammary tissue, so they don't get in baby's way as she latches.

NIPPLE TILTING is a shaping strategy that makes it easier for baby's lower working jaw to land further back on the areola for a deeper latch. Here's how this technique works.

- With the baby's body pulled in close to the parent and her chin touching the gland, parents press on the gland just above the nipple with a thumb or finger running parallel to the baby's upper lip. This causes the nipple to point up and away from the baby (Figure C.4).
- The touch of the gland on baby's chin triggers a wide-open mouth (gape).
- Parents then use the top thumb or finger to press into the gland and roll the underside of the areola into baby's wide-open mouth.
- As the areola enters the baby's mouth, parents can use the top finger or thumb to gently push the nipple inside the baby's upper gum before removing their finger.

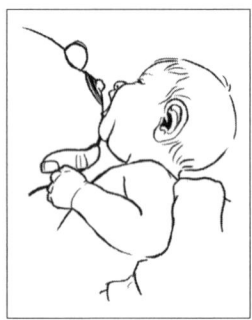

Figure C.4 Nipple tilting.
©2021, Nancy Mohrbacher Solutions, Inc.

APPENDIX D

MILK-EXPRESSION TECHNIQUES

HAND EXPRESSION is a useful skill every nursing parent should have. When storing milk for the baby, prepare to hand express by finding a relaxing setting, such as a private, comfortable area with good body support, and wash hands thoroughly with soap and warm water. Have on hand a clean collection container, either one with a wide mouth, such as a cup, or during pregnancy or the first days after birth—when milk volumes are small—a syringe or a clean spoon.

FINGER PLACEMENT Effective hand-expression techniques vary from person to person. What's most important is finding the "sweet spot" on the mammary glands for best milk flow. Using the areola as a guide can be misleading because of the large variation in areola size. Those with very large areolae may find their sweet spot within the areola and those with small areolae may find their sweet spot well away from it. During the early learning stages, apply small circle band-aids to these sweet spots to make finding them easier the next time. Use comfort and milk flow as a guide.

INSTRUCTIONS FOR HAND EXPRESSING vary by instructor. This technique combines several, including one from the World Health Organization:

1. Before expressing, spend some time gently massaging the glands with hands and fingertips, a soft baby brush, or a warm towel. This video demonstration shows possible massage techniques, including fingertip tapping: **bit.ly/ BA2-BolmanMassage**.

2. Sit up, leaning slightly forward to allow gravity to help with milk flow.

3. At the first expression, to find the sweet spot, start by putting thumb on top of the gland and fingers below about 1.5 inches (4 cm) from the nipple. Apply steady pressure into the gland toward the chest wall a few times. If no milk comes, shift finger and thumb placement farther away or closer to the nipple and compress again a few times. Repeat, moving finger and thumb until slightly firmer tissue is felt and pressure yields more milk. At future hand expressions, skip the "finding" phase and place fingers directly on this area.

4. Apply steady pressure into the gland toward the chest wall, not toward the nipple. The idea is to put pressure on areas of milk within the gland.

5. As this inward pressure is applied, compress the pads of the thumb and fingers together (pushing in, not pulling out toward

the nipple), finding a good rhythm of press-compress-relax, like a baby's sucking pattern.

6. Alternate sides every few minutes (5 or 6 times in total at each expression), rotating finger position, so that all areas of the mammary gland are expressed and feel soft, which usually takes about 20 to 30 minutes.

Avoid sliding the fingers along the skin. See a video demonstration of one version of this technique at **bit.ly/BA2-Stanford HandExpress**.

If parents feel pain or discomfort, they may be compressing too hard, sliding their fingers along the skin, or squeezing the nipple itself, which can be both ineffective and painful. Ask them to describe what they are doing to determine what changes will make expression more comfortable.

To hand-express milk while baby is nursing, some use pillows or cushions to support the baby's body, so they have both hands free. Some learn to hand-express milk from both sides simultaneously, with the right hand expressing the right side and the left hand expressing the left side, with collection containers on a stable surface just below nipple level.

HAND-EXPRESSING DURING PREGNANCY Learning to express milk during the last month of an uncomplicated pregnancy is safe and recommended. If the pregnant parent's healthcare provider considers it safe to have sex (which releases the same hormones as milk expression), then it is also safe to express milk.

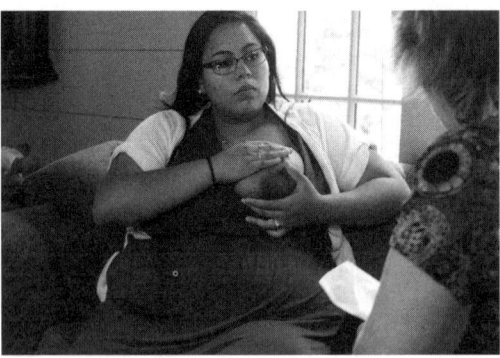

Figure D.1 After warming her breast, this pregnant mother uses massage to help stimulate milk flow before hand expressing.

Around the 36th or 37th week of pregnancy is a good time to begin. Start by warming the mammary glands. If the milk is not going to be collected and stored, expressing in the shower or bath may be a good start. If the plan is to collect and store the colostrum, expressing after a shower or bath may make the process easier. After warming the glands, use massage (Figure D.1) to stimulate the release of oxytocin, which triggers milk flow. Then follow the instructions for hand expression in the previous section. If any pain or discomfort is felt, suggest stopping and evaluating what needs to change. Ideally, hand expression should always be done gently enough to feel comfortable.

If the plan is to collect and store the expressed colostrum, the drops can be sucked up into a syringe or collected in a small, clean cup (Figure D.2) or vial. Plan to hand-express milk from both sides for about 5 minutes per side. Some parents do this just once each day. Others do it more often, depending on the situation. The collected colostrum can be stored in the refrigerator between collections. If a syringe is used, avoid overfilling it to allow room for expansion during freezing. Once the syringe is full enough, put on the cap and freeze. If the colostrum will be used to supplement the newborn during the first days after birth, plan to freeze it in volumes of no larger than 10 to 20 mL, (0.3 to 0.5 oz.).

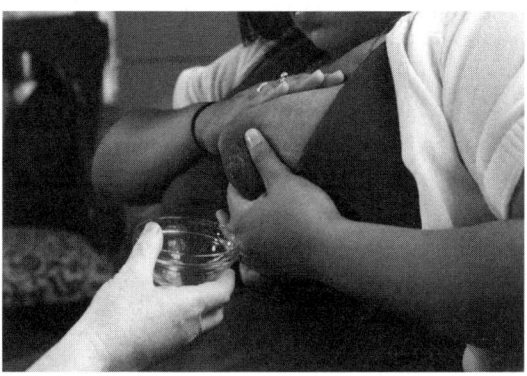

Figure D.2 Depending on the volume of colostrum expressed, it may be collected in a small cup, vial, or syringe.

BREAST PUMP SUCTION, SPEED, AND FIT When parents start pumping, most are unsure about how to use the pump's suction and speed controls to their best advantage. Some guidance can shorten their learning curve for better milk yields more quickly.

SETTING THE PUMP'S SUCTION/VACUUM Many mistakenly assume "more is better" when it comes to pump suction. But expressing milk with a breast pump is not like sucking a drink through a straw. For the highest milk yields, milk ejections are necessary. When suction levels are so high as to be uncomfortable, this may actually inhibit milk ejection, resulting in less milk expressed. When starting to pump, set its suction to the highest level that is truly comfortable, both during and after pumping. Unlike many other medical devices, the best setting will vary from person to person. For some, it may be at the highest suction setting and for others, it may be at the lowest, or anywhere in between.

To find the highest comfortable suction level, suggest parents:

- Turn up the pump suction until they feel a slight discomfort.
- Then turn down the suction slowly, just until it feels completely comfortable.

Avoid starting at a low suction setting and gradually increasing it throughout the pump session. Instead, increase milk yields by 33% by setting pump suction to its highest comfortable setting before the first milk ejection, which occurs on average about 2 minutes into the pump session.

SETTING THE PUMP'S CYCLES/SPEED The term **cycles per minute** (or **cpm**) refers to the number of times each minute the pump's suction builds, peaks, and releases. For comfort and effectiveness, pumps need to generate a cycle speed of at least 30 to 60 cpm. Slower speeds—which involve a longer pull on the tissue—can cause discomfort and even skin damage.

Many pump brands and models now use what some call 2-phase pumping. These pumps automatically start at the high-speed setting of about 120 cpm. After 2 minutes, they automatically shift to a slower speed. This is supposed to mimic a nursing baby's suck, which is faster at first to trigger a milk ejection and then slower to drain the milk faster. If parents use a pump with this feature, encourage them to press its "let-down" button as soon as their milk flow begins. If the first milk ejection occurs before 2 minutes, staying longer at the fast 120 cpm may reduce milk yield. Most users express no milk at all during this very fast first phase. Taking maximum advantage of that first milk ejection—when the most milk is expressed—is key to higher milk yields.

If the pump has separate suction and speed controls, encourage parents to experiment and use whatever settings produce the best results. As a starting point, suggest they:

- Start pumping at the fastest speed
- When milk flow starts, turn it down to a slow speed.
- As milk flow slows, return to a fast speed to more quickly trigger the next milk ejection.
- Repeat, alternating between fast and slow speeds (like a nursing baby) for the fastest and highest milk yields

GETTING A GOOD PUMP FIT is vital, especially for parents who pump often and whose pump's nipple tunnel is made of rigid plastic. Pump fit affects both nipple comfort and milk flow. A poor fit can lead to pain, skin trauma, and less milk expressed.

Pump fit is based on how well parents' nipples fit into the pump's **nipple tunnel** (Figure D.3), the opening the mammary gland is drawn into during pumping. Pump manufacturers call this pump part by different names (flange, breastshield). Parents often refer to it as the "horn" or "funnel."

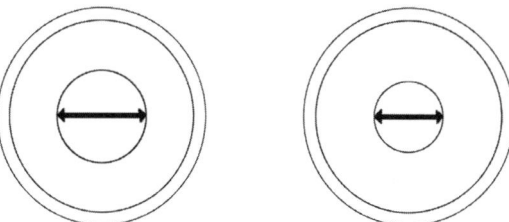

Figure D.3 Pump nipple tunnels come in different diameters.
©2021 Nancy Mohrbacher Solutions, Inc.

Nipple tunnel diameter varies slightly by brand, with 24 or 25 mm the standard size of many pumps. A different size nipple tunnel may be needed if parents feel pain or discomfort while pumping on or near the lowest suction setting. Because nipple sizes can vary, some parents get better results by using one size on one side and another size on the other side.

If pumping is comfortable with good milk flow, parents probably have a good fit. If in doubt, suggest parents compare what they see while pumping with the line drawing at this link **bit.ly/BA2-PumpFit**. Depending on the pump brand, larger or smaller nipple tunnels may be available to purchase separately.

How common is the need for larger or smaller nipple tunnels? Depending on the pump brand, between about 25% and 50% of users benefit from using a size other than standard. Keep in mind, too, that regular pumping increases nipple size, so pump fit may change over time.

Here are signs parents may need a larger or smaller nipple tunnel.

Suggest a larger nipple tunnel if parents report:

- Discomfort, even on low suction settings
- Nipple rubs along the tunnel, despite efforts to center it
- Nipple blanches, or turns white
- Nipple does not move freely in the nipple tunnel
- Slow milk flow or less milk expressed than expected

Suggest a smaller nipple tunnel if parents report:

- Discomfort, even on low suction settings.
- More than about 1/8 inch (3 mm) of the areola is pulled into the nipple tunnel
- Nipple bounces in and out of the tunnel
- Difficulty maintaining an air seal

APPENDIX E

NIPPLE SHIELDS

Unlike hard plastic breast shells, flexible silicone nipple shields are worn over the nipple during nursing, with the baby getting milk through holes in the tip. Most consist of a thin ***brim*** that covers all or part of the areola and a firmer, protruding ***tip*** that fits over the nipple. Like any tool, nipple shields can be used appropriately or misused. In some situations, nipple shields can support and preserve direct nursing, while in others, they can undermine it.

INDICATIONS FOR USE Nipple shields are used most often to overcome latching struggles due to engorgement, infant anatomy issues, flat/inverted nipples, birth trauma, oral aversion, or the use of feeding bottles. Many parents use nipple shields to reduce nipple pain, but they do not address the root cause of the pain, and there are other, better strategies (p. 221).

Nipple shields may also improve nursing effectiveness in babies with a weak or uncoordinated suck, due to tongue-tie, recessed or receding jaw, cleft palate, high, bubble, or grooved palate, prematurity, or airway abnormality. In babies with high or low muscle tone, the firm tip of the shield may push past baby's tongue to reach the area that triggers active sucking.

DISADVANTAGES OF NIPPLE SHIELDS It is currently unknown if nipple shields negatively impact milk production and infant weight gain. Their use complicates direct nursing, and they are often difficult to wean from. For these reasons, nipple shields are almost never a good first strategy. Whenever possible, solve a nursing problem by improving feeding dynamics.

IS IT NECESSARY TO PUMP AFTER NURSING? More research is needed. But there is cause for concern about the effect of nipple-shield use on milk production, because it reduces the sensation of nursing. Each situation needs to be considered individually. It makes sense to express milk after nursing with a shield post-delivery to support early milk increase, when milk production is low, or if parents are unsure about whether milk transfer with the shield is effective. Regular weight checks are recommended until it is clear that regular milk expression is not needed. Pumping after nursing might not be needed if the baby transfers milk well with the nipple shield. In this case, watch the baby's energy levels, diaper output, and signs of satiety after feeds. If the baby is sleepy, has scant diaper output during the early weeks, or seems unsettled, pumping after feeds may be wise.

FOLLOW-UP IS VITAL Sending nursing parents home from the hospital with a nipple shield without scheduled follow-up is a recipe for failure. When nipple shields are used, the nursing couple needs to be seen regularly to make sure the baby is feeding effectively and the family has the support they need to meet their nursing goals. If a hospital does not offer outpatient help for nursing families, they can instead provide referrals to local lactation specialists who can see families shortly after discharge, so that they can be evaluated and assisted in weaning from the shield.

NIPPLE SHIELD STYLES, SHAPES, AND SIZES If a nipple shield is not the right size or shape for a nursing couple, it may not be an effective tool. These are some options.

REGULAR OR CONTACT STYLE The two basic nipple shield styles are both made of ultra-thin silicone and have a firm, protruding tip surrounded by a soft brim that lays flat on the areola. The **regular** nipple shield has a completely circular brim and is preferred by some because in some cases, it stays in place more securely during feeds. The **contact** nipple shield has a cutout area on its brim that can be positioned for skin-to-skin contact with the baby's nose or chin. Some prefer this second style because of this increased skin-to-skin contact and because aligning the cutout with the baby's nose prevents the shield brim from bending back into baby's face during nursing. It also allows the baby to smell the parent's skin during feeds. Because the anatomies and preferences of parents and helpers vary, one option is to start with one of each style and see which works better.

NIPPLE SHIELD SHAPES vary by brand. The most common shapes are conical and cherry-shaped. As with the other variations, some babies respond better to one shape than another.

NIPPLE SHIELD SIZES The size measurement listed on many packages is the diameter of the tip opening. The length of the nipple shield tip varies very little among brands. A nipple shield will only be an effective tool if it is a good fit for both parent and baby. If the shield is too large for the baby, it can cause gagging (which can lead to feeding aversion), and if his jaws close on its tip rather than its soft brim, it can prevent effective milk transfer. A too-small shield may fail to stimulate baby to suck actively because it doesn't extend deep enough into his mouth.

Some lactation specialists fit nipple shields primarily to the parent, some to the baby, and some to a mix of both. When fitting a shield to the baby, many recommend the narrower tip openings (16 mm and 20 mm) for preterm babies and newborns. Those with wider tip openings (24 mm) are most often chosen for term or older/larger babies.

But the size of the baby is unrelated to the width of his parent's nipple, which means the nipple shield that is a good fit for a baby may not be a good fit for the parent, and vice versa. The parent's nipples may not fit comfortably into the shield tip (which can slow milk flow like a too-small breast-pump nipple tunnel) and the shield that fits the parent may not fit comfortably in the baby's mouth. In this case, a nipple shield will not be a helpful tool.

APPLYING A NIPPLE SHIELD can be done in different ways. Some simply center the nipple inside the tip and place the shield on the mammary gland. Using this method, to keep the shield in place during nursing, the parent places a thumb on one side of the brim's border and fingers on the other side. The following application method draws the nipple farther into the tip, reducing the suction baby needs to generate and making it easier to keep the shield in place:

1. Turn most of the shield tip inside out.
2. Place the shield tip over the nipple.
3. When the shield is slowly turned right side out and smoothed into place, the nipple is drawn into the tip.

Other ways to keep a nipple shield in place during nursing include running hot or warm water over it before putting it on or applying a small amount of USP-modified lanolin to the inside borders of the brim to help it stick to the skin.

LATCH DYNAMICS WITH A NIPPLE SHIELD In addition to a well-fitted shield and its effective application, parents need to be sure the baby latches deeply to the shield for effective nursing. If the baby's jaws close on the shield's tip instead of its brim, the shield is less likely to trigger active sucking. A shallow latch with a nipple shield can also be painful, as the nipple is compressed in the tip. Just like when latching without the shield, the baby needs to open wide and latch deeply. If parents can see any part of the firmer tip of the shield while the baby nurses, suggest unlatching the baby and trying again, making sure his mouth is open very wide as he latches.

ASSESSING FEEDING EFFECTIVENESS WITH THE NIPPLE SHIELD After the first feeds with the nipple shield, suggest looking for signs of effective feeding, such as milk in the tip of the shield and a decrease in mammary fullness. The baby's behavior can also provide clues. A satisfied baby will release the nipple when he's full. He may rest his head on the gland or be quietly alert, hands relaxed and not immediately fuss when laid down. As a precaution, arrange for baby's weight to be checked after a day or two on the shield and weekly after that to be sure he is getting enough milk and is stimulating adequate milk production.

WEANING FROM THE NIPPLE SHIELD is influenced by several variables.

WHEN TO WEAN FROM THE NIPPLE SHIELD will depend largely on the reason it was used. For example, if it is used to help a baby who was bottle-feeding recognize the mammary gland as a source of milk, it may only be useful at one feed. But if they were struggling with nursing for some time and the baby associates the parent's chest with frustration, a longer time of easier nursing to build positive associations may be better. The preterm baby using the nipple shield to improve milk intake may need to mature for several weeks before he can feed well without the shield.

HOW TO WEAN FROM THE NIPPLE SHIELD depends in part on the situation. A baby may need the shield for one feed, a few feeds, a few days, a few weeks, or rarely, a few months. It was once recommended to gradually cut off more and more of its tip until it was gone. But this strategy is not recommended for the ultra-thin silicone shields used today, because when they're cut, this creates rough edges that can irritate the baby's mouth. So what to do instead? Suggest starting nursing with the shield on. After milk ejection (listen for swallowing), try removing the shield quickly, allowing baby to latch immediately. If baby latches, use this strategy whenever needed to move from shield to bare nipple. Usually, as baby becomes more coordinated, the shield will be needed at fewer and fewer feeds.

If this strategy doesn't work, suggest parents continue using the shield throughout the feed and try again a few days later, when parent and baby are feeling relaxed and the baby is not too hungry. Suggest avoiding the stress of trying to nurse without the shield at every feed. Encourage parents to use the shield as long as it helps the baby nurse. With more practice and more positive associations with direct nursing, the easier weaning from the shield will be. If the baby is unable/unwilling to nurse without the shield, the problem that caused the nipple shield to be needed may not yet be fully resolved. Follow the baby's cues, but keep trying to nurse without the shield every few days.

APPENDIX F

REVERSE PRESSURE SOFTENING (RPS)

Developed by U.S. lactation consultant and nurse Jean Cotterman, reverse pressure softening (RPS) can help any time a nursing parent's areola is so firm that latching or milk expression is challenging. This technique is used most often during the early days after birth when the mammary glands become swollen from excess IV fluids given during labor or when a nursing parent becomes engorged (p. 27). RPS can also be used at any stage of lactation to trigger milk ejection before expressing milk or whenever the glands are so full that the areola needs to be softened.

Reverse pressure softening involves applying gentle pressure to the areola to soften it by moving the swelling (edema) farther back into the mammary tissue. With the areola soft and the swelling out of the way, the baby can latch deeper and nursing parents have easier access to their milk during milk expression.

REVERSE PRESSURE SOFTENING FOR HELPERS

Developed by K. Jean Cotterman, RNC-E, IBCLC

Try this if pain, swelling, or fullness creates problems during the early weeks of learning to nurse.

The key is making the areola *very soft* right around the base of the nipple for better latching.

- A softer areola protects the nipple deep in baby's mouth, helping his tongue remove milk better.
- Parents say curved fingers work best (Fig. F.1 or F.2).
- Press inward toward the chest wall and *count slowly to 50*.
- Pressure should be *steady and firm*, and *gentle enough to avoid pain*.
- If desired, someone other than the nursing parent may help, using thumbs (Fig. F.5).
- For long fingernails, try another way shown below (Fig. F.4, F.5, or F.6).
- If glands are quite large or *very* swollen, count *very* slowly, with parents *lying down on their back*.
- This delays return of swelling to the areola, giving more time to latch.
- Soften the areola *right before each feeding* (or pumping) till swelling goes away.

- For some, this takes 2-4 days.
- Make any pumping sessions short, with pauses to re-soften the areola if needed.
- Use medium or low vacuum, to reduce the return of swelling into the areola.

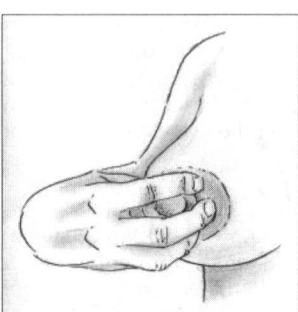

Figure F.1

One-handed "flower hold:" Fingernails short, fingertips curved, placed where baby's tongue will go.

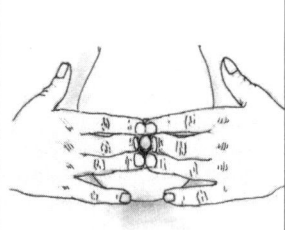

Figure F.2

Two-handed, one-step method: Fingernails short, fingertips curved, each one touching the sides of the nipple.

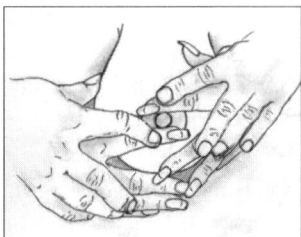

Figure F.3

You may ask someone to help press by placing fingers or thumbs on top of yours.

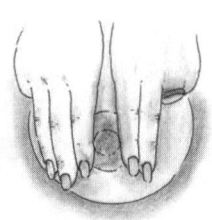

Figure F.4

Two-step method, two hands: Using 2 or 3 straight fingers each side, first knuckles touching nipple, move 1/4 turn, repeat above and below nipple.

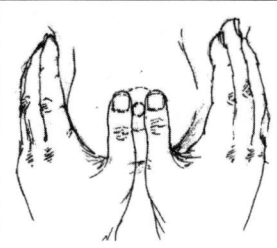

Figure F.5

Two-step method, two hands: Using straight thumbs, base of thumbnail at side of nipple, move 1/4 turn, repeat, thumb above and below nipple.

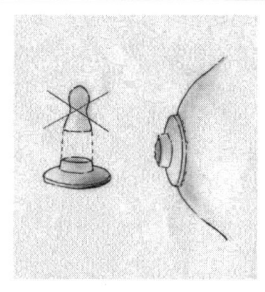

Figure F.6

Soft-ring method: Cut off bottom half of an artificial nipple to place on areola to press with fingers.

INDEX

Note: b. indicates box; f. indicates figure; t. indicates table

A

abscess, 33–34
acid (drug, aka LSD), 247–248
adjustments to starter positions
    baby, 8–9, 9f.
    body, 7–8, 7f., 8f.
    breast, 9, 10f.
adoptive parents, 276–277. *see also* induced lactation
AIDS, 142. *see also* HIV
airway abnormalities, 60, 111–112
alcohol consumption during lactation, 186, 243, 264
alertness, 3
allergies, 65, 117, 118
allodynia, 35–36
all-purpose nipple ointment (APNO), 224
alveoli, 179
anesthesia, 162
angel dust, 247–248
anorexia nervosa, 240
antibiotics, 29, 31, 32, 33
antidepressants, 149
areola, 180
Assessment Tool for Lingual Frenulum Function (ATLFF), 102
asymptomatic tongue-tie, 101. *see also* tongue-tie
at-breast supplementers. *see* nursing supplementers

B

baby blues. *see* postpartum depression
bait and switch strategy, 73, 267
bed-sharing, 25–26
Bilicam app, 173
bilirubin, 170. *see also* bilirubin levels; jaundice
bilirubin encephalopathy, 172
bilirubin levels
    dangers of high, 171–172
    monitoring, 172–173
    nursing and, 170
Bili-ruler, 173
biopsies, 38
birth practices
    and early nursing, 17
    and low milk production, 193
    and non-latching, 70–71
    and slow weight gain, 302
biting, 223–224
blebs, 32, 231–232
blisters, 32, 231–232
block feeding
    full drainage and (FDBF), 203–204
    modified, 204, 204t.
    one side per feed, 203
blood, in milk, 39, 225
blood sugar. *see* diabetes; hypoglycemia
bone health, 239
bottle-feeding
    bait and switch strategy, 73, 267
    and cleft palate, 109–110
    introducing, 93
    and milk expression volumes, 208
    and nursing reinforcement, 200
    paced, 312–313, 313f.
    preterm babies, 267
    pros and cons, 311t.
    strategies, 94
    transitioning to nursing, 278
breast augmentation, 46–48
breast cancer. *see* cancer
breast compression, 309–310
breast crawl, 1, 18t.
breast development
    extra nipples/glands, 40–41
    gestational gigantomastia, 42–43
    insufficient glandular tissue (IGT), 41–42
breast infection, 29
breast pumps. *see* pumps and pumping

breast reduction, 48–49
breast shaping, see mammary shaping
breast shells, 28, 224, 233
breast-binding, 294
breast/chest injuries, 43–44, 50, 182
breast/chest surgery
    abscess, 33
    augmentation, 46–48
    basics, 44–45
    deep breast pain, 36
    lift/mastopexy, 46
    milk production, 43–44, 182
    reduction, 48–49
    and slow weight gain in baby, 302
    supplementation, 45–46
    top surgery, 49–50, 191
breastfeeding self-efficacy (BSE), 3
bright light therapy, 149
Bristol Tongue Assessment Tool (BTAT), 102
bromocriptine, 294
bubble palate, 104–105
buccal-ties, 104
bulimia nervosa, 240

C

cabergoline, 205
caffeine, 239
calcifications, 38
calcium, 239
cancer, 37, 145–147
Candida albicans, 66, 226
cannabis use, 186, 245–246
carbohydrates, in human milk, 122
cardiac issues
    baby, 118–120
    parent, 147
carpal tunnel syndrome, 163
CAT scans, 38
cervical caps, 77
cesarean birth
    early nursing interventions, 17
    pain, 60
    positioning, 8, 14
challenges, nursing
    after the early weeks, 63–64, 63b.
    early weeks, 54–56, 55b., 57b.
    non-latching, 70–71
    one-sided nursing, 68–70
cheeks, baby, 104
chemotherapy, 146
chest. see breast/chest entries
chestfeeding, 191, 281
chickenpox, 140
child care, 94
chocolate, 239
cholecystokinin (CCK), 202
chronic conditions, in baby
    allergies, 118
    cardiac issues, 118–120
    cystic fibrosis, 120–121
    diabetes, 121–122
    Down syndrome, 122–124
    galactosemia, 124–125
    neurological impairments, 126–130
    PKU (phenylketonuria), 124, 125–126
chronic conditions, in parent
    cystic fibrosis, 151–152
    diabetes mellitus type 1, 152–153
    galactosemia, 154
    gestational diabetes, 153–154
    lupus, 156–157
    multiple sclerosis (MS), 155
    PKU (phenylketonuria), 154
    polycystic ovary syndrome (PCOS), 155–156
    rheumatoid arthritis, 156–157
    thyroid disease, 157–160
    type 2 diabetes, 153
circumcision, 58
cleft lip, 105–106
cleft palate, 14, 105, 106–110
clothing, work, 96–97
clustering feeds, 20, 301
cocaine, 247
coconut oil, 225
cold sores, 140–141, 229
colds
    baby, 112–113
    parent, 137
colic, 65
colic hold, 127, 127f.
color
    colostrum, 39, 188
    expressed milk, 39, 218
    jaundiced skin, 172

colostrum
  color, 188
  expressing, 28, 44, 50, 107, 152, 211, 325, 325f.
  intake amounts, 18
  and nursing during pregnancy, 252
  spoon-feeding, 28, 44, 168
  storing, 152, 325
condoms, 77
congenital heart disease (CHD), baby, 118–120
congestion
  baby, 65, 112–113
  parent, 137
contraception
  barrier methods, 77
  cultural and religious values, 76–77
  emergency, 82
  estrogen-containing methods, 81–82, 205
  hormonal, 79–82
  intrauterine devices (IUDs), 78
  lactation amenorrhea method (LAM), 77
  long-acting reversible (LARC), 80
  natural family planning methods, 77–78
  progestin-only methods, 79–81
co-nursing, 190–191, 252, 280–282. see also induced lactation
coughing, 60, 62, 64, 67
COVID-19, 137–138
cow's milk, 117
cultural beliefs and practices
  contraception, 76–77
  feeding and sleeping schedules, 21
  milk production, 275–276
  obesity, 240–241
  weaning, 289
cup feeding, 312t., 313–314, 313f.
curcumin, 31
cystic fibrosis
  baby, 120–121
  parent, 151–152
cysts, ovarian, 154–156
cytologic studies, 38
cytomegalovirus (CMV), 141, 263–264

D

dairy elimination, 238–239
Dancer Hand position, 108, 109f.
deep breast pain, 35–37
dehydration, infant, 303
depression, postpartum, 147–149
dextrose gel, 169
diabetes
  baby, 121–122
  gestational, 153–154
  type 1, 152–153
  type 2, 153
diagnostic tests
  abscess, 33
  breast lumps, 38
  cancer, 145–146
  hyperthyroidism, 159–160
  hypothyroidism, 158–159
  intraductal papilloma, 39
  postpartum thyroiditis, 158
diaper output, 45, 53–54, 300. see also stools
diaphragms, 77
diarrhea, 113–115
diet and nutrition
  basics, 237
  milk composition, 188–189
  milk production, 184, 199
  nursing during pregnancy, 251–252
  with preterm babies, 264
  reactions to foods in parent's diet, 237–239
  supplements, 237, 284–287
  vegetarian/vegan diets, 239
  weight and weight loss, 239–242
disabilities. see physical limitations
distractibility, infant, 66
domperidone, 197, 198
donor milk, 219–220, 262
Down syndrome, 122–124
dry nursing, 191, 281
Duarte galactosemia, 125
ducts and ductules
  anatomy, 179
  ductal candidiasis, 37
  ectasia, 36, 40
  intraductal papilloma, 39
  lactiferous duct infection, 35, 36

mastitis, 29
milk production, 182
positioning for plugged, 14–15
dummies, 23
dynamics, nursing. *see also* positioning
basics, 3–5
and low milk production, 193–194
and nipple pain, 45
and slow weight gain, 299, 301–304
dysphagia, 129
dysphoric milk ejection reflex (D-MER), 181

E

ear infections, infant, 112–113
eating disorders, parent, 240
e-cigarettes, 245
ecstasy, 247–248
eczema, 229–230
edema, 27
ejection. *see* milk ejection
emergencies and natural disasters
formula-feeding risks, 83, 85–87
optimal practices, 83–85
emergency contraception, 82
employment
access to baby, 96
milk expression strategies, 90–93, 97–99
parental leave priorities, 89–90
returning to work, 89, 96–97
work schedules, 94–95
worksite lactation support, 95–96
engorgement
areolar, 27
breast/chest surgery, 44–45
deep breast pain, 35
peripheral, 27
strategies, 28
swelling, 27, 61
treatment, 28–29
vascular, 39
environment, nursing
during hospitalization, 132
and milk expression, 210
and nursing strikes, 72
preterm babies, 257–258
epilepsy, 163–164
establishing nursing
challenges, 55–56, 55b., 57b.
during first 2 hours after birth, 18, 18t.
during first 40 days after birth, 20–21
rooming-in, 19
strategies, 72–74
estrogen, 79, 81–82, 205
exercise, 149, 242
expression. *see* milk expression

F

face masks, 135, 138
failure to thrive, 299
family planning. *see* contraception
fat-soluble vitamins, 286
feedback inhibitor of lactation (FIL), 185, 203
feeding behaviors
alertness, 3
breast crawl, 1, 18t.
ending feeds, 15–16
primitive neonatal reflexes (PNRs), 1
rooting, 1–2
sucking, 1–2
swallowing, 2
triggers, 2
feeding methods. *see also* bottle-feeding; supplementation systems
and cleft palate, 109
comparison chart, 311t.–312t.
cups, 312t., 313–314, 313f.
finger-feeding, 312t.
and high/low tone, 129–130
nursing supplementers, 46, 200, 311t., 315–318
preterm babies, 264
for slow weight gain, 304
spoon feeding, 313, 314, 314f.
spoons, 312t.
syringes, 312t., 314
feeding patterns, 22
feeding schedules, 21
feeding-tube devices. *see* nursing supplementers

fenugreek, 198
fertility, 75–76. *see also* contraception
fever, from engorgement, 27
finger-feeding
    basics, 314–315
    pros and cons, 312t.
    for short/recessed jaw, 111
"finish the first side first," 301, 304
flat nipples, 61, 232, 233–234
flu
    baby, 112–113
    parent, 137–138
fluids, 237
fluoride supplements, 285
food intolerances, baby, 65, 118
food poisoning, 135–136
foremilk, 22
formula-feeding. *see also* bottle-feeding; supplementation
    emergencies and natural disasters, 83, 85–87
    intake amounts, 23
    jaundice, 174–175
    night feeds, 24
    with nursing supplementers, 316
    during phototherapy, 177
    preterm babies, 262
fortified milk, 262–263
fractionated milk, 120
frenotomy, 103
frequency days, 21, 188
"full glands make milk slower" dynamic, 203

G

galactoceles, 36, 38
galactogogues, 196–199, 274
galactorrhea, 200
galactosemia
    baby, 124–125
    parent, 154
gas, 201, 237–238
gasping, 64
gastroesophageal reflux disease (GERD), 64, 65, 112, 116–117
gender dysphoria, 49, 191
genital herpes, 140–141, 229
gentian violet, 227, 228
German measles, 144
gestational ovarian theca lutein cysts, 154–155

glands. *see* mammary glands
Goldfarb, Lenore, 275
group B streptococcus (GBS), 136, 199
growth. *see also* weight gain, baby
    after 12 months, 298
    birth to 12 months, 297–298
growth charts, 53, 298
growth spurts, 21, 188
gulping, 62

H

hair care products, 242
hallucinogenic drugs, 247–248
headaches, 160
health issues. *see* chronic conditions, in baby; chronic conditions, in parent; illnesses, in baby; illnesses, in parent
hepatitis A, B, C, D, E, G, 138–139
herbal remedies
    anti-galactogogues, 204–205, 295
    depression, treatment, 149, 159
    galactogogues, 198–199
herbal teas, 239, 295
herpes viruses, 140–142, 229
hindmilk, 22
hip dysplasia, 58
HIV
    mastitis, and, 29
    parent, 142–143
homeopathic remedies, 205
hormones
    estrogen, 79, 81–82, 183
    for induced lactation, 275
    milk production, 182–184, 184t., 195t.
    and obesity, 240–241
    oxytocin, 1, 3, 8, 73, 75, 180, 325
    progesterone, 79, 183
    prolactin, 183–184, 184t.
    testosterone, 49, 154–155, 156, 191
hospitalization. *see also* preterm babies
    of baby, 130–132
    of parent, 160–161
    postpartum psychosis, 150
    and stored milk, 218, 219
HTLV-1, 143
hydration

"drinking to thirst," 237
vomiting, 115–116
hypersensitivity, 65, 118
hypertension, parent, 147
hyperthyroidism, parent, 159–160
hypoglycemia, newborn, 167–169, 169t.
hypothyroidism, parent, 158–159
hysterectomies, 77

I

illnesses, in baby. *see also* chronic conditions, in baby
   colds/flu/congestion, 112–113
   ear infections, 112–113
   gastrointestinal, 113–117
illnesses, in parent. *see also* chronic conditions, in parent
   bacterial, 135–137
   cancer, 145–147
   cardiac issues, 147
   mental health, 147–151
   and preterm babies, 264
   and slow weight gain in baby, 302, 303
   viral infections, 137–145
imaging scans, 38
immunizations, 283
impetigo, 226
induced lactation
   considerations, 272
   defined, 271
   goals, 271–272
   milk production strategies, 272–276
   physical and emotional changes, 276
   protocols, 274–275
   transitioning to nursing, 276–278
ineffective nursing, 59
Infant Sleep Info app, 25
infections
   bacterial, 135–137, 226
   ear, 112–113
   fungal, 6, 37, 226–229
   preventing, 225
   viral, 112–113, 137–145, 229
inflammation, 148
influenza. *see* flu
injuries. *see* breast/chest injuries
instinctive feeding position, 2, 320
intake volumes
   by age, 54t., 208t., 305t.
   calculating, 122
   colostrum, 18
   first 40 days after birth, 20–21, 188
   first days after birth, 18–19, 187
   low, 58
   measuring, 300–301
   1 to 6 months, 22–23
   preterm babies, 266
   relactation/induced lactation, 278–280
intrauterine devices (IUDs), 78
inverted nipples, 61, 232–234
involution, after weaning, 189
iron supplements, 285, 286

J

jaundice
   bilirubin levels, 170–173
   causes of, 170
   exchange transfusions, 177–178, 177t.
   formula-feeding and, 174–175
   hepatitis A, 138
   medications, 178
   nursing and, 170, 173–174
   pathological, 170–171
   phototherapy, 175–177, 176t.
   physiological, 170
   prolonged, 171
   sleepiness, 57
   treatments to avoid, 178
jaw, 110–111

K

kangaroo care. *see* skin-to-skin contact (SSC)
kernicterus, 172

L

lactation aid, 315
lactation amenorrhea method (LAM), 77
lactation help and support
   approaches to, 3–5

breast/chest surgery, 44
emergencies and natural disasters, 83–85
labor medications, 17
worksite, 95–96
lactation inhibitors, 186
lactogenesis I, 183
lactogenesis II, 183
lactose intolerance, 114–115
lanolin, 224
laryngomalacia, 60, 111
latch
    asymmetrical, 11, 12, 319–321, 319f.
    baby-driven approach, 128
    challenges, 68
    "comfort zone," 319
    depth, 2, 11, 319–321
    nipple shields and, 331
    non-latching, 70–71
    and nursing supplementers, 317
    one-sided, 68–70
    reverse pressure softening (RPS), 28, 333–334, 334f.
    and slow weight gain, 301, 302
lecithin, 33
LGBTQ nursing, 190–191, 280–282
lip flanging, 103
lip-ties, 103–104
lobes and lobules, 179
long-chain omega-3 fatty acids, 149
LSD, 247–248
lumps
    breast, 37–38
    mastitis, 30
lupus, 156–157
Lyme disease, 136

M

magic number, 98
Making More Milk (Marasco & West), 199
male lactation, 281
malnutrition, 240
malunggay, 198–199
mammary dysbiosis, 30, 35, 36
mammary glands
    anatomy, 179–180
    deep breast pain, 37
    engorgement, 27
    extra, 40–41
    fibrocystic changes, 38, 39
    firmness, 68
    hyperplastic, 182
    hypoplastic, 182
    insufficient glandular tissue (IGT), 41–42
    large, 62
    mastitis, 29–30
mammary shaping
    basics, 9, 10f., 13
    breast sandwich, 321–322, 321f.
    flat/inverted nipples, 234
    nipple tilting, 322, 322f.
mammograms, 38
mastitis
    abscesses, 33–34
    basics, 29
    causes, 29–30
    recurring, 32–33
    symptoms, 30
    treatment, 30–31, 33
    weaning, 31–32
maternity leave. *see* employment
measles, 143–144
medications
    antibiotics, 29, 31, 32, 33
    antidepressants, 149
    anti-galactogogues, 205
    labor, 17
    lactation inhibitors, 186
    parent's use of, with preterm babies, 264
    sleepiness, 57
    thrush, 225–228
menstruation, 67, 75–76
mental health
    postpartum depression, 147–149
    postpartum psychosis, 149–150
    sexual abuse and childhood trauma, 150–151
    substance use disorder (SUD), 248–249
    weaning, 295
metabolic syndrome, 153
metformin, 156, 198
methamphetamine, 247
methicillin-resistant Staphylococcus aureus (MRSA)

abscesses, 34
mastitis, 30
nursing and, 136–137
metoclopramide, 197–198
micrognathia, 111
migraines, 160
milk composition, 188–189
milk ejection
    basics, 180–181
    breast/chest surgery, 45
    challenges, 55–56, 64
    deep breast pain, 35
    delayed, 181
    dysphoric milk ejection reflex (D-MER), 181
    during milk expression, 209–210, 209t.
    preterm babies, 259
    triggering, 209–210
milk expression. *see also* milk storage; pumps and pumping
    after radioactive procedures, 146–147
    basics, 207
    to boost yields, 211–212
    engorgement, 28
    flat/inverted nipples, 234
    by hand, 210–211, 323–324
    induced lactation, 273–274
    milk ejection during, 209–210, 209t.
    during pregnancy, 324–325, 324f.
    for preterm babies, 255, 261, 263
    to protect production, 54
    returning to work strategies, 90–93, 97–99
    volumes, 207–209, 209t.
    as a weaning comfort measure, 294
milk flow
    and airway abnormalities, 111–112
    fast, 62, 67, 68–69, 201–202
    for high/low tone, 129
    positioning, 56
    slow, 62
    through nursing supplementers, 317–318
milk production
    autocrine control, 20
    basics, 181–185, 184t.
    birthing parent's, 281–282
    breast/chest injuries, 50
    breast/chest surgery, 43–44, 45–46
    cultural beliefs and practices, 275–276
    decreasing, 203–205
    emergencies and natural disasters, 84
    engorgement, 28
    exclusive pumping, 213–216
    expressing to protect, 54
    first 40 days after birth, 20–21
    first days after birth, 19, 20
    galactogogues, 196–199, 274
    increasing, 193–194, 196
    induced lactation, 272–276
    insufficient glandular tissue (IGT), 41
    lactation inhibitors, 186
    LGBTQ nursing, 190–191
    low, 62, 191–193, 195t.
    magic number, 98
    mastitis, 30
    milk removal and, 184–185, 187
    misconceptions about, 186–187
    for multiples, 189–190
    nipple shields and, 329
    norms, 187–189
    overabundant, 62, 67, 200–205
    pacifier/dummy use, 23
    physical and emotional changes, 276
    during pregnancy, 252
    preterm babies and, 262
    pumping and, 90
    relactation, 272–276
    storage capacity, 22, 24, 185–186
milk sharing, 219–220, 262
milk stasis, 27
milk storage
    colostrum, 152, 325
    containers, 219
    exclusive nursing, 212–213
    guidelines, 216, 217t.
    handling and preparing expressed milk, 217–219

for preterm babies, 261
returning to work, 90–91
Montgomery glands, 180
mouth sores, 66
MRIs, 38
multiple sclerosis (MS), 155
multiples. *see also* tandem nursing
  milk production, 189–190
  positioning, 15, 15f.
  preterm, 269–270
muscle tone. *see also* Down syndrome
  high, 60, 126–127
  ineffective nursing, 59
  low, 60, 123, 127–128
  nursing strategies, 128–130

N

nasogastric (NG) tubes, 110
natural disasters. *see* emergencies and natural disasters
necrotizing enterocolitis (NEC), 262
neonatal abstinence syndrome (NAS), 246–247
Neonatal Behavior Assessment Scale, 3
Neonatal Tongue Screening Test (NTST), 102
neurological impairments, 60, 126–130
newborns, syncing with, 3
Newman-Goldfarb induced lactation protocols, 275
nicotine, 186, 243–245
night feeds
  multiples, 190
  sleep patterns and, 24–25
  weaning, 293–294
nipple creams and ointments, 66, 224
nipple everters, 233
nipple pain. *see also* nipple trauma
  biting, 223–224
  breast/chest surgery, 45
  comfort measures, 224
  early, 221–222
  inverted nipples and, 234
  latch, 56
  normal, 221
  teething, 222–223

nipple shields
  applying, 331
  basics, 329
  contact style, 330
  disadvantages, 329
  engorgement, 28
  flat/inverted nipples, 234
  for high/low tone, 128–129
  indications for use, 329
  latch dynamics, 331
  mastitis, 32
  milk flow, 62
  and milk production, 329
  nursing effectiveness, 330, 331
  for pain, 225
  and preterm babies, 260
  regular style, 330
  shapes, 330
  for short/recessed jaw, 111
  sizes, 330–331
  and slow weight gain, 301
  for tongue-tie, 102
  weaning from, 332
nipple trauma
  blood in milk, 39, 225
  deep breast pain, 35, 36
  infection prevention, 225
  mastitis, 29–30, 32
  treatment, 224–225
nipples
  accessory/supernumerary, 40–41, 235
  anatomy, 179
  blebs, 32, 231–232
  blind, 236
  blisters, 32, 231
  dimpled, 233
  discharge, 39–40
  double/bifurcated, 236
  flat, 61, 232, 233–234
  infection, 35
  inverted, 61, 232–234
  latch challenges, 68
  pierced, 33, 235–236, 243
  skin problems, 229–230
  taste of, 66
  tilting, 322, 322f.
nisin, 31
nursing pillows, 11
nursing strikes
  causes, 71–72
  strategies, 72–74
nursing supplementers, 46, 200, 311t., 315–318
nutrition. *see* diet and nutrition

O

obesity, 240–241, 307
olive oil, 225
omega-3 fatty acids, 287
one-sided nursing, 68–70
opioid use, 246–247
oral anatomy, baby
    airway abnormalities, 60, 111–112
    cheeks, 104
    cleft lip, 105–106
    cleft palate, 105, 106–110
    jaw, 110–111
    lip flanging, 103
    lip-ties, 103–104
    palate shapes, 104–105
    and slow weight gain, 302
    tongue size and tone, 103
    tongue-tie, 59–60, 101–103
ovulation, 75–76
oxytocin
    breast crawl, 1
    cannabis and, 246
    low thyroid function and, 159
    milk ejection, 75, 180
    nicotine and, 186
    skin-to-skin contact, 3, 73, 75
    stimulating release of, 8, 325
    synthetic, 17, 45, 182

P

pacifiers
    contraindications, 23
    and palate shape, 105
    and slow weight gain, 301
    and Sudden Infant Death Syndrome (SIDS), 23
Paget's disease, 230
pain. *see also* nipple pain
    baby's, during nursing, 58
    birth-related, 60
    circumcision, 58
    deep breast, 35–37
    nursing to relieve, 132, 283
    premenstrual, 37
palatal obturators, 110
palate shapes, 104–105
parental leave. *see* employment
PCP, 247–248
perceived insufficient milk, 84
phototherapy
    for jaundice, 175–177, 176t.
    for nipple pain, 225
physical limitations
    carpal tunnel syndrome, 163
    epilepsy, 163–164
    spinal cord injuries, 164
    strategies, 162
    stroke, 164
    visual impairment, 165
pierced nipples
    mastitis and, 33
    nursing and, 235–236, 243
PKU (phenylketonuria)
    baby, 124, 125–126
    parent, 154
placentophagy, 199
plugged ducts
    mastitis, 29
    positioning, to alleviate, 14–15
polycystic ovary syndrome (PCOS), 155–156, 194
poor fit, 56, 61–62
positioning
    for airway abnormalities, 112
    all-fours dangle, 14–15, 15f.
    baby adjustments, 8–9, 9f.
    basics, 5
    body adjustments, 7–8, 7f., 8f.
    body dynamics, 11–12
    breast adjustments, 9, 10f.
    for cleft palate, 107–108, 108f.
    for high/low tone, 127, 128
    for hip dysplasia, 58
    instinctive feeding position, 2, 320
    and large mammary glands, 62
    and latch depth, 319–320
    over-the-shoulder hold, 14, 14f.
    preterm babies, 258
    for reflux, 116–117
    self-attaching, 319–320, 320f.
    semi-reclined, 5, 6–7, 6f., 6t., 108f.
    for short/recessed jaw, 111
    side-lying, 12, 13f.
    slide-over, 69
    stability, 2

starter, 5, 6–7, 6f., 6t., 10t., 56
straddle hold, 14, 14f.
tandem, 15, 15f.
for torticollis, 58
upright, 5, 6t., 13
post-delivery practices
and blood sugar, 168
and low milk production, 193
postpartum depression, 147–149
postpartum psychosis, 149–150
postpartum thyroiditis, 158
posttraumatic stress disorder (PTSD), 17
preemies. see preterm babies
pregnancy
hand expressing during, 324–325, 324f.
nursing during, 251–252
preoperative fasting, 132–133
preterm babies
bilirubin levels, 172, 176
bottle-feeding, 218–219, 267
cheeks, 104
cytomegalovirus (CMV), 263–264
developmental lactase deficiency, 114
direct nursing, 257–258, 260
donor milk for, 262
early nursing, 259–260
early term, 269
fortification, 262–263
going home, 267–268
hindmilk feeding, 262–263
intake volumes, 266
latching, 258
late-preterm, 268–269
milk expression for, 218, 255
milk production challenges, 262
multiples, 269–270
nursing effectiveness, 259
nursing phases, 256, 256b.
pacifiers, 23
parental illnesses, 264
positioning, 258
primitive neonatal reflexes (PNRs), 1
skin-to-skin contact, 255, 259
slow weight gain, 302
supplementation, 260, 261, 264
transitioning to full nursing, 265–267
weight gain, 120, 260–261, 266, 267–268
primitive neonatal reflexes (PNRs), 1
probiotics, 31, 287
progesterone, 79
progestin, 79–81, 82
proinflammatory cytokines, 148
prolactin, 183–184, 184t., 195t.
pseudoephedrine (Sudafed), 205
psychosis, postpartum, 149–150
psychotherapy, 149
pumps and pumping. see also milk storage
to boost yields, 211–212
exclusive, 213–216
fit, 326–328, 327f.
flat/inverted nipples, 234
hands-on, 211–212, 212f.
increasing milk production, 196
induced lactation, 274
mastitis, 32
nipple pain, 222
relactation, 274
selection considerations, 90
speed, 326
suction, breaking, 325–326
volumes, 208
pyloric stenosis, 115

R

race, and jaundice, 172, 173, 175, 176
radiation therapy, 146–147
radioactive procedures, 145–147, 160
Raynaud's phenomenon, 36, 157, 221
reflux. see gastroesophageal reflux disease (GERD)
relactation
considerations, 272
defined, 271
emergencies and natural disasters, 85
goals, 271–272
milk production strategies, 272–276

physical and emotional changes, 276
transitioning to nursing, 276–278
respiratory issues, 60, 111–112
retrognathia, 111
reverse cycle nursing, 95
reverse pressure softening (RPS), 28, 333–334, 334f.
rheumatoid arthritis, 156–157
RhoGAM, 283
rooting, 1–2, 265
rubella, 144
rubella vaccine, 283
rusty-pipe syndrome, 39

S

sage, 205, 295
scientific mothering, 21
secretory activation, 183
secretory differentiation, 183
seizure disorders, 163–164
semi-demand feeding, 266
sexual abuse, 150–151
sexual desire, 75
shingles, 142
SIDS. *see* Sudden Infant Death Syndrome (SIDS)
silicone, 47–48
skin problems, 229–230
skin-to-skin contact (SSC)
    cesarean birth, 17
    feeding behaviors, 2, 19
    oxytocin release, 3
    preterm babies, 255, 259
sleep patterns, 20, 24–25
sleep training, 25
sleepiness, baby
    as a nursing challenge, 57–58
    Down syndrome, 123
    jaundice, 174
    slow weight gain, 301
sleeping arrangements, 19, 25–26
smallpox vaccine, 283
Smillie, Christina, 204
solid foods
    fertility effects of introducing, 75–76
    and weight gain, 307–308
spermicides, 77
spinal cord injuries, 164

spoon feeding, 312t., 313, 314, 314f.
sputtering, 60, 62, 67
St. John's Wort, 149, 159
sterilization, surgical, 77
stools
    blood/mucus in, 238–239
    diarrhea, 113–115
    first days after birth, 20
    gauging milk intake, 45, 53–54
    green, watery, 115, 202
storage. *see* milk storage
storage capacity, 22, 24, 185–186, 207
stress, 66
stridor, 60, 111
stroke, 164
submucous cleft, 106
substance use, 186, 243–249, 264
substance use disorder (SUD), 248–249
sucking, 1–2, 265
suction, breaking, 223, 224
Sudden Infant Death Syndrome (SIDS)
    formula-feeding, 24
    pacifier/dummy use, 23
    sleeping arrangements, 25
    tobacco use, 244
supplementation
    amounts by age, 54, 54t.
    breast/chest surgery, 45–46
    for cardiac issues, 120
    decreasing, 279–280
    determining need for, 53–54
    feeding methods, 54
    insufficient glandular tissue (IGT), 41
    and milk production, 199–200
    preterm babies, 260, 261
    for slow weight gain, 304–306, 305t.
    unnecessary newborn, 19–20
    weaning from, 306
supplements, 237, 284–287
support. *see* lactation help and support
surgery. *see also* breast/chest surgery; hospitalization
    cancer, 145–146

cleft lip, 106
cleft palate, 110
parent, 161–162
preoperative fasting, 132–133
pyloric stenosis, 115
weight-loss, 242
swaddling, 301
swallowing
 effective vs. ineffective nursing, 59, 300
 instinctive feeding position, 2
symptomatic tongue-tie, 101. see also tongue-tie
syringe feeding, 312t., 314

T

tail of Spence, 27
tandem nursing
 basics, 253
 and cleft palate, 109
 defined, 252
 emotional adjustments, 253
 milk production, 189–190
 positioning, 15, 15f.
tanning beds, 242
teething, 66, 222–223
testosterone, 49, 154–155, 159, 191, 195t.
thawing milk, 218
THC, 245–246
thickeners, 117
thrush
 recurring, 228–229
 symptoms, 226–227
 treatment for baby, 227
 treatment for parent, 228
thyroid disease, 157–160
tobacco use, 186, 243–245, 264
tongue-tie
 assessment tools, 102
 Coryllos Classification System, 101–102
 frenotomy, 103
 nursing problems associated with, 60, 101
 nursing strategies, 102–103
 positioning, 7
Tongue-Tie and Breastfeed Baby (TABBY) assessment tool, 102
top surgery, 49–50, 191
torticollis, 58, 69
tracheomalacia, 60, 111
transcutaneous bilirubinometry (TcB), 172–173
transgender men and nursing, 191, 281
transgender women and nursing, 191, 281
trauma. see also nipple trauma
 birth-related, 17, 60
 breast/chest, 39
 childhood, 150–151
triplets. see multiples
tubal ligation, 77
tube-feeding devices. see nursing supplementers
tuberculosis (TB), 137
twins. see multiples

U

ultrasound for diagnosis, 38
ultrasound therapy, 33
underfeeding, 58

V

vaccines, 283
vaping, 245
vasectomies, 77
vasospasm, 36, 221
vegetarian/vegan diets, 239
visual impairment, 165
vitamin B_6, 295
vitamin B_{12}, 284–285, 286
vitamin D, 284, 285–286
vitamin E, 225
vitamins, 225, 284–287. see also specific vitamins
vocal cord paralysis, 60, 111
vomiting, 115–116

W

warming milk, 218–219
water-soluble vitamins, 286
weaning
 abrupt, 294
 basics, 290–291
 comfort measures, 294–295
 cultural beliefs and practices, 289
 from exclusive pumping, 215–216
 gradual, 291–292

mastitis, 31–32
natural, 292–293
night, 293–294
from nipple shields, 332
from nursing supplementers, 318
parent-child dynamics, 290
partial, 91–92, 293
physical and emotional changes, 295
postpartum psychosis, 150
during pregnancy, 251–252
reasons for, 289–290
recommendations, 289
from supplementation, 306
weight gain, baby
airway abnormalities and, 60
average volumes, 45, 57–58, 297–298
cardiac issues and, 120
cleft palate and, 109–110
increasing, 303–304
and loss, 299–300
nursing dynamics and, 301, 302, 303
overabundant milk production, 203
preterm babies, 260–261, 266, 267–268
rapid, 306–308
relactation/induced lactation, 278–279
slow, 298–303
supplementation for, 304–306, 305t.
WHO Child Growth Standards, 53, 298
weight loss, baby
engorgement, 28
during first days after birth, 45, 297
gain and, 299–300
weight loss, parent, 239–242
West Nile virus, 144
WHO Child Growth Standards, 53, 298
work. *see* employment

X

x-rays, 38

Y

yeast infections
candidiasis, 37, 226
thrush, 6, 226–229
yellow fever vaccine, 283

Z

zika virus, 144–145

ABOUT THE AUTHOR

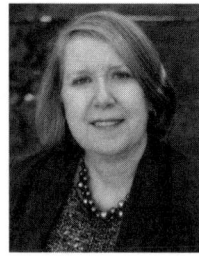

Nancy Mohrbacher, IBCLC, FILCA has worked with nursing families for nearly 40 years. Board-certified as a lactation consultant in 1991, she worked in private practice and corporate lactation, developed training courses for aspiring lactation consultants in the U.S. and China, and is currently contracted by hospitals to help improve breastfeeding practices. Her mission is to simplify breastfeeding for parents and professionals by creating innovative lactation education and tools.

Nancy's 2020 textbook for lactation specialists, *Breastfeeding Answers, Second Edition* is used worldwide. Her Natural Breastfeeding Professional Package provides digital resources for professionals for staff training and one-on-one work with families.

Her books for parents include *Breastfeeding Made Simple: Seven Natural Laws for Nursing Mothers,* which she co-authored with Kathleen Kendall-Tackett, *Working and Breastfeeding Made Simple,* and *Breastfeeding Solutions: Quick Tips for the Most Common Nursing Challenges.* Its companion Breastfeeding Solutions app is used internationally and is available on the App Store and Google Play. Her YouTube channel is viewed by millions of families.

In 2008 the International Lactation Consultant Association officially recognized Nancy's contributions to the field of lactation by awarding her the designation FILCA, Fellow of the International Lactation Consultant Association. Nancy was one of the first group of 16 to be recognized for their lifetime achievements in breastfeeding.

For more, visit **NancyMohrbacher.com**